Society & Medicine

Festschriften Series by Transaction

Joseph L. Blau
History, Religion, and American Democracy
Maurice Wohlgelernter, ed.

Herbert Blumer
Human Nature and Collective Behavior
Tamotsu Shibutani, ed.

Werner J. Cahnman
Ethnicity, Identity, and History
Joseph B. Maier and
Chaim I. Waxman, eds.

Rose Laub Coser
Social Roles and Social Institutions
Judith R. Blau and
Norman Goodman, eds.

Gray Dorsey
Law, Culture, and Values
Sava Alexander Vojcanin, ed.

Abraham Edel
Ethics, Science, and Democracy
Irving Louis Horowitz and
H. Standish Thayer, eds.

James W. Fesler
The Costs of Federalism
Robert T. Golembiewski and
Aaron Wildavsky, eds.

Raymond Firth
Leadership and Change in the Western Pacific
Richard E. Feinberg, ed.

Eli Ginzberg
The Economist as a Public Intellectual
Irving Louis Horowitz, ed.

John Hicks
John Hicks: His Contribution to Economic Theory
K. Puttaswamaiah, ed.

George C. Homans
Behavioral Theory in Sociology
Robert L. Hamblin and
John H. Kunkel, eds.

Irving Louis Horowitz
The Democratic Imagination
Ray C. Rist, ed.

Ian Kidd
The Passionate Intellect
Lewis Ayres, ed.

Georg Lukacs
Georg Lukacs: Theory, Culture, and Politics
Judith Marcus and
Zoltan Tarr, eds.

Joseph B. Maier
Surviving the Twentieth Century
Judith Marcus, ed.

Robert K. Merton
Robert K. Merton and Contemporary Sociology
Carlo Mongardini and
Simonetta Tabboni, eds.

Hans J. Morgenthau
Truth and Tragedy
Kenneth Thompson and
Robert J. Myers, eds.

George L. Mosse
Political Symbolism in Modern Europe
Seymour Drescher, David Sabean,
and Allan Sharlin, eds.

Gwynne Nettler
Critique and Explanation
Timothy F. Hartnagel and
Robert A. Silverman

Karl Popper
Critical Approaches to Science and Philosophy
Mario Bunge, ed.

Earl Raab
American Pluralism and the Jewish Community
Seymour Martin Lipset, ed.

Paul Samuelson
Paul Samuelson and the Foundations of Modern Economics
K. Puttaswamaiah, ed.

Pitirim Sorokin
Sorokin and Civilization
Joseph B. Ford, Michel P. Richard,
and Palmer C. Talbutt, eds.

Aaron Wildavsky
Budgeting, Policy, and Politics
Naomi Caiden and Joseph White, eds.

Hans L. Zetterberg
Sociological Endeavor
Emil Uddhammar and
Richard Swedberg, eds.

Essays in Honor of Renée C. Fox

Society & Medicine

Carla M. Messikomer
Judith P. Swazey
Allen Glicksman
editors

Routledge
Taylor & Francis Group
LONDON AND NEW YORK

First published 2003 by Transaction Publishers

Published 2017 by Routledge
2 Park Square, Milton Park, Abingdon, Oxon OX14 4RN
711 Third Avenue, New York, NY 10017, USA

Routledge is an imprint of the Taylor & Francis Group, an informa business

Library of Congress Catalog Number: 2002020274

Library of Congress Cataloging-in-Publication Data

Society and medicine : essays in honor of Renée C. Fox / Carla M. Messikomer, Judith P. Swazey, and Allen Glicksman, editors.
p. cm.— (Festschriften)
Includes bibliographical references and index.
ISBN 0-7658-0156-6 (cloth : alk. paper)
1. Social medicine. 2. Bioethics. 3. Medicine—Philosophy. I. Fox, Renée C. (Renée Claire), 1928- II. Messikomer, Carla M. III. Swazey, Judith P. IV. Glicksman, Allen. V. Series.

RA418 .S6723 2002
306.4'61—dc21 2002020274

ISBN 13: 978-0-7658-0156-2 (hbk)

Contents

Introduction ix
Carla M. Messikomer, Judith P. Swazey, and Allen Glicksman

I. Health and Medicine: Social and Cultural Dimensions

1. Longing for Certainty: The Modern American Experience of Pregnancy 3
Elizabeth M. Armstrong

2. Healthy Beliefs: Wellness in Action at Company X 23
Jacqueline Hart

3. Gods, Living and Dead: Generativity Among Soviet Born Elders in the United States 43
Allen Glicksman

4. It Couldn't Hurt: An Ethnographic Study of a Ritual for Healing 59
Gail G. Glicksman

5. Overused and Underappreciated: Culture in an Academic Medicine Merger 69
Carla M. Messikomer and Judith P. Swazey

6. Transplanting the Transplant: Japanese Sensitivity to American Medicine as an American Mission 87
William R. LaFleur

7. Forty Years of Fieldwork: Renée Fox and Belgium/Belgium and Renée Fox 109
Yves Winkin

II. Becoming and Being a Physician

8. Responding to a Poor Evaluation: What Constitutes an "Honest" Response in the Eyes of Residency Program Directors — 117
Virginia Adams O'Connell and Charles L. Bosk

9. On the Sociological Anxiety of Physicians — 135
Nicholas A. Christakis

10. The Transplant Surgeon, the Sociologist, and the Historian: A Conversation with Thomas E. Starzl — 145
Renée C. Fox

11. What if Food Were a Medicine? The Pediatrician and Childhood Hunger — 161
Deborah A. Frank

12. Uncertainty and Changing Trust Relationships in Medicine — 169
David Mechanic

13. The Social and Moral Commitments of a Physician-Writer — 183
Robert Klitzman

III. Bioethics, Sociology, and Medicine

14. Renée Fox, Human Experimentation, and Therapeutic Innovation: A Career of Values and Observations — 193
Victor Lidz

15. Religious Sources for Debates in Bioethics — 211
Jonathan B. Imber

16. Sociology and the De-moralization of Bioethics — 227
Howard L. Kaye

17. The Moral and the Medical: The Stakes of Social Experience 243
Arthur Kleinman

IV. Postlude

18. Exploring the Moral and Spiritual Dimensions of Society and Medicine 257
Renée C. Fox

About the Contributors 273

Index 279

Introduction

Carla M. Messikomer, Judith P. Swazey, and Allen Glicksman

Society and Medicine grew out of a conference held in November 1999 under the auspices of the University of Pennsylvania's Center for Bioethics, Graduate School of Arts and Sciences, and Department of Sociology to pay tribute to the achievements of Renée C. Fox, and recognize her becoming Annenberg Professor Emerita of the Social Sciences.[1] To celebrate the dedication and talents she has displayed in her vocation as a teacher, the influential role she has played as a mentor to many students and younger associates, and the richness and power of her research and writing, the conference brought together many of her colleagues and current and former students from medicine, sociology, nursing, and bioethics for two days of presentations, lively discussions, and shared appreciations of the teacher, scholar, and friend who forged a common bond among the participants. The conference, at Dr. Fox's request, was dedicated to the memory of Dr. Herbert W. Nickens (1947-1998), who studied with her as an undergraduate at Harvard College and subsequently at the University of Pennsylvania while concurrently earning his MD and an MA in sociology, and then as a Robert Wood Johnson Clinical Scholar.[2]

The title of this book, and of the conference, reflect the interrelated leitmotifs in Renée Fox's work: her studies of and teaching about the nature of medicine and medical research, the training and work of their practitioners, the interrelationships between medicine and the societies and cultures of which it is a part, and, above all, the moral and spiritual dimensions of the healing arts. Implicitly, and in some cases explicitly, the essays bear the imprint of her scholarship and teaching upon their authors. The majority of the contributors have been her students at some point in their education and training as physicians and social scientists, ranging from their undergraduate studies to fellowship work as Robert Wood Johnson Clinical Scholars. These former students, many of whom have become colleagues who have collaborated with her, include Elizabeth Armstrong, Nicholas Christakis, Deborah Frank, Allen Glicksman, Gail Glicksman, Jacqueline Hart, Jonathan Imber, Howard Kaye, Robert Klitzman, Carla Messikomer, and Virginia O'Connell. The other authors—Charles Bosk, Arthur Kleinman, William LaFleur, Victor Lidz, David Mechanic, Judith Swazey, and Yves Winkin—are social science colleagues who have not been Renée Fox's students in a conventional sense. But their work, too, reflects the influence of her scholarship in terms, variously, of the subjects they have pursued, the methodologies they have employed, and the conceptual and analytic frameworks they have used.

The enduring impact Renée has had upon those who have studied and worked with her was captured by Belgian social scientist Yves Winkin, a specialist in social communications, in the talk he gave at the conference. Professor Winkin has been a friend and colleague of hers since they met in the 1970s, and later arranged to have her book, *In the Belgian Château*, published in French and took an active part in its translation. "On a personal level," he said, recognizing the mentor-like role she has played in his career, as well as in the careers of many others, "she taught me much about my country and about the ways I could be an ethnographer in my own country."

Though the conference, and subsequently this volume, was inspired by the desire of colleagues and students to honor Renée Fox, in the editors' view *Society and Medicine* is not a "festschrift" in the conventional sense of the term (Monaghan 2001). That is, although many of the papers explicitly address the influence of her work, it is not a collection of tributes or discussions about the corpus of her writings and their influence. Rather, in accord with our request that the contributions be substantive papers, the topics addressed by the authors are connected, in various ways, to the themes Renée has explored over the years in her own "journeys into the field" (Fox 1988), or the journeys she has inspired others to make.

With two exceptions, the papers in *Society and Medicine* were developed from presentations their authors made at the conference. The first exception is William LaFleur's "Transplanting the Transplant," a paper that cross-culturally analyzes the translation of Fox and Swazey's book, *Spare Parts*, into Japanese and its reception in Japan, which we invited him to contribute to the book after he shared a draft manuscript with us. The second exception—which we realize is unusual for a book such as this—is an essay by Renée Fox herself, in the section titled "Becoming and Being a Physician." It is based on a "conversation" she had with transplant surgeon Thomas Starzl, who attended the conference dinner to pay a tribute to the honoree, but, due to other commitments, could not give a paper. In characteristic fieldworker fashion, Renée persuaded Dr. Starzl to come back to Philadelphia so that she could interview him about his work and the three-decades-long relationship that she and Judith Swazey developed with him during their firsthand research on organ transplantation.

The papers in this volume have so many interrelated, crosscutting themes that it was difficult to decide how to order them. In the end, we settled on four parts: social and cultural dimensions of health and medicine; becoming and being a physician; bioethics, sociology, and medicine; and a postlude in which Renée Fox reflects on the nature and meaning of her work.

The seven papers in Part I explore various social and cultural dimensions of health and medicine, and the interrelationships between them. In "Longing for Certainty," Elizabeth Armstrong examines the phenomenon of pregnancy in modern American society. Drawing, in part, on the plethora of lay publications and websites for pregnant women, she explores contemporary social and individual attitudes towards risk and responsibility in pregnancy, particularly what she calls the "longing for certainty" that now characterizes the experience of gestation. As her study shows, Armstrong writes, "pregnancy has so much cultural salience not only because it is a profoundly meaningful experience in individuals' lives...but also because of [its] usefulness and richness as a deeply resonant social metaphor" that embodies risk and, "literally, the future as well."

The "wellness ethic," an ideology and a set of practices that intertwines psychological, moral, spiritual, medical, and economic elements is becoming an important part of many corporate health programs. Based on her study of the wellness division of an international company, Jacqueline Hart's "Healthy Beliefs" delineates the ways that the organization's institutionalization of the wellness ethic became a form of medical social control in the workplace. By conceptualizing health as a condition shaped primarily by a person's innate character, personal belief system, and moral fiber, and holding that individuals can and should be accountable for their health, sickness was de-legitimized for the employees of company X. The wellness ethic approach to health and illness, Hart argues, is "potentially socially destructive."

Ethnographically-based perspectives on the experiences of very different groups from those studied by Armstrong and Hart are provided in the papers by Allen Glicksman and Gail Glicksman. Drawing on data from a study of access and barriers to community-based long term care for elderly immigrants, Allen Glicksman's "Gods, Living and Dead" describes how two groups of elderly Soviet immigrants—Jews and Ukrainian Baptists—dealt with issues of "generativity," or their desire to pass on their faith traditions and a cultural legacy to their families. For the Jewish refugees, life in the Soviet Union left them with little of their faith or culture to transmit, whereas the continuity of the Ukrainians' faith provided them with a link between generations.

Another rich ethnographic picture is provided by Gail Glicksman in "It Couldn't Hurt." Dipping into her experience as a participant observer during the five years that she served as rabbi to a group of predominantly elderly congregants, she examines the coping strategies that they developed to deal with an often bewildering increase in morbidity and mortality among their families and friends. Those strategies, Glicksman found, centered on creative elaborations of the ritual surrounding the recitation of a prayer for the restoration of health—a means of coping with illness that also revealed much about the social dynamics of the congregation.

A different dimension of the role of cultural factors in medicine—their critical importance in an organizational merger—is addressed by Carla Messikomer and Judith Swazey in "Overused and Underappreciated." Based on their study of the Allegheny Health, Education and Research Foundation's acquisition of Hahnemann University and its merger with the Medical College of Pennsylvania, they explore the ways in which the failure to appreciate the importance of the differing academic and corporate cultures affected the union of the two medical schools and their faculty and staff, and created a series of shock waves that slowed and often derailed the merger process.

The preceding five papers are based on research conducted in the United States. The next two papers, by William LaFleur and Yves

Winkin, take us into different countries and cultures—Japan and Belgium. LaFleur's cross-cultural analysis of "Transplanting the Transplant" has two interrelated foci. First, how the 1999 Japanese translation of Fox and Swazey's book, *Spare Parts*, was intended to serve as a "telescope" for the Japanese, making them more aware of the cultural and religious ramifications of the initiation of cadaveric transplants in their country. Secondly, as LaFleur writes, he turns that telescope around, examining how aspects of the process of introducing the book to a Japanese audience has significance for North Americans, and a more generalized relevance for thinking about how medicine is involved in the interaction between cultures.

Part I ends with Yves Winkin's "Renée Fox and Belgium/Belgium and Renée Fox." Beginning with her first trip to this country in 1959 to study its medical research enterprise, he reflects on Fox's forty years of fieldwork in that small, socially and culturally intricate country, what he called in his conference presentation her "journeys into the soul of a society." As part of his perspective, he examines the complex, ongoing, shifting nature of the reactions of many groups in Belgium to her research and writings, and why the attitude of most Belgian social scientists to her work has remained critically dismissive through the years, despite the fact that certain of her publications created something akin to a national furor.

The six papers in Part II address another major theme in Fox's research and teaching: the nature of medical education and the roles and work of physicians. The first paper in this set, Virginia Adams O'Connell and Charles Bosk's "Responding to a Poor Evaluation," draws on data from a study of attrition in surgical residency training programs. They examine what program directors mean by "honesty," which the directors rated as the most important trait a resident could possess, the variables affecting assessments of it in terms of how residents responded to faculty criticisms of their performance, and how those assessments determined whether trainees were retained, terminated, or defined as "problematic completers."

Moving from training to the work of physicians and the role strains that work entails, Nicholas Christakis' "On the Sociological Anxiety of Physicians" examines the nature and sources of the anxiety engendered by prognosis, and its meaning for medical care. The task of prognosis, as his research on "foretelling" death has shown, is a source of psychological anxiety, and poses a threat to a physician's "sociological existence and security," primarily because of concerns about the "self-fulfilling prophecy" consequences of making a negative prognosis.

Turning to the "experiment perilous" world of therapeutic innovation that has been one major focus of her research, Renée Fox's "The Transplant Surgeon, the Sociologist, and the Historian" offers insights into the work and beliefs of a transplantation pioneer, Thomas E. Starzl. Through talking with him about the reasons why he has engaged in an ongoing, thirty-plus year dialogue with her and Judith Swazey about the nature of his clinical, technical, and scientific contributions, and about the field of organ transplantation more generally, she draws a vivid sketch of a leading and often controversial figure in the evolution of organ replacement. And, turning the tables on the sociologist, when Tom Starzl becomes the interlocutor, he elicits insights into what Renée Fox sees as the meaning of her work.

A picture of what seems in many ways to be a very different world of medicine, yet one that has commonalities with the arena in which a Thomas Starzl works, is painted by Deborah Frank in "What if Food Were a Medicine?" In it, she conveys the passionate convictions and concerns that she brings to her work as a practicing inner city pediatrician who cares for children diagnosed with "failure to thrive," a condition often due to malnutrition. She shares with us the "grubby experience" of what it is like for her and her anti-hunger colleagues to fund and stock an emergency food pantry as they shoulder the day-to-day "responsibility of caring for poor children without adequate resources to assure them the quality of life we want for our own children."

David Mechanic, in turn, takes up the topic of trust—"the expectation that others will act as expected consistent with status and role and meet their responsibilities to us"—which physicians like Deborah Frank know well is a vital element of their work. Some reasonable level of trust, Mechanic observes, is requisite for the effective functioning of social institutions and interpersonal relationships, and trust has had particular salience in medical care. Drawing on various exploratory studies, he examines the evidence and reasons for the erosion of the public's trust in both medical institutions and physicians, and various attempts to develop health care programs that seek to build and maintain trust.

The last paper in this section, by Robert Klitzman, takes us back to the personal level of a physician's work. Klitzman is both a psychiatrist trained in the social sciences and a literary nonfiction writer, and in his essay he eloquently shares the social and moral commitments that have shaped his latter vocation as a participant-observer author since his medical student years. Klitzman tells us that he writes for many reasons: to remember and give voice to patients who cannot speak; to make himself and his readers more aware of the larger social issues he and others face; to reveal how we construct disease, and the assumptions embedded in those constructions; and to provide an antidote to medicine's empiricism.

The four papers comprising Part III, authored by three sociologists and a physician-medical anthropologist, deal with the frequently contentious relationships between bioethics, sociology, and medicine. In his essay, "Renée Fox, Human Experimentation, and Therapeutic Innovation," Victor Lidz traces how the personal and professional values and observational skills Fox has brought to her work have been manifested in her studies of therapeutic innovation. Within their sociological framework, these studies contain deep-structured skeins of ethical themes and issues, many of which antedate the development of bioethics. He also uses that thematic analysis to examine strengths and weakness of the now extensive regulatory system for the protection of human research subjects. Fox's research, his account shows, belies the view of many involved with the protection of human subjects that clinical research before the era of IRBs was a "completely unregulated," "wild and woolly" enterprise.

Readers of Jonathan Imber's "Religious Sources for Debates in Bioethics" will find a number of topical linkages to David Mechanic's analysis of trust relationships in medicine. Protestant and Catholic inheritances, Imber holds, account for the contemporary force of "what remains of trust in doctors," and for the diminished authority of physicians that has created uncertainty about "the meaning of their vocation." He goes on to analyze the roles of religious belief, doctrine, and debates in bioethics in relation to sociological characteristics of both the discipline of sociology and the field of philosophical bioethics, and why there has been such an uneasy relationship between them.

The connections, or lack thereof, between sociology and bioethics are also explored by Howard Kaye in his essay "Sociology and the De-moralization of Bioethics." Over the past thirty years, Kaye contends, as bioethics has been successfully routinized and professionalized, the field has undergone "a paradoxical change in its approach to ethical issues." Using the National Bioethics Advisory Commission's report on cloning as an example, Kaye argues that this change has involved bioethics becoming both increasingly secularized, "as the price for its wider acceptance," and "increasingly amoral, "preferring to develop purportedly value-neutral procedural compromises instead of persuasive moral guides. Sociology, Kaye avers, can play a perhaps unexpected role in helping bioethics to counteract such tendencies.

The final paper in Part III, Arthur Kleinman's "The Moral and the Medical: The Stakes of Social Experience," was presented as the keynote address at the November 1999 conference. In his essay, Kleinman holds that "the moral, the political, and the medical are inseparably bound together through the stakes of collective and subjective experience." This recognition, which involves differences between moral processes and ethical deliberations, is one of anthropology's, sociology's, and social history's "more salient contributions" to the study of health and medicine. Understanding the stakes of social experience, he goes on to argue, is a major challenge to the "old" bioethics and a reason for the development of a "new" bioethics. In a new form, Kleinman holds, the social sciences and history would complement philosophy, the study of religion, and clinical ethics, and bioethics would find the means to accommodate both moral processes and ethical discourse in its framework.

This volume, as did the conference, concludes with an essay by Renée Fox. In Part IV, which we have titled "Postlude," she reflects on the topics and themes around which the meeting was structured, and how they are connected to her career as a sociologist and her relationship to the conference participants. It seems fitting to end this Introduction by letting Renée speak, in her own eloquent way, about what her work has signified to her, and, we would add, to her students and colleagues. "I hope that I do not sound either sanctimonious or self-congratulatory," she writes,

> in saying that my career has been a "vocation" in Max Weber's sense of the term: an "inward calling" to do social scientific work; questing after knowledge and understanding of what Weber described as the "pulsating...reality" of human life and human relations; trying to impart that knowledgeable understanding, and a way of thinking

about it, through teaching and writing, with "intellectual integrity" that does not preclude vividness; believing that what is conveyed can contribute to greater clarity and insight about our own lives and the lives of others, and to a "sense of responsibility" and of compassionate caring that extend beyond the particularistic enclaves in which we dwell. It is essential to "the very *meaning* of science as a vocation," Weber wrote, that "we cannot work without hoping that others will advance further than we have." This is not only "our common fate" but "our common goal," he declared. Many of you who have participated in this conference personify for me the fulfillment of that hope and goal.

Notes

1. Carla Messikomer and Allen Glicksman co-chaired the conference program committee, aided by Robin Heller, M.S.S.W., who at the time of the conference was senior administrator at the University of Pennsylvania's Center for Bioethics, and Tricha Shivas, who was a degree candidate in the master's program in bioethics. Currently, Ms. Heller is the Director of Grants Development at Jewish Family and Children's Services of Philadelphia and Ms. Shivas is a doctoral student in philosophy at Michigan State University. Ms. Deborah Putnam Thomas provided administrative support, and Charles Bosk and Nicholas Christakis assisted the committee in the early phases of planning.
2. Dr. Nickens, who trained as a psychiatrist, became the first director of the Office of Minority Health at the Department of Health and Human Services in 1986, and then joined the American Association of Medical Colleges in 1988, serving as its first Vice President for Community and Minority Programs until his sudden death from a heart attack at age fifty-one. Dr. Nickens was deeply committed to redressing the limited opportunities for minorities in health care and the development of minority academic physicians as part of his broader convictions about issues of social justice and equity in health care.

References

Fox, Renée C. 1988. *Essays in Medical Sociology. Journeys into the Field.* Second, enlarged edition. New Brunswick, NJ: Transaction Publishers.

Monaghan, Peter. 2001. "The festschrift is dead. Long live the festschrift." *Chronicle of Higher Education* 13 (April):A20-21.

I

Health and Medicine: Social and Cultural Dimensions

1

Longing for Certainty: The Modern American Experience of Pregnancy

Elizabeth M. Armstrong

"I am just allowing myself to comprehend what is going on in my body. I basically have been floating along with this pregnancy in a pool of uncertainty."
—From Melanie's pregnancy journal, Week 6: Overcoming Fears, at www.ePregnancy.com

To be pregnant is to be expectant. Pregnancy is a time of waiting and uncertainty, a time of doubt, of wondering, a time of longing. As a biological process, pregnancy has probably been invariant through human history. Yet as a social process, pregnancy is subject to endless permutations through time and place. In the past, the process and outcome of pregnancy seemed idiosyncratic, variable and unpredictable to women and doctors alike in the Western world. Pregnancy might as likely end in the mother's premature death, or the delivery of fantastical "monsters and marvels," as described by Ambroise Paré in the sixteenth century, or in the famous 1726 case of Mary Toft, a litter of rabbits, as in the birth of a baby. Likewise the duration of gestation: Hippocrates wrote of both the "seven months child" and the "ten months child," and even longer gestations were reported as late as the eighteenth century. A pregnant woman's craving for strawberries might "impress" the unborn child with a birthmark; the sight of a rabbit hopping across her path might cause the child to be born with a harelip. The experience of pregnancy has always been the experience of uncertainty, particularly a deeply embodied and visceral uncertainty. Will the baby be "normal" or not? Will it be a girl or a boy? Will it look like its mother or father, both or neither? Will the mother and the child even survive birth and infancy?

Women today may be able to answer many of these questions more definitively and with greater confidence than in the past. The range of possible variation is greatly reduced, as is the risk of pregnancy and childbearing. Although reproduction in the United States poses less threat to life and limb than ever before, the experience of pregnancy—both individual and social—remains fraught with uncertainty. This enduring uncertainty itself seems to be an ever-greater source of social and individual anxiety—one that we wish to tame or manage. We want to know—and expect that we can know—"What to Expect When You're Expecting," as the commercial success of the best-selling pregnancy guide by this title attests.

The contours of modern pregnancy reflect not only individual worries and expectations, but social norms and social anxieties as well. We live in an aggressively pronatalist society—the average number of children borne by American women is about twice that in Europe and Japan—and the proliferation of pregnancy media and cultural artifacts and practices around pregnancy partly attests to America's besotted love affair with babies (and mothers). But the ubiquity of pregnancy in our social life today also is a testament to its power to capture and refract such social norms, values, and preoccupations as individualism, consumerism, faith in the expert, and the virtue of self-improvement.

The experience of pregnancy today is characterized by a longing for certainty that exists at both a personal and societal level. We attempt to assuage this longing according to the best principles of Enlightenment rationality; that is, by pursuing knowledge and precision. In doing so, pregnant women are subject to a quantification and abstraction of their experiences of pregnancy. This paper examines three manifestations of the longing for certainty. First, the impact of medical technology on pregnancy, especially the "mirage of certainty" that technologies such as ultrasound and prenatal testing seem to offer. Second, the intellectual preparation that is now *de rigeur* for pregnancy, particularly as it is exhibited in books, magazines, and on the Internet. Third, the commodification of pregnancy through which babies are not only transformed into "products" of their mothers' labor, but are expected to be "perfect" products. The consequence of these trends is an immersion in the experience of pregnancy, particularly for pregnant women, so that pregnancy becomes the most salient aspect of a woman's social identity, subjecting her to a wide range of behavioral prescriptions and proscriptions. Pregnancy in effect becomes, in Goffman's terms, a master status (Goffman 1963).

In demonstrating the longing for certainty that characterizes pregnancy today and responses to it, I will draw primarily on the lay literature about pregnancy. For the cultural sociologist, our cultural pursuit of knowledge about, in, of, and during pregnancy provides a treasure trove of written, visual, and electronic materials: books, magazines, websites, newsletters, TV programs, prenatal care protocols, and medical routines and practices.

What is it that makes this individual and collective longing for certainty in pregnancy so acute today? In the last decades of the twentieth century, pregnancy was transformed into embodied risk. The medicalization of pregnancy, not just labor and delivery, and the universalization of prenatal care highlight the transformation of pregnancy into *routine risk*. The very idea that medical surveillance of all pregnancies is necessary to ensure good outcomes—an article of faith in the U.S. today—presupposes that pregnancy is a risky endeavor, one that must be carefully managed by professionals and also requires active involvement of the pregnant woman herself to manage and contain risks. Merely to be pregnant in our society today is to be classified by medicine and society alike as being "at risk." Therefore, it is to experience an uncertainty that is at once physical, emotional, and existential.

Prenatal Tests: Training for Uncertainty

Responses to the uncertainty and risk inherent in modern pregnancy exhibit some of the same characteristics that Reneé Fox first noted over forty years ago in relation to physicians' training for uncertainty (Fox 1988). These include striving to "achieve cognitive command of the situation," adopting "quantitative thinking," emphasizing "probablistic logic," and banding together in a "little society" of insiders who share a common language, brand of humor, and set of problems. Pregnant women, like the medical students and apprentice doctors described by Fox, employ each of these general strategies as they cope with the existential uncertainty of gestation.

Testing the Pregnancy

Medical verification and supervision of pregnancy have become central to the modern experience of pregnancy. Passing the pregnancy test, which was invented only in the 1920s and was not widely available until mid-century, is today a rite of passage for all pregnant women. Moreover, the pregnancy test in the doctor's office has become domesticated in the form of home pregnancy tests, readily available in drugstores or over the Web. Total sales of home pregnancy tests, which typically cost less than $15, top $200 million annually; one in three pregnant women has used a test at home to verify a pregnancy before heading to the doctor (Bastian et al. 1998). The widespread use of home pregnancy tests has three significant effects. First, such tests increase the medicalization of pregnancy. Even before a woman has set foot in a doctor's office or clinic, she has taken a laboratory test. Second, because women often purchase and use several home pregnancy tests at once, these kits contribute to the commercialization of pregnancy by establishing that it is something for which one must buy special products. Third, home tests, which may be accurate as soon as ten days after conception, contribute to the increasing length of pregnancy as a social status—women reveal their pregnancies at much earlier stages than were possible, or considered appropriate, in the past. Thus, women are publicly pregnant for much longer, and a "longer" gestation contributes to the emergence of pregnancy as a master status.

Yet the home pregnancy test is only the first and in many ways the least morally complicated of the many diagnostic tests that pregnant women face today. These include the maternal alpha-fetoprotein screening (the AFP test), which serves as a very non-specific screen for fetal abnormality; routine blood and urine tests throughout pregnancy; amniocentesis; chorionic villus sampling (CVS); ultrasound; and occasionally fetoscopy, percutaneous umbilical cord sampling, MRI, or fetal echocardiography. Probabilistic logic is necessary both to explain the risks to the fetus inherent in many prenatal tests and to interpret their sometimes cryptic results. Maternal serum screening (AFP), for example, has a very high false positive rate. Because a positive AFP is not indicative of abnormalities itself but rather is used to decide whether to pursue amniocentesis or CVS, among 100 women who test positive on the AFP, only two to four will turn out to have a fetal abnormality.

Although the existence and sheer abundance of prenatal tests reflect the longing for certainty about pregnancy, the tests themselves may offer only a "mirage of certainty." Information about prenatal testing abounds in the lay literature on pregnancy. A significant subcategory of pregnancy advice books is devoted solely to helping expectant parents face these tests and whether to undergo them, and an omnipresent feature of general pregnancy advice books and magazines is the chapter or article billed as "a complete guide to prenatal testing." Most commonly, tests are presented in a positive way, as "helpful" and as antidotes to uncertainty. "The best reason for prenatal diagnosis is the reassurance it almost always brings,"[1] states the popular book *What to Expect When You're Expecting* (Eisenberg, Murkoff and Hathaway 1996:42). At the same time, much of the literature acknowledges that prenatal testing can exact a toll on pregnant women. "You probably haven't thought about taking tests since you left the classroom behind. Guess what—they're back, and the high anxiety you experienced over algebra and the SATs is going to seem like nothing compared to that from some of these prenatal exams" (Reigel 1999:23). Whether to undergo certain prenatal tests—particularly those that diagnose chromosomal anomalies or neural tube defects for which there is no remedy other than abortion—is a source of tremendous anxiety for many women. Yet prenatal tests clearly represent a means of coping with uncertainty. They allow doctors and women to quantify possibilities that are both unthinkable and ineffable. They impose a structure of ordered probabilities on the unknown.

Seeing is Believing: Picturing the Fetus

One prenatal procedure that is universally seen as beneficent is the ultrasound. On pregnancy chat boards women often express disappointment when they cannot have an anticipated ultrasound because the procedure is not reimbursable or because their doctor decides it is not necessary at this visit. Like the pregnancy test, the ultrasound has become a prenatal rite of passage for most women. Just as the pregnancy test offers "proof positive" that the pregnancy exists, visualization of the fetus/baby on the ultrasound monitor provides evidence that the pregnancy continues to exist, and moreover that all is proceeding normally, as expected. Seeing is believing in our culture. This trend towards visual perception of the baby in utero represents an unacknowledged but profound shift in the experience of pregnancy. Until the 1800s, quickening—the woman's first perception of fetal movement, usually around 12-14 weeks gestation—

was the legal definition of the beginning of pregnancy (Reagan 1997), as well as a primary tactile marker. For the woman, physical sensations of pregnancy—nausea, swollen breasts, and quickening—were the primary sense apprehensions of pregnancy. These physical feelings, along with cessation of menses, were how a woman identified that she was pregnant. Moreover, throughout pregnancy, they remained the primary source of connection between the woman and the fetus. Until very recently, it would have been impossible for women to visualize any stage of embryonic or fetal development in the way we do today, although surely women must have carried pictures of the baby in their mind's eye. Because images of the fetus are so ubiquitous today and because we are able to conjure a mental image of various stages of embryonic and fetal development instantly, the fetus has become an everyday image in our society.

Two of the most significant forces driving this visualization are the tremendous power of visual images in the culture at large and the ubiquity of fetal images in popular, political, and religious culture. The fetus is visible today not just through graphic representations or stylized depictions such as line drawings, but the thing itself, rendered with photographic veracity. This veracity sets the fetus apart from almost every other part of the interior body, with the possible exception of the skeleton and the skull. We have seen graphic representations of the interior organs, like the heart and the liver. We know their basic contours, their shapes, we may even visualize them in color, but rarely do we see photographs of these viscera. When we experience a stomach cramp, our primary sensation is still kinesthetic, not visual. We do not "picture" our stomach when it feels sick. Pregnancy is different. It is a bodily process that takes place inside the body and that yields abundant physical sensations, but today it is a visual phenomenon as much as a visceral one. The visualization of pregnancy is another way of addressing the need for certainty. It is also a way of socializing pregnancy, of making the experience commonly accessible to all, not just a private, interior experience of the pregnant woman alone. Since we can all "see" the fetus, we all "know" what pregnancy is.

While pregnancy is visible to all of us, pregnant women are particularly encouraged to think of their pregnancies in visual rather than sensate terms. Websites like "The Visible Embryo" present detailed photographs and pictures of all stages of development—from fertilization and implantation, to forty weeks gestation. A particularly stunning depiction of development can be seen at "First 9 months," which offers a "multimedia journey through the first, second and third trimesters of an unborn child's life," including ultrasound images and the sound of a beating heart. Women are trained through prenatal care to think of their baby in visual terms. Ultrasound technicians produce grainy images labeled "Baby's first picture" or they write bubble captions like "Hi Mom!" before they print out the pictures. Many women speak of ultrasound as a transformative moment in their pregnancies—the moment the baby became "real" to them. This transformation seems to be the modern equivalent of quickening—a shift in the pregnant woman's emotional relationship with the fetus/baby. The "Make-a-Sono Portrait" computer software package enables expectant parents to "make a pre-portrait of your baby-to-be using sonogram enhancement." The irony of the importance ascribed to ultrasound is that it so often yields blurry images, all but inscrutable to the layperson. Yet despite its technical and erudite nature, the fetal sonogram has rapidly become another visual icon in our society, appearing even in an advertisement for Volvo.

Learning to be Pregnant: What Every Woman "Needs to Know"

The ubiquity of images and descriptions of the fetus and fetal development in lay materials for pregnant women reflects the information imperative that accompanies the experience of pregnancy in our society today. Pregnancy makes not only physical demands on women, but mental ones as well. Various forms of education are deemed necessary, whether it comes in the form of childbirth education classes, prenatal classes, parenting classes, or self-tutoring through reading, surfing the web, or watching instructional videos. Women are expected to master a wide variety of facts and information, and rules and regulations that pertain to pregnancy. "Good" prenatal behavior (and by extension good mothering) has expanded to include not only seeking medical prenatal care, but also learning. Pregnancy is no longer only physical work—it is a cognitive mental task as well. Ignorance is no longer blissful; it is inappropriate, even dangerous. Women are expected to know a lot about pregnancy and about how to be pregnant the right way. As Carol Brooks Gardner notes, there is now a "pregnancy scholarship" for women to "train" themselves to be pregnant by reading and absorbing vast quantities of information (Gardner 1994, 1995). In Fox's terms, they are striving to "achieve cognitive command" of their situation.

There is no shortage of materials to draw on. In June 2001, *Books in Print* listed over 2000 books on pregnancy, including such titles as *What to Expect When You're Expecting* (Eisenberg et al. 1996), *125 Things You Must Know About Being Pregnant* (Landi 1998), *The Girlfriends' Guide to Pregnancy: Or Everything Your Doctor Won't Tell You* (Iovine 1995) from one side of the aisle, and *Advice from a Pregnant Obstetrician: An Insider's Guide* (Brasner and Wolitzer 1998) from the other. In addition, there are some half-dozen pregnancy magazines on sale at newsstands or available as give-aways in doctors' offices. Pregnancy is prominent on the Internet as well. Pregnancy websites typically offer information, charts of fetal growth and maternal weight gain, products to buy, chat rooms, Frequently Asked Questions, pregnancy journals, and message-boards.[2]

Many of the pregnancy advice books encourage women to make pregnancy a cognitive task: *Conscious Pregnancy: Enhance Your Physical, Emotional, Mental and Spiritual Experiences* (Bancroft 1999) and *Mindful Maternity: Loving your Unborn Child to Health and Happiness* (Wirth 2001) are but two examples. The March of Dimes sponsors the "Think Ahead!" campaign, producing posters and brochures that exhort women to "Think ahead! Is there a baby in your future?" Why should thinking and thoughtfulness be such crucial components of pregnancy? Pregnancy, after all, is a physiological process controlled by hormones, not by consciousness. Thought assumes such importance because it becomes a way of attacking uncertainty. Particularly in our largely secular modern culture, rational thought and logic are seen as the way to overcome fear and to master uncertainty.

Although these materials make overt the injunction to think during pregnancy, by far the largest category of pregnancy publications and websites position themselves as repositories of information, as the source of what women "need to know" during pregnancy. They presume that women need and want a detailed encyclopedia of pregnancy. *The Everything Pregnancy Book: What Every Woman Needs to Know Month-by-Month to Insure a Worry Free Pregnancy* (Brinley 1999) and *The Unofficial Guide to Having a*

Baby (Douglass and Sussman 1999) exemplify this genre. There is also *The Complete Idiot's Guide to Pregnancy* (DiGeronimo and Gliksman 1999), and even the popular series in the bright yellow covers has an entry in the pregnancy genre: *Pregnancy for Dummies* (Stone and Murray 1999). The exemplar of the lay pregnancy guides and one of the bestsellers of the genre is *What to Expect When You're Expecting* (Eisenberg et al. 1996), which positions itself as the "pregnancy bible." First published in 1984, with a second edition published in 1991 and revised in 1996, *What to Expect*, written by a mother and her two daughters, strives to project an aura of folksy coziness. The cover depicts a pastel drawing of a pregnant woman in a rocking chair, book balanced on belly, against the backdrop of a pink and yellow quilt. The subtitle on the cover claims that the book "reassuringly answers the concerns of mothers- and fathers-to-be..." (The cover of the 1996 printing also boasts that 9 million copies have been sold to date.)

Yet reassurance is coupled with constant reminders of risk in *What to Expect When You're Expecting*. The authors portray pregnancy as the ultimate gamble—a venture in which risks are many and the "pay-off" far from certain. A section on "Playing baby roulette" (p.76) discusses exposure to potential teratogens during pregnancy and describes genetic counselors as "a sort of heredity bookmaker" (p. 41). The book recommends that women follow the "Best-Odds" diet to "improve the odds significantly, to come as close as possible to guaranteeing your baby not just good health, but excellent health" (p.80). One of the precepts of this diet is that "every bite counts."

> You've got only nine months of meals and snacks with which to give your baby the best possible start in life. Make every one of them count. Before you close your mouth on a forkful of food, consider, "Is this the best bite I can give my baby?" If it will benefit your baby, chew away. If it'll only benefit your sweet tooth or appease your appetite, put your fork down. (p. 81)

The Best-Odds diet and the metaphor of pregnancy as a wager or a gamble capture several dimensions of modern pregnancy. The notion of pregnancy as a wager expresses both risk *and* hope that one can "beat the odds" by playing the game right or smartly. These metaphors vividly express the uncertainty surrounding pregnancy, yet they also rely on probabilistic logic to manage that uncertainty. They also imply a moral imperative on the part of the pregnant woman to act in ways that beat the odds. In short, such metaphors foster the notion of pregnancy as a master status. In fact, the Best Odds diet makes explicit what many other books imply: that the entire and only point of eating during pregnancy is to feed the fetus—a woman's own appetite or sweet tooth be damned.

The proliferation of information about pregnancy promises to remove much of the uncertainty from the nine months of waiting. Women can know precisely what is happening inside them everyday—or at least have the comforting illusion of knowing. The popularity of *What to Expect* attests to the fact that many women do in fact want detailed knowledge. Yet many women rebel against the tyranny of information that such books represent, a tyranny which assumes on the one hand that every woman wants to be an expert in fetal development, although some women do not. As one woman wryly notes, "Did I really need to know when my firstborn developed an anus?" (Kelley 2000). On the other hand, pregnancy scholarship is not essential. If a woman does not show interest in this kind of detailed knowledge, is she somehow insufficiently maternal? In fact, many women reject the tyranny of information and react strongly to the hectoring, moralistic tone in which it is often delivered. The Amazon.com website lists 309 readers' comments on *What to Expect When You're Expecting*; they are about evenly divided between positive and negative reviews. The negative reviews describe the book as "preachy," "scary," "alarmist," "negative," "puritanical," and "condescending." "Who needs to be belittled and berated when pregnancy is supposed to be a happy time?" asks one reader. Another declares, "Maybe this was written for a previous generation. I can't help but feel as though this book is trapped in some kind of mysterious time warp, where modern obstetrical technology meets the social values of the 1950s." Indeed, one of the primary lessons the book imparts is that women ought to expect their doctors to be in control. One indignant reader, partly in reaction to the highly medicalized view of birth presented in the book writes that it "should be re-titled 'What to Expect When You Are a Lamb Being Led to Slaughter.'" As these women vividly express, not all pregnant women find information necessary or even desirable. Nevertheless, such information is omnipresent for the pregnant woman and more often than not she is made to feel that if she ignores it, she does so at her own peril. "This book was my Bible," writes another reader. "I was completely clueless about pregnancy and what to expect. I don't think there was a day that went by that I didn't look up something in this book... I don't think I could have made it through without it" (Amazon customer reviews 2001).

Counting the Days: The Quantification of Pregnancy

What to Expect When You're Expecting is organized by month of pregnancy. Each chapter of the book focuses on a particular month and explains in sections "what you can expect at this month's checkup," "what you may be feeling," "what you may be concerned about," and "what it's important to know." This organization reflects another aspect of modern pregnancy. It is—like the life span in general—being broken into smaller and smaller discrete stages. Pregnancy is an experience of constant physical change, and the rapidity with which the transformations of pregnancy unfold introduce yet another kind of uncertainty: 'what will happen to my body *today*?' the pregnant woman wonders. Thus, the measurement of time's passage has become central to the modern experience of pregnancy. Time's passage and the quantification of accompanying change are evident in both the scrupulous monitoring and recording of a pregnant woman's changing weight and the estimation of her due date, which serves as a marker around which the experience of pregnancy is ordered. Pregnancy thus becomes an arithmetic experience as much as a physiological metamorphosis. Like visualization of the fetus, this chronological quantification of pregnancy has occurred in stages over the last several decades. First women and doctors learned to think of pregnancy in terms of trimesters, then in terms of months of gestation (Arney 1982). Now many pregnancy materials discuss pregnancy in terms of weeks, informing women exactly what is happening and should happen in each week. And some—particularly websites and computer software programs such as "InfanTime"—encourage women to think of their pregnancies in days. Every day, for example, InfanTime offers the woman a counter that works both backwards and forwards in time; it tells her both how many days since she conceived and how many days left until her due date. InfanTime estimates fetal weight and length daily and daily offers a new fact about fetal development in that period of pregnancy.[3]

Pregnancy has thus been transformed from a seamless flow of experience into a discrete, discontinuous experience of trimesters, months, weeks, and days. The milestones become less memorable as they proliferate. Fragmenting pregnancy chronologically enables women and doctors to pinpoint with greater and greater precision just "what is happening." This precision serves as another defense against uncertainty. How comforting to turn on the computer every morning and learn just how much your fetus/baby weighs *that day*. Like the due date—a wide estimate that may be as much as two weeks off in either direction—this chronological measurement of pregnancy offers women a mirage of certainty.

Pregnancy Journals and Navel-Gazing

Pregnancy also is meant to be self-consciously introspective. Many books and websites encourage women to keep journals or diaries throughout their pregnancies. This introspection and navel-gazing reach their extreme in the many Internet chat-rooms that encourage women to communicate with others who are pregnant, often grouping those with common due dates together so they can reflect on their own experiences with others who mirror them. This self-reflection combined with literal reflection in others is perceived as reassuring, offering the comfort of the comrade-in-arms. There is a whole genre of books geared towards helping women record their pregnancy experience, such as *My Pregnancy Record Book: A Treasured Keepsake for a Special Time* (DK Publishing 1999) and *Expecting You: My Pregnancy Journal* (Kranz 2000). Many websites also allow women to keep their pregnancy diaries or journals online, posting a new installment every week. Readers can follow the woman's experience of pregnancy and often can post comments or questions on a special message board for the journal writer. These electronic media and such books as *The Everything Pregnancy Organizer: Monthly Checklists, Calendars, Schedules and More* (Smolen 2000) blur the traditionally female adolescent activity of keeping a diary with the traditionally male activities of keeping a campaign record or a ship's log. They make pregnancy at once an introspective experience and a bureaucratic one. The notion of record keeping also echoes the process of medical prenatal care.

All of these products and books encourage women both to self-identify as pregnant and to socialize with other pregnant women. They make pregnancy the central salient aspect of a woman's individual identity and they also construct "being pregnant" as a kind of collective group identity. There are pregnancy books for single women, black women, Jewish women, lesbian women, New Age women, older women, Christian women, New York City women, and "thinking" women. It is on the many websites devoted to pregnancy that this "little society" of pregnant women finds its fullest expression. In chat rooms, on message boards, and through shared online pregnancy journals, women self-consciously identify themselves as pregnant to strangers, form intimate relationships with other women who share their due date, and establish a community in which they can safely joke with each other about the travails of pregnancy. Many of the websites provide glossaries for newcomers, parsing the insider abbreviations such as DPO (days past ovulation), TTC (trying to conceive), HPT (home pregnancy test), and EW (egg white, i.e. cervical mucus) employed in chat rooms and on message boards. Curiously, these virtual communities of pregnant women—in particular, the popular online pregnancy journals—blend and blur the private experience of pregnancy into a social and public activity. Online, women share a lingo and a culture, markers of an insider culture, yet their world online is transparent and accessible to anyone. Pregnancy is at once private and intimate, public and social.

Buying into Pregnancy and Perfecting Production

That there are thousands of books on pregnancy for sale reflects another aspect of pregnancy today: its commodification and commercialization. These trends reflect broader patterns in our social life generally, especially the intense consumer ethic of modern American culture. The commodification of pregnancy occurs along two dimensions. The first is the emergence of the pregnant woman as a special market niche, with a wide array of products targeted just at her. The second is the notion of the baby as a "product," and pregnancy as a production process that a woman can control to produce an optimal, preferably even a "perfect" product. The notion of pregnancy and birth as production processes is not new (Martin 1992), but the entrenchment of the idea is perhaps deeper than is commonly acknowledged. Indeed, the quantification and record keeping that have become accepted aspects of pregnancy are regular features of the industrial production process, used in part to insure quality.

A *de rigeur* feature of pregnancy and parenting magazines is the article on what you need to buy for baby. In America, these consumer products are treated as essentials: "How can one little baby need so much stuff?" runs the typical headline. Of course, "one little baby" does not in fact "need so much stuff." The need is socially constructed, but constructed in such a way that to deprive one's little baby of all this stuff seems neglectful. Pregnancy also increasingly seems to require consumer spending for the woman herself: on maternity clothes, pregnancy scholarship materials, special teas and foods and vitamins, pregnancy exercise videos, and things like the pregnancy awareness bracelet, a stainless steel bracelet that warns "Baby in Waiting" in case of an emergency. There are products like the BébéSounds Prenatal Heart Listener, a small monitor and a set of headphones, which enable parents to recreate a medicalized experience of pregnancy at home. "Now you can listen to the wonderful sounds of your unborn baby, months before birth, in your own home. The BébéSounds Prenatal Heart Listener amplifies the sounds of your developing baby so you can hear the kicks, hiccups, and most miraculously, as early as your fifth month, the precious sounds of your baby's heartbeat."

In addition to the myriad consumer products targeting pregnant women, babies themselves are turning into commodities. Many prenatal products are geared towards improving the quality of the child that will result from the pregnancy (Blank 1990; McGee 1997). Indeed, pregnancy today is marked not only by an information imperative, but by a perfection imperative as well.[4] Pregnant women can perfect their "product" through quality control, facilitated by prenatal testing, and by increasing their inputs into the production process. Special headphones can be bought that are worn on the abdomen to play Mozart for the fetus. The BébéSounds Prenatal Teacher claims it will "stimulate your unborn baby's intellectual and emotional development," enabling women to "Have a smarter baby!" Books promote special diet regimens designed to optimize fetal development. *Program Your Baby's Health: The Pregnancy Diet for Your Child's Lifelong Wellbeing* (Luke and Eberlein 2001), for example, echoes the precepts of the Best-Odds diet and fosters the moral obligation on the part of the pregnant woman to "program" her future child correctly.

Pregnancy as Master Status

All of these trends—the increasing medicalization of pregnancy, prenatal testing, fetal visibility, the information imperative, and the transformation of the fetus into a "product"—accrete to change dramatically the position of the pregnant woman in society. All encourage the pregnant woman herself, as well as all those around her, to see her primarily as pregnant. The consequence of these trends is the evolution of pregnancy into a "master social status" (Goffman 1963) that trumps all other aspects of a woman's social being. Although we do not think of pregnancy as stigmatizing in the way that race or deviance or criminality may be, it nevertheless has the power to color social perceptions of its bearer and to govern all her social interactions. And like other master statuses, pregnancy can result in the objectification of those who bear it. Even cultural artifacts as innocent as the popular maternity t-shirt bearing the slogan "Baby on Board" or the special "stork parking" places reserved for "moms to be" (Levey 2001) contribute to this objectification of pregnancy and pregnant women. Pregnancy as a master status makes women essentially reproductive rather than social beings. It emphasizes women's biological identities over their social ones. When a woman's master status is pregnancy, it is all too easy to conceive of her as a "walking womb," a "life support system," or a "fetal container"—a mere vessel rather than a social actor.

Women joke about "the pregnancy police," yet the phenomenon is a very real one and almost every pregnant woman has stories of being scolded, chastised, harangued, or denied service by a stranger in public, merely because she was visibly pregnant (Balsamo 1996). A regular topic of discussion on pregnancy websites and in magazines is what is often called "pregnancy etiquette"—or how to handle the rude, inappropriate, and insensitive comments, queries, and actions of strangers in public (Spencer 2001). These interactions are precipitated in part by the sense that the pregnant woman "belongs to all of us." She is a kind of public trust, something like our national parks, and the public has a stake in the outcome of her pregnancy—and thus in her actions *during* pregnancy.

By facilitating the separation of the woman and the fetus into two distinct entities, the evolution of pregnancy into a master status, along with the iconic status of the fetus, contributes powerfully to the notion of the maternal-fetal conflict, which pits the pregnant woman against the fetus she carries. Increasingly, our laws, public policies, and medical practices presume that the pregnant woman may have interests in opposition to the fetus she carries, that in fact the fetus may need to be "protected" from its mother (Cole 1990).

Conclusion

The longing for certainty manifest in these cultural forms suggests that the lesson of uncertainty writ large in pregnancy is an especially vexing one in today's world of instant gratification and heightened expectations of personal control. Uncertainty and its management have been central themes in Reneé Fox's work and she has demonstrated again and again the need to be attentive to the moral and spiritual dimensions of social and individual psychic states. As the case of pregnancy shows, uncertainty in the realm of health and illness is a central problem not only for the practitioners of medicine involved in the care of patients, but also for the patients themselves. The burden of uncertainty shouldered by the pregnant woman, like that assumed by the physician, looms especially large because the well-being of another life is deeply implicated in her actions and because a personal sense of responsibility for an unforeseeable outcome seems inescapable. Pregnant women bear the burden not only of their own individual worries, but of collective anxiety as well. Pregnancy, moreover, demonstrates that, as more and more dimensions of human experience become medicalized, patients and lay persons face pressures to adopt strategies similar to those of physicians and medical professionals to make sense of their experiences of uncertainty.

Finally, pregnancy has so much cultural salience not only because it is a profoundly meaningful experience in individuals' lives, a voyage from one stage of life to another, but also because of pregnancy's usefulness and richness as a deeply resonant social metaphor. Pregnancy embodies not only risk; it embodies, literally, the future as well. Hence society's collective sense of having a stake in individual women's pregnancies. As the Association for Pre- and Perinatal Psychology and Health puts it on their website, "Womb ecology has a way of becoming world ecology" (APPPAH 2001). Pregnancy holds our collective future, and as a society entering a new millennium, we are deeply anxious and uncertain about what that future holds.

Notes

1. Yet the real purpose of prenatal tests like amniocentesis and CVS is not to provide reassurance to the vast majority of women whose fetuses suffer no defects, but rather to identify precisely those who do.
2. The Storksite helps parents to choose names and includes a feature called Babygram, which describes the specific stage of fetal development according to the woman's due date. The BabyZone includes a "due date club" and ePregnancy offers due date buddies, recipes, message boards, pregnancy diaries, and news. On the Labor of Love site women can read pregnancy poetry, pregnancy journals, correspond on message boards, or enter their newborn in a photo contest. The BabyCenter site offers surveys and polls, special chat rooms for women pregnant for the first time or on bed rest, as well as ample opportunities for online shopping. Women can also create a "baby name poll" or send out electronic birth announcements. The Parent Time site offers advice columns from an ob/gyn and a midwife, the opportunity to find a pregnant "pen pal" who shares a woman's due date, and interviews with celebrity parents.
3. Books such as *Pregnancy Week-by-Week: Everything You Need to Know about Yourself and Your Developing Baby* (MacDougall and Jennings 2000), *Perfect Pregnancy Week by Week: Practical Handbook* (MacKonochie 1999), and *The Pregnancy Calendar: Your 40-Week Guide to Prenatal Care and Fetal Development* (Jones, Rumbach and Frazier 2001) make pregnancy comprehensible by breaking it down into small units. The Pregnancy Daily Calendar website promises to help women "find out what's happening to your body and your baby every day." Many websites offer a "Due Date Calculator" to "determine the milestones during your pregnancy." Once women subscribe to "Pregnancy Weekly," the service sends weekly updates "on how your baby is developing and the changes within your body" via email.
4. Later, when their new product proves recalcitrant or mystifying, women can turn to articles with titles such as "Owner's manual for new moms."

References

Amazon customer reviews. 2001.

Arney, William Ray. 1982. *Power and the Profession of Obstetrics*. Chicago: University of Chicago Press.

Association for Pre- and Perinatal Psychology and Health (APPPAH). 2001. "Welcome to Birth Psychology," http://www.birthpsychology.com/birthpsychology/.

Balsamo, Anne. 1996. "Public pregnancies and cultural narratives of surveillance," in *Technologies of the Gendered Body: Reading Cyborg Women*. Durham: Duke University Press.

Bancroft, Mark. 1999. *Conscious Pregnancy: Enhance Your Physical, Emotional, Mental and Spiritual Experiences.* Visalia, CA: EnSpire Press.

Bastian, Lori A., Kavita Nanda, Vic Hasselblad, David L. Simel. 1998. "Diagnostic efficiency of home pregnancy test kits." *Archives of Family Medicine* 7:465-469.

Blank, Robert H. 1990. *Regulating Reproduction.* New York: Columbia University Press.

Brasner, Sheri and Meg Wolitzer. 1998. *Advice from a Pregnant Obstetrician: An Insider's Guide.* New York: Hyperion.

Brinley, Maryann B. 1999. *The Everything Pregnancy Book: What Every Woman Needs to Know Month-by-Month to Insure a Worry Free Pregnancy.* Avon, MA: Adams Media Corporation.

Cole, Helene M. 1990. "Legal interventions during pregnancy." *Journal of the American Medical Association* 264(20):2663-2670.
Conkling, Winifred. 2000. *The Expectant Mother's Checklist.* New York: St. Martin's Press.
DiGeronimo, Theresa Foy and Michele Isaacs Gliksman. 1999. *The Complete Idiot's Guide to Pregnancy.* New York: Macmillan USA.
Douglass, Ann and John R. Sussman. 1999. *The Unofficial Guide to Having a Baby.* New York: Hungry Minds, Inc.
Eisenberg, Arlene, Heidi E. Murkoff and Sandee E. Hathaway. 1996. *What to Expect When You're Expecting.* New York: Workman Publishing.
Fox, Reneé C. 1988. "Training for uncertainty," pp. 19-50 in *Essays in Medical Sociology: Journeys into the Field.* New Brunswick: Transaction Publishers.
Gardner, Carol Brooks. 1994. "Little strangers: Pregnancy conduct and the twentieth-century rhetoric of endangerment," pp. 62-92 in *Troubling Children: Studies of Children and Social Problems,* edited by Joel Best. New York: Aldine de Gruyter.
Gardner, Carol Brooks. 1995. "Learning for two: A study in the rhetoric of pregnancy practices." *Perspectives on Social Problems* 7:29-51.
Goffman, Erving. 1963. *Stigma: Notes on the Management of Spoiled Identity.* New York: Simon & Schuster Inc.
Iovine, Vicki. 1995. *The Girlfriend's Guide to Pregnancy: Or Everything Your Doctor Won't Tell You.* New York: Pocket Books.
Jones, Marion Finholm, Beth Rumbach and Julie Linden Frazier. 2001. *The Pregnancy Calendar: Your 40-Week Guide to Prenatal Care and Fetal Development.* Denver: Linholm Corporation.
Kelley, Tina. 2000. "You can't speed up the stork, but you can track him online." *New York Times* December 13: H22.
Kitzinger, Sheila and Vickey Bailey. 2001. *Pregnancy Day by Day: The Expectant Mother's Diary, Record Book and Guide.* New York: Alfred Knopf.
Kranz, Linda. 2000. *Expecting You: My Pregnancy Journal.* Cambridge, MA: Fisher Books.
Landi, Nina D. 1998. *125 Things You Must Know About Being Pregnant.* New York: Owl Books.
Levey, Bob. 2001. "The latest controversy: 'Stork Parking.'" *Washington Post,* Nov 14:C13.
Luke, Barbara and Tamara Eberlein. 2001. *Program Your Baby's Health: the Pregnancy Diet for Your Child's Lifelong Well-Being.* New York: Ballantine Wellspring.
MacDougall, Jane and Madeleine Jennings, eds. 2000. *Pregnancy Week-by-Week: Everything You Need to Know about Yourself & Your Developing Baby.* Collingdale, PA: DIANE Publishing Company.
MacKonochie, Alison. 1999. *Perfect Pregnancy Week by Week: Practical Handbook.* New York: Anness Publishing.
Martin, Emily. 1992. *The Woman in the Body: A Cultural Analysis of Reproduction.* Boston: Beacon Press.
McGee, Glenn. 1997. *The Perfect Baby: A Pragmatic Approach to Genetics.* New York: Rowman & Littlefield.
"Melanie and Pete's Pregnancy Journal." 2001.http://www.epregnancy.com/features/journals/melanie/week6.htm.
My Pregnancy Record Book. 1999. New York: Dorling Kindersley Publishing, Inc.
Reagan, Leslie J. 1997. *When Abortion was a Crime: Women, Medicine, and Law in the United States, 1867-1973.* Berkeley: University of California Press.
Reigel, Margaret. 1999. "Testing, testing." *Healthy Pregnancy* 1(2):23-25.

Rosen, Lynn, ed. 2000. *My Pregnancy Journal: A Guided Journal.* Mt. Vernon, NY: Peter Pauper Press.

Smolen, Marguerite. 2000. *The Everything Pregnancy Organizer: Monthly Checklists, Calendars, Schedules, & More.* Avon, MA: Adams Media Corporation.

Spencer, Paula. 2001. "Maternity manners." *BabyTalk* 66(1):50-55.

Stone, Joanne and Mary Murray. 1999. *Pregnancy for Dummies.* New York: Harper Books.

Wirth, Frederick. 2001. *Mindful Maternity: Loving Your Unborn Child to Health and Happiness.* New York: Harper Collins.

2

Healthy Beliefs: Wellness in Action at Company X[1]

Jacqueline Hart

"The Good News: Chalk up another point for healthy living. Half of all fatal cancers are linked to diet, smoking and lack of exercise—all factors that individuals can control" (*Time* 1996:16). Why is this good news? Health and illness are viewed as being in our control, based on the choices we make about how we live our lives—through what we eat, how much we exercise, and what substances we smoke and drink. This understanding relies on the belief that an individual's health behaviors (e.g. diet, engaging in physical activity, smoking, drinking) literally produce that person's health. Further, this implies that we each have an equal opportunity to *choose*[2] good health. A corollary of this view, sometimes explicitly stated, is that we must take responsibility for our health through living healthier lives, so as not to tax the common good.[3] Virtually everywhere we turn in the contemporary United States, we are confronted with warnings about the unnecessary disease and premature death that will result from a lack of personal vigilance over our health. We are a society that produces and consumes sound bytes of health information about risk, lifestyle, and the promise of freedom from disease and aging.[4]

The current stress on prevention (cultural, personal, medical, economic, and political) and the identification and control of risk factors through lifestyle or health behavior changes, will be referred to as the wellness ethic, or wellness. The wellness ethic is powerful and pervasive because it highlights dominant American ideals of individualism, self-fulfillment, equality of opportunity, freedom, and the importance of work and productivity (Tocqueville 1984 [1840]; Weber 1991 [1930]; Lasch 1979; Sennett 1992 [1974]; Bellah et al. 1985). Wellness serves as a cultural myth, or morality tale, much like the Horatio Alger story. Good health is equally available to each and every one of us, and our success in achieving it depends only on our desire and effort. Wellness is presented, and often understood, as a strategy that is beneficial to both the individual, in the form of a long and disease-free life, and to society through the reduction of health care costs and increases in productivity. Current economic and political agendas are served well by such an ethic in American society because it removes the responsibility for achieving good health from the public to the private sphere. Through invoking the wellness ethic, health interventions emphasize the cultural value of equal opportunity, individualizing and normalizing high standards of self-care and good health, while ignoring the increasing social stratification that leads to health and health care disparities in the United States.

Previous work on wellness has, for the most part, focused on its felicitous aspects and impact both individually and collectively. In an effort to provide a more balanced view of the wellness ethic, I have been particularly attentive to the unintended, and possibly negative, consequences of its uses. One driving concern of my research is how a well-entrenched belief that we are each responsible for our own health supports practices that maintain that we each have the *duty* to be well (Crawford 1979, Skrabanek 1994), which in turn might lead to social and economic exclusion based on health behaviors and health (Nelkin and Tancredi 1989). I view wellness as an ideology, as well as a set of practices, and ask how such a trenchant individualistic approach (Fitzgerald 1994, Skrabanek 1994) to health in the United States is created in the face of evidence that shows how the economy, community, workplace, and environment are so important to an individual's state of health. This ideology precludes any real possibility for conceiving of health in a truly psychosocial way that better addresses the complex ways in which social and individual factors interact to create health.

While "healthist" discourses, such as wellness, have been studied (Crawford 1979, Conrad 1994, Ehrenreich 1995), previous analysts have not studied the *creation* of wellness. My research shows the dynamic process of the institutionalization and creation of wellness ideology and discourse, as well as what the implicit and explicit messages about individual attributes are in the information, programs, and individual understandings about health behaviors. A fundamental aspect of my work is to ask, what is wellness in practice? What does wellness action tell us about who we are and what we value? In analyzing the explicit and implicit meanings of health and illness, and being attentive to the interpretive process that continually shapes and changes them, what do we learn about where we as a society are going? What does wellness ideology highlight?

The research on which this paper draws focuses on wellness professionals as the critical actors, and the worksite as the central arena, for the implementation of wellness ideology. Wellness professionals are the crucial actors who put wellness discourse into action, especially those who develop worksite-based wellness programs. The worksite is an especially important place to view the wellness ethic as it is a milieu where dominant American cultural values concerning health have been made explicit and have been invested with human and material resources. The analysis is based on data gathered through ethnographic observation and in-depth interviews in the wellness division of an international health maintenance organization (HMO) and insurance company, Company X.[5] The field work focused on observing the development of a new wellness program called *Winning.* I argue that the importance of wellness, as created by wellness professionals at Company X, lies in the meanings given to health and illness, and not in the literal reduction of disease in the workplace. In this paper I demonstrate how the wellness division staff understood health to be primarily shaped by an individual's innate character, moral fiber, and individual choice. This conceptualization of health was important to what I argue was the de-legitimization of sick leave. In analyzing what health and illness came to mean in the institutionalization of wellness in the corporate setting of Company X, we can begin to see the implications of this ideology for the meaning and uses of health and illness, not only at the workplace but in society at large as well.

The Wellness Division

The research is based on data gathered over a two-year period, from September 1996 to July 1998, in the wellness division of the international headquarters of Company X. The company has been nationally recognized as a leader in wellness programming. Company X has 36,000 domestic employees, 14,000 international employees, and 500 offices worldwide. According to its 1997 Annual Report, the company has assets of 100 billion dollars and a net income of $1 billion. Company X is self-insured,[6] and 90 percent of their employees have the company's HMO-based health plan.

The wellness division, with a budget of $4 million in 1997, is comprised of three sub-divisions: the statewide health centers (including an onsite care facility in the headquarters); the national wellness programs; and the fitness center, the headquarters' onsite fully-equipped gym. The division had twenty-nine full-time staff members and one temporary full-time nurse during my time there. Four staff members, Elizabeth, Carol, Tara, and Alice, were in charge of developing all of the wellness programs at Company X. In addition, Cindy, a nurse at an onsite care facility in one of Company X's field offices, was part of the program planning committee for *Winning*. With one exception (Tara, who holds an MS in worksite health), all were registered nurses (RNs).

A New Direction: *Winning*

The wellness division's response to their new mandate of making wellness integral to corporate goals was to develop *Winning*,[7] a behavior and lifestyle management program with the goal of reducing short-term disability costs. According to *Winning*'s project manager, the aim of the program was not just to get employees back to work faster from short-term disability, but also to return them to the worksite at a "higher productivity level."[8] The program's goal of "...improving the functional status of returning individuals" was also conceived of as a way to prevent the incidence of short-term disability.

The conviction that individuals can prevent illness through health behavior modification guided the development of *Winning*. Staff believed that short-term disability claimants' diagnoses could be traced back to, and therefore prevented by, health behaviors. As explained in an internal company report on *Winning*, "It is widely accepted that obesity, sedentary lifestyles, stress, smoking and high cholesterol are risks for one or more of the targeted diagnoses. [*Winning*] focuses on those five areas through weight management, exercise, stress management, smoking cessation, and cholesterol management." These five categories of change became what the staff termed the *change tracts* of *Winning*, and focused on health behavior modification. In reports to upper management, staff did not attempt to demonstrate, or prove, the connection between employee health behaviors, the change tracts, and their short-term disability categories; rather they relied on what they viewed as general knowledge about the correlation, and causality, between health behaviors and illness. The causal relationship between behaviors, risk, and illness were accepted as facts, and therefore did not warrant further investigation.

Based on an analysis of short-term disability claims data at Company X, *Winning* staff defined six short-term disability categories as the targets of their program: breast cancer, back pain and injury, respiratory illness/asthma, hypertension/cardiac disease, diabetes mellitus, and a catch-all category, short-term disability repeaters. Some of these categories are themselves a product of the wellness ethic. Aronowitz, in a discussion of the implications of the risk factor approach, argues that the use of risk factors "has ushered in a new era of diseases fashioned from risk" (1998:140). For example, in the 1960s, before the risk factor era, hypertension was only considered a disease when it was associated with acute or chronic organ damage. Now, hypertension has been re-defined as something associated with the increased risk of developing a disease or condition (e.g. heart attack). Following this argument, to be a "short-term disability repeater" is to have a condition that needs to be treated because it means you are at "risk" of taking short term disability leave—taking short term disability leave then becomes an illness.

The staff viewed their new claims-based health behavior method for program targeting as the best way to create an innovative and effective wellness approach that would serve the business goals of the company. The stated goal of the program—the reduction of short-term disability costs through health behavior change—is, in the words of the wellness division director, "the last frontier" of wellness. The staff chose an existing model known as the *stages of change* (Prochaska and DiClemente 1992) as the guiding theory for their new program. They believed it would enable them to achieve their goal of producing a new kind of worksite health promotion and disease prevention program that would rigorously focus on individual behavior change.[9]

The Wellness Ethic in Action

The development of *Winning* reflected the ways in which notions of health and illness had been re-conceptualized in wellness ideology, and the ways in which these meanings have been institutionalized at Company X. The staff generally displayed a highly individualized, psychological, and moralistic approach to their understanding of health and illness at Company X. Their conceptualization of health indicated an understanding of "normal" health that emphasized a kind of hyper health, one that was characterized by healthiness, self-reliance, and productivity. Health and illness were seen as almost entirely due to individual attitude and choice. One ramification of this view was that it tended to de-legitimize sick leave.

Individual Attitude = Health and Illness

Wellness is a particular way of defining and approaching health and illness, the individual and society. As a concept of health, wellness tends to generate specific approaches with respect to how society should treat people with different diseases, who is helped, and how that help is delivered and experienced. A fundamental wellness staff belief, buttressed by their use of the stages of change model, was that there is a mind-body connection. Their understanding of health was based on the World Health Organization's (WHO) definition of health, which has become the core definition used by proponents of wellness: "a state of complete physical, mental, and social well being, and not merely the absence of disease or infirmity (Fitzgerald 1994: 196)."

The way that the wellness staff at Company X used the WHO definition in their own conceptions of health provides insight into how they approached the meaning of health in the workplace, and the development of wellness programs. Elizabeth, the Assistant Vice President of Employee Health and director of the wellness division, first gave a definition of health that was a synopsis of the WHO definition. She then added the concept of normality with respect to biomedical measures, and the idea that managing the exigencies of life in a positive manner was integral to health:

Elizabeth: "Health being a dimension of physical, emotional, and spiritual well being."

Jacqueline: "What does well being mean, when you say well being?"

> Elizabeth: "Well, having a sense of homeostasis where everything is sort of within normal range, having energy and vitality to tackle new things and also to weather adversity, having capacity to feel joy and sadness, being realistic in one's expectations about life." (Elizabeth interview. 7-23-97)

Alice, the *Winning* project manager, in her definition of health, said that independence and self-reliance were important parts of health:

> Alice: "Health, to me, is a place that someone feels that they are at their optimum level. What I mean by that is I'm thinking of people who have a stroke, so they're never going to be as they were prior to the stroke perhaps. But, their optimum level may be that they can feed themselves, and that they can go to the bathroom by themselves. So that would be their optimum level, whatever it is at that point in time. So, to me, health is really an individual thing. I don't think there is a common definition of what it would be for every person because the circumstances are so different. But, to me, it's where the person is, I guess, feeling at their best or at their highest level of well being, if you want to use the lingo." (Alice interview. 11-23-98)

In every case, staff defined *health* as if they had been asked to define *healthy*. Their definitions referred to a kind of *hyper-health*, one that was taken to be the new standard and expectation for "normal" health. They all defined health partly with respect to being able to function independently and productively in the world. An essay in the *New England Journal of Medicine* noted that both the lay public's and the medical profession's use of the WHO's new definition for health has started to "confuse the ideal of health with the norm for health" (Fitzgerald 1994: 196).

Staff viewed this mind-body understanding of health as the hallmark of their new wellness approach. According to proponents of the wellness ethic, the physical aspects of health have been overstressed by western medicine, and it is only by re-integrating the body and the mind that progress can be made in the area of health promotion and disease prevention. In the process of institutionalizing the wellness understanding of health, the staff almost entirely abandoned the body in favor of the psyche, understood as "attitude." In addition, their efforts at improving health were ultimately directed exclusively inward, to an individual's outlook, as opposed to the structural arrangements of the workplace or society.

This focus may have both status implications and religious dimensions. A psychological and individualistic approach to health may be associated with a certain amount of material and social privilege. Blair (1993) found class differences in how people communicate the experience of illness. When asked about the cause of cancer, middle class respondents mentioned mental factors and the role of the self, such as stress and anxiety, while working class respondents referred to physical and environmental factors such as pollution and safety.[10]

In addition, focusing on the mind, specifically outlook, is something of a religious component. As Thomas noted in commenting on the association between moral well being and physical health, the Protestant belief in health regimens necessitates "peace of mind." "[I]nner cheerfulness and confidence were thus essential psychological attributes. They could be induced by religious faith and a clear conscience" (1997:23). Similarly, in the context of Company X, subscribing to the wellness message meant believing not only that one has the ability to over-come the exigencies of life, but also that crisis and calamity are opportunities for self-improvement. Health was viewed as being determined by a deeply held worldview, and there was a belief that the signs of an individual's *outlook* would be reflected in health behaviors and attitudes:

> Well I guess as you get older, I think you expect certain things to happen, and as long as you can take it in stride and don't get all upset about every little thing, I would say you're still healthy. You still have a good state of health... Attitude, I think, plays the biggest part of your state of health. (Sara interview. 11-24-97)

Wellness calls for a particular kind of attitude, one that is optimistic, positive, and even cheery.

Tara, the national director of wellness programs, and the initial project manager of *Winning*, emailed a story to colleagues and friends as a New Year's motivational message. The story described a man she knew, Joe, who consistently displayed a positive attitude. Joe explained to her how he maintained his positive attitude: "Each time something bad happens, I can choose to be a victim or I can choose to learn from it. I choose to learn from it." Joe was shot in a robbery and was in intensive care for weeks recovering. She asked him how he handled what must have been a frightening experience. Joe replied that as he lay on the floor after being shot, "...I remembered that I had two choices. I could choose to live or choose to die. I chose to live." Tara wrote in reference to the example Joe had set for her:

> I learned from him every day we have the choice to live fully. Attitude after all is everything...there is a big wellness message in this story—we all choose whether we are going to take care of ourselves or not, physically, emotionally, spiritually, socially. Don't blame external forces for your own well being or lack thereof. Take charge and choose to live a happy and healthy life (Tara email message. 12-30-98).

This sense of self-efficacy and empowerment is avowedly hopeful. At the same time, the wellness message, as Tara put it, is clear: you are responsible for everything that happens to you, there is no room for external excuses, and you are the locus of control.

One should not blame external forces for one's sickness or health—that much is clear. But what are the implications for such concepts as empathy or altruism? What does being told not to blame "external forces" for sickness or health, fortune or misfortune, mean for how we treat people who are viewed as "unsuccessful," or who are unhappy or sick? During an annual two-day wellness division meeting, a nurse psychotherapist was brought in to do a staff training on weight control and eating disorders. At one point she commented, "So many people think poverty creates obesity, but obesity creates poverty (Field notes. 10-14-97)." This, she said, was because obesity limits opportunities. Peter, one of the wellness division staff, took the reasoning of individual responsibility even further, disagreeing with the statement because he felt it implied "blaming the external world," instead of putting responsibility for weight and poverty, or failure, on the individual. This individualistic approach is explicitly devoid of more traditional notions of the common good: since the unfortunate choose their misfortune, there is no reason they should be helped.

Efforts towards leading a healthier life through good health behaviors were taken as signs of being a reasonable and rational person, and as an indication that someone had the right belief system. Some employees who were not willing to strive to be healthier were called "aggressive," "irrational," and even "suicidal." To be "well" was viewed as depending on an individual's worldview, or personal philosophy, rather than physical state:

> I think wellness...can be looked at as a philosophy where a person believes that they have the power and the ability to make certain changes in their life, or to have an impact on their life by doing certain behaviors, and that that is wellness, that can be considered wellness. Even a person with a disease can be considered well as far as being in a group that is controlling that disease or minimizing that disease. So, I guess, I see wellness as a little more than just absence of illness. I think it's a philosophy and an active desire and translated into behavior that moves towards trying to be well. And that includes spiritual wellness, psychological wellness, as well as the functioning of our body. (Alice interview. 3-20-98)

According to this logic, a person with a terminal illness but resigned to the condition, and nonetheless still striving for a healthy lifestyle, might be considered healthy and well. The right attitude that leads to good health was considered important in part because it indicated that the person could be as self-sufficient as possible. *Winning*, after all, targeted individuals on short-term disability leave, who, by definition, relied on the company to take care of them. Despite the fact that short-term disability leave was a legitimate recourse for a sick employee, the implication was still that it was a base form of reliance on others, a state brought on by an individual's unwillingness to take responsibility for themselves.

An important belief, expressed by staff and operationalized by the materials and consultants they chose to use in *Winning*, was that a person's health attitudes are determined by his/her values. Tara expressed a strong belief in the link between values and health. She described to me her frustration over the process of crafting school health policy as a member of the local school board's health legislation committee: "...They won't let you teach values," she said, "but that's what it is."

This belief in the connection between health and values was reinforced by the programs and consultants who were hired to help create *Winning*. For example, for the weight change tract, a consultant was brought in for three days to conduct a staff training called, "Stages of Change and THINK LIGHT!" to teach the staff the philosophy and tools of the "Lowfat Living Plan." This training focused on how the staff could use the stages of change theory to help employees change their eating habits. The consultant told the staff that this program is not about healthy eating, rather it is about teaching clients a new outlook: "...It's rarely about nutrition, [it's about] behavior, attitudes, values..." (Field notes. 6-30-97). At the beginning of the Think Light! training manual, key terms and their definitions were provided. The first word on the list was values, defined as "Ideals and standards used to guide and determine acceptable behavior. They are our most important measure for rights and wrongs. They represent our deepest aspirations and our understanding of what gives life meaning." By highlighting values, the Think Light! program stressed the idea that a person's health behaviors reflect their deepest values and their moral compass. During the training, a message that was often repeated was that values underlie the choices we make about how to live our lives, what we eat, and as a result quite literally who we are. In this way the adage "you are what you eat" is flipped: according to this program, "you eat what you are." Through *Winning*, Company X could discuss and outline a vision of an acceptable personal belief system for employees.

An individual's desire to be healthier was taken as an indication of "…not just lifestyle, but who we are..." According to Dorothy, a senior staff nurse, the difference between people who try to pursue a healthy lifestyle and those who don't was, "Motivation, how they see themselves. People that look at themselves in a positive [way] certainly probably do better than people who get caught up in a lot of negative things in their lives." (Dorothy interview. 10-30-97) She doubted the usefulness of health risk appraisals in wellness programs because they rely on self-reports of health behaviors. She believed that people were likely to lie because, "…why would you want to tell somebody that you're a failure, that you really don't care enough about yourself to do it [healthy behaviors]?"

One's attitude towards life was viewed as so important to health that a consultant was brought in to do a staff training on "learned optimism." The goal of the training was to teach staff how to teach employees to "adopt stress-reducing techniques to gain personal control, feel energized, achieve goals, and promote physical health." The consultant told us, "If we think in terms of health and wellness we won't get colds, flus...psychosomatic illnesses people bring to work, we need to give people control" (Field notes. 10-13-97). The consultant did not provide evidence for this amorphous connection between individual outlook, control, and health, but as with many other statements made by consultants and wellness staff, these kinds of correlations were simply assumed to be true and did not warrant justification.

Illness De-legitimized

The belief that one literally creates one's health through values, attitudes, and behaviors leads to another conclusion: illness was often understood in terms of character flaws. This sentiment was expressed by the director of the wellness division who said "…we already know they have a bad attitude because they are repeat STD [short-term disability] people." Having identified the basis for short-term disability as being an individual's attitude, *Winning*'s treatment for short-term disability was then largely a retraining of the employee's attitude.

As Dr. Miller, the consultant who was hired to help design *Winning*, said in reference to sick employees who did not volunteer for the program, "You already know there's an attitudinal problem; that's why they said no [to the opportunity to participate in *Winning*]" (Field notes. 4-30-98). Because results of the program are based almost entirely on employee self reports, and because the stages of change model so heavily emphasizes an individual's intent as a crucial part of the change process, the goal of the program became to train employees to think about their health and health behaviors in a self-responsible and risk-averse way. As a ramification of the belief in attitude as the basis for health, a sick employee's choice not to participate in *Winning* was, for the staff, even further evidence that they had a character problem.

One consequence of viewing an individual's attitude as a powerful predictor of his/her health was that illness in turn was viewed as almost entirely preventable and unnecessary. Illness, in effect, was viewed in this prism as *illegitimate*. This is an interesting twist on Parsons' (1951) insights into the sick role. His conception of the sick role rests on the important understanding that a sick person is not to be held morally responsible for their illness, that they are legitimately excused from normal obligations, and that they are not expected to get well solely on the power of their own desire. Rather they must seek expert help from the medical profession in order to recover. Most fundamentally, Parsons' concept of the sick role is based on the fact that people will get sick, something that is not allowed for in Company X's approach to illness. Company X's wellness approach to sickness emphasized culpability and illegitimacy to a significant degree. The institutionalization of wellness at Company X tended to de-legitimize the sick role, with employees morally responsible for illnesses that conflicted with their work obligations.

Freedom from the traditional patriarchal doctor-patient relationship, where patients must cede control over their care to doctors, is widely considered to be a positive result of the self-care movement. However, an emphasis on self-care can also be used to de-legitimize the medical sanctioning of sick leave. For example, Elizabeth intervened on behalf of an employee for the right to go back to work (Field notes. 4-30-98). The man wanted to return to work, but his manager, following his doctor's advice, wanted him to stay at home.

Elizabeth and the employee were successful. When Elizabeth was telling this story, she presented it as a case where the patient knows his needs best, and should be the one who decides on returning to work. In this instance Elizabeth saw a patient's self-knowledge as superceding the advice of medical professionals. She applauded the employee's initiative and desire to return to work. However, it is doubtful that patient self-knowledge would have been so valorized had the employee requested a longer leave than suggested by his doctor. She invoked both the wellness ethic, challenging the medical model with the patient's unique knowledge of himself, and the business ethic, supporting a good employee who wanted to work and take responsibility for himself.

The themes outlined so far with respect to the treatment of illness at Company X find corroboration in other settings. In a study of white collar workers in France, Dodier (1985) found that moral evaluation by co-workers, as opposed to the clinical evaluation by the medical professional, played a key role in the social control of sickness at work. In particular, he found that the professional medical evaluation of sick leave that excused people from work, in extreme cases, was ignored and an "implicit scale of morbidity" (p. 126) was used instead. This meant that an employee's ability to perform his or her job was the most important, if not only, criteria used by co-workers in the social control of a sick employee.

Company X institutionalized the ideal of self-care and individual responsibility for health and illness, to the point that absence from work due to illness, particularly a prolonged absence, was seen as the result of individual actions. Their approach to sick days mirrored their management of the behavior change process, where there are "no days off" from striving to be healthier (Field notes. 7-14-97). This understanding of illness is clearly reflected in the company's lack of official sick days. Sick days are monitored at the manager level, and after five days of sick leave "it [absence] becomes a management issue." The employee is then faced with the obligation to apply to exercise their short-term disability benefit. The implicit reasoning underlying the lack of sick days was that, because health and illness are products and reflections of an individual's health attitudes and behaviors, these individuals could legitimately be held responsible for their ill health, and sick days should not be an entitlement.

There is some evidence that Company X's approach to sick leave is becoming widespread in the United States. A *New York Times* article entitled "A Plan for Unplanned Absences: New Policies Improve Attendance," describes the new approach to "unplanned absences." Worksite policies range from awarding employees with extravagant gifts, such as a $40,000 Ford Explorer, for never taking an unplanned absence, to giving employees "time-off banks" where days off can be used for any reason, but are planned for ahead of time. The thinking behind this is that sick days can be prevented. Continental Airlines, for example, holds a raffle twice a year as part of their "perfect attendance program" for employees at the manager level or below who have not missed a day of work in six months. Employees get various raffle prizes as gifts to reward them for their "devotion." One of the employees at Continental Airlines commented on his award: "It's a great incentive. It creates excitement among all of us, and people really strive to come to work and achieve" (Wells 1998: 8).

As described in the article, traditional sick leave policies are increasingly seen as "being out of step with the times." This is driven by a perceived need to make the American workforce more productive. As the vice-chairwoman at Fannie Mae said, "It's a more mature approach to the workplace. The need is recognized up front...rather than being ignored until the worker calls in to say he or she will not be coming in to work that day" (p. 8). The language used to describe sick leave, an "unplanned absence," indicates that taking a day off from work due to illness is irresponsible. The terminology implies that people have control over when they get sick, and can actually time their illness. Further, describing sick leave as "unplanned absence" does not indicate a legitimate reason for not going to work, while "sick leave" does. By changing the very language used to describe sick leave, the act of being absent from work due to illness is de-legitimized.

Conclusion

Wellness serves to direct attention to individuals, while directing attention away from the social contexts that in part create and impinge on individual well being. Proponents of the wellness ethic purport to increase individual healthiness, prevent illness, lower health care costs, and increase the productivity of the American workforce.

However, this goal is not neutral or innocuous. It requires that a host of understandings be established regarding definitions of what is "normal" health, what we should expect as a minimal level of self-care, and introducing new notions of "acceptable" vs. "unacceptable" illness.

Whether or not most Americans actually follow the prescriptions and proscriptions for healthy living found in the wellness ethic is in some ways beside the point. Currently, wellness is a dominant ideology, one that is supported and utilized by key institutions, and therefore has the ability to impact American society through the meanings we impute to health and illness, how we allocate our resources, and our notions of privacy in the workplace.

Corporate wellness activities are viewed as an effective and laudable way to cut medical costs in general. "This campaign against illness marks a crucial second phase in corporate America's war on medical costs. The first was the shift over the past few years to managed care.... The second and newest phase is improving employees' health habits so there's less chance they'll get sick to begin with" (Tully 1995: 99). The process of developing *Winning* at Company X demonstrates new directions for health promotion and disease prevention in the workplace that hinge on the belief that individuals can and should be held accountable for their health. This was accomplished by re-defining health to focus on individual attitudes and behaviors. The meaning and expectations for health at Company X became both more personal and more standardized in the process.

The interpretation and use of the stages of change model in the wellness division made the foci of *Winning* individual attitudes and behaviors. Health was partially redefined as an outlook, or attitude, demonstrated by the way employees talked about health behaviors and lived their lives. As a result, the new expectation for wellness became the employees' willingness to take complete responsibility for their health, and to act appropriately on the knowledge given about health risks by changing their health behaviors.

Caring for and empathizing with people who are sick is part of what binds us together. Sickness provides opportunities for us to give love and reassurance, and to reaffirm commitments to each other. When wellness teaches us that illness is to a large degree self-inflicted, it may discourage valuable social phenomena. This approach to health and illness is potentially socially destructive.

In the wellness ethic the bar of normal health has been raised. Health is understood as a kind of hyper-health, where what is minimally expected of individual health becomes more perfect, and where the possibility for never becoming ill is at the least an implied possibility. This ethic has implications for how we view the allocation of medical resources. If health care is in part supposed to treat and cure people, what can we expect if more and more attitudes and activities are viewed as risky and unacceptable? Wellness programs may be viewed as not just an avenue to the enhancement of personal health, but may become treatments that are seen as required components of the health care system. If this is coupled with strict notions of individualism and autonomy, then people who have chosen not to adhere to wellness may be viewed as ever more culpable for their poor health.[11]

With health promotion and disease prevention in the workplace as a national public health goal, and as more employers and health insurance companies make health behaviors the basis for insurance premiums, it becomes increasingly important to understand the new meanings of and expectations for health behaviors, health, and illness. While the goal of improving health is undoubtedly praiseworthy, implementers of health promotion and disease prevention programs in the workplace will need to be attentive to the possibly coercive, discriminatory,[12] and moralistic aspects of the interpretation and institutionalization of wellness ideology. At worst, judgments about who is worthy of a job or a medical resource[13] may increasingly be based on the kinds of health behaviors that are targeted by wellness programs. As a consequence of an ideology based so heavily on the belief that individuals can, and should, control their health through attitudes and behaviors, it is possible that a survival of the fittest mentality, linked to health and health behaviors, will result in a new constellation of factors necessary to be a successful participant in today's society and economy (Martin 1994).

Notes

1. I would like to thank Charles L. Bosk, Renée C. Fox, and Ewa Morawska for their guidance, support, and inspiration in completing the dissertation on which this paper is based. I also thank the Department of Veterans Affairs for the Postdoctoral Fellowship in Health Services Research.
2. The belief that we have free and unfettered choice over health behaviors, and health, obscures the socio-political limits on choice, and negates the socioeconomic dimensions of health and illness. There is an "illusion of choice" (see Rothman 1986). A

discussion of the rhetoric of choice in health care consumerism, and wellness, is developed elsewhere.

3. Bellah et al (1985) provide a useful definition of the common good: "In the individualist tradition, the public good is usually identified with the sum of private benefits. In the republican tradition, the public good is that which benefits society as a whole and leads to what the founders of the American republic called public happiness. It includes everything from adequate public facilities to the trust and civic friendship that makes public life something to be enjoyed rather than feared. Also called the common good" (p. 335). When I use the term common good, it refers to the latter (republican tradition) definition.
4. We are also increasingly exposed to information about the role that genes play in our health and illness. Wellness might appear to be at odds with the increasing use of genetics as a way to understand the causes of illness. While wellness identifies the causes of illness to be modifiable individual behavior, genetics identifies the gene, a purportedly immutable individual trait. However, the increasing use of genetics in health care appears to support an even more finely tuned use of the wellness ethic, as it serves to re-enforce the individualization and de-politicization of health and illness by helping to identify those individuals who are most in need of behavior change (see Lippman 1998).
5. For both methodological and legal reasons the company where I did my research is anonymous. In addition, all of the names for the individuals and institutions connected to Company X, with the exception of mine, are fictitious.
6. The fact that most of Company X employees have the company's own insurance plan has implications for the uses of health and illness in the workplace that were institutionalized in the creation of *Winning*. As Light (1992) noted, "About 81 million people under the age of 65 have chronic problems that self-insured employers can drop" (p. 2504).
7. The budget for the pilot phase of *Winning*, excluding staff salaries, was $100,000 (*Winning* memo, Oct. 1997).
8. Although beyond the scope of this paper, the ways in which the wellness ethic was used to teach and support the business ethic is an important dimension of the uses of wellness at Company X.
9. The stages of change was a natural model for the new wellness program, as it reflected staff's belief in individual responsibility for health. The model was developed by psychologists as part of a larger theoretical framework for health promotion (Prochaska, Norcross, and DiClemente 1994). The model posits that individuals progress through a series of stages when they change a behavior: *pre-contemplation*, *contemplation*, *preparation*, *action*, *maintenance*, and *termination*. Briefly: *Pre-contemplators* do not acknowledge that they have a problem, such as an unhealthy behavior; *Contemplators* acknowledge that they have a problem and express the possibility of changing in the future. This is the point on the stages of change continuum where individuals are in danger of getting stuck. Often individuals require a "teachable moment" or "emotional arousal" (such as having a heart attack) to get them to the next stage. In *preparation*, the individual plans to take action within the next thirty days, and starts to visualize a "positive self-fulfilling prophecy"; in *action*, the individual is engaged in changing the unhealthy behavior; in *maintenance*, the individual has maintained the change for one year and they no longer think about the behavior. The entire process of moving from one stage to another is called the "spiral model of change" (Prochaska, Norcross, and DiClemente 1994: 47).

10. As others have shown, socio-cultural context also plays a role in definitions of health. The Europeans I interviewed tended to view the socioeconomic circumstances of life as being the most important influences on an individual's state of health.
11. Because wellness ideology governs the way we think about health and illness, about what is good and what is bad, the positive impact of "unhealthy" behaviors is not given space to be considered. For a notable exception to the lack of studies on this topic see Graham, 1987. In addition, as Klein (1993), among others, has pointed out, if we take perfect health and longevity as the principal measures of a good life, what becomes of the inherent worth of unhealthy pleasures? Wellness zealots would have little patience for the argument that they are proscribing ways of living that have some intrinsic worth for the pleasures they provide.
12. As the title of a *New York Times* article declared, "For Good Health, It Helps to be Rich and Important" (Goode 1999).
13. In a study of public judgments about transplant allocation, the authors found that people were unwilling to give organs to patients with controversial health behaviors, despite being told that the behavior was unrelated to both the cause of the organ failure, and the prognosis for the success of the transplant (Ubel, Baron, and Asch 1999).

References

Aronowitz, Robert A. 1998. *Making Sense of Illness: Science, Society, and Disease.* Cambridge: Cambridge University Press.

Bellah, Robert N., Richard Marsden, William M. Sullivan, Ann Swidler, and Steven M. Tipton. 1985. *Habits of the Heart: Individualism and Commitment in American Life.* New York: Harper and Row Publishers.

Blair, A. 1993. "Social Class and the Contextualization of Illness Experience," pp. 27-48 in *Worlds of Illness: Biographical and Cultural Perspectives on Health and Disease*, edited by Alan Radley. London: Routledge.

Conrad, Peter. 1994. "Wellness as Virtue: Morality and the Pursuit of Health." *Culture, Medicine, and Psychiatry* 18: 385-401.

Crawford, Robert. 1979. "Individual Responsibility and Health Politics in the 1970s," pp. 247-268 in *Health Care in America: Essays in Social History*, edited by Susan Reverby and David Rosner. Philadelphia: Temple University Press.

Dodier, Nicolas. 1985. "Social Uses of Illness at the Workplace: Sick Leave and Moral Evaluation." *Social Science and Medicine* 20(2): 123-128.

Ehrenreich, Barbara. 1995. "The Naked Truth About Fitness," pp. 59-64 in *The Snarling Citizen.* New York: Harper Perennial.

Fitzgerald, Faith T. 1994. "The Tyranny of Health." *New England Journal of Medicine* July 21:196-198.

Goode, Erica. 1999. "For Good Health, It Helps to be Rich and Important." *New York Times* 1 June: F1, F9.

Graham, Hilary. 1987. "Women's Smoking and Family Health." *Social Science and Medicine* 25(1): 47-56.

Klein, Richard. 1993. *Cigarettes Are Sublime.* Durham: Duke University Press.

Lasch, Christopher. 1979. *The Culture of Narcissism: American Life in an Age of Diminishing Expectations.* New York: Norton.

Light, Donald W. 1992. "The Practice and Ethics of Risk Rated Health Insurance." *Journal of the American Medical Association* 267(18): 2503-2508.

Lippman, Abby. 1998. "The Politics of Health: Geneticization Versus Health Promotion,"

pp. 64-82 in *The Politics of Women's Health: Exploring Agency and Autonomy*, edited by Susan Sherwin. Philadelphia: Temple University Press.
Martin, Emily. 1994. *Flexible Bodies: Tracking Immunity in American Culture from the Days of Polio to the Age of AIDS.* Boston: Beacon Press.
Nelkin, Dorothy and Laurence Tancredi. 1989. *Dangerous Diagnostics: The Social Power of Biological Transformation*. New York: Basic Books.
Parsons, Talcott. 1951. *The Social System.* New York: Free Press.
Prochaska, James O. and Carlo DiClemente. 1992. "Stages of Change in the Modification of Problem Behaviors," pp. 184-218 in *Progress in Behavior Modification*, edited by M Hersen, RM Eisler, and PM Miller. Indiana: Sycamore.
Prochaska, James O., John C. Norcross, and Carlo DiClemente. 1994. *Changing for Good: A Revolutionary Six-Stage Program for Overcoming Bad Habits and Moving Your Life Positively Forward.* New York: Avon Books.
Rothman, Barbara Katz. 1986. *The Tentative Pregnancy*. New York: Viking.
Russsell, Louise B. 1986. *Is Prevention Better Than Cure?* Washington, DC: The Brookings Institution.
Sennett, Richard. 1992 (1974). *The Fall of Public Man*. New York: Knopf.
Skrabanek, Petr. 1994. *The Death of Humane Medicine and the Rise of Coercive Healthism.* Great Britain: The Social Affairs Unit.
Thomas, Keith. 1997. "Health and Morality in Early Modern England," pp. 15-33 in *Morality and Health*, edited by Allan M. Brandt, and Paul Rozin. New York: Routledge.
Time. 1996. 2 December: 16.
de Tocqueville, Alexis. 1984 (1840). *Democracy in America.* New York: Mentor.
Tully, Shawn. 1995. "America's Healthiest Companies." *Fortune.* 12 June: 98-106.
Ubel, Peter A., Jonathon Baron, and David A. Asch. 1999. "Social Acceptability, Personal Responsibility, and Prognosis in Public Judgments about Transplant Allocation." *Bioethics* 13(1): 57-68.
Weber, Max. 1991 (1930). *The Protestant Ethic and the Spirit of Capitalism.* London: HarperCollins *Academic*.
Wells, Susan J. 1998. "A Plan for Unplanned Absences: New Policies Improve Attendance." *New York Times* 5 July: 8.

3

Gods, Living and Dead: Generativity Among Soviet Born Elders in the United States

Allen Glicksman[1]

It has been suggested that the desire to pass on something of value to future generations is part of what it means to be human. Leaving a legacy, either to one's own offspring, to some larger group, or to humanity in general, is a desire that transcends class, race, gender, and nationality. It has also been suggested that the desire to pass on something to future generations becomes a more central concern as one ages. A sense of one's own mortality, as well as a desire to pass on some of what one has learned in life, contributes to this feeling. Erikson, in his discussion of the developmental stages of the individual, speaks of this desire, which he calls "generativity" (Erikson 1980).

In traditional societies, where most knowledge is gained through years of experience, being old means that one has survived and learned much, and therefore has much to teach to younger generations. In modern society, more dependent on technological knowledge, not only does the wisdom that comes from long life play a less important role in daily activities, but the young, who feel more comfortable with technological innovations, may be the ones to teach their elders about the social and cultural changes fostered by these innovations.

Even elders in technologically advanced societies such as the United States still express the need for generativity and find ways to do so. This desire can be expressed in many ways, but it often appears in the role grandparents can play in teaching grandchildren about their family's culture and faith. This is important because the ability to preserve a living connection to faith is also a way of maintaining a connection to family tradition. Being the teacher of family traditions can also enhance the lives of older persons by giving them an important role in the family. Many older persons say that they want to feel needed as well as loved. Passing on faith traditions provides a role for the grandparent that makes her or him a contributing member of the family. The faith that sustained the elder is passed on both as a legacy to the grandchild and as a tool for the grandchild to use to maintain his or her own identity.

But what happens when the elder has no spiritual or cultural legacy to provide? Does the desire for generativity simply disappear, or can it be expressed in another way? This question is critical because it speaks to the nature of the human condition: is the need for generativity so innate that if the normal path for its expression is blocked, individuals will find other outlets for this desire? Using data from a study of older refugees, this paper explores the meaning of generativity among two groups of elders. The first group feels at a loss in identifying something to pass on to future generations; the second group is proud of their heritage and has a clear sense of what they can teach the young. A comparison of the two groups provides insight into the experience of generativity and its social and psychological dimensions.

Objectives and Methods

The central question addressed in the study was whether refugee status alone created barriers to access or whether minority status added additional problems.[2] To accomplish this goal we decided to examine access and barriers to health and social services in four refugee communities: Vietnamese and Cambodian (minority communities), and Soviet Jewish and Soviet Ukrainian (non-minority communities). Thirty Cambodian, Vietnamese, and Soviet Jewish caregivers each were interviewed, along with fourteen Ukrainian caregivers. In half the cases the elder was interviewed as well. The caregivers ranged in age from twenty to seventy-one years, the care receivers ranged from ages fifty-five to ninety-four. Most of the Asian respondents arrived in the early 1980s, while most of the respondents from the former Soviet Union arrived since 1988. Most of the data presented here come from this study, augmented by additional materials collected by the author.

The Asian communities were selected for study because they represented two of the largest minority refugee groups in Philadelphia and in the United States. The Soviet populations were selected for two reasons. First, Soviet refugees were a large non-minority group in the Philadelphia area. Second, the author of this paper and the project manager for the Soviet side of the study had significant previous experience working with Jewish and Ukrainian immigrants. This paper focuses only on the two Soviet groups in our study.[3]

To accomplish the goal of the study we decided to interview an adult child who was responsible for the care of a parent or a parent-in-law, as adult children are usually the individuals in families who negotiate such services, and a sample of the elders themselves. All the respondents were refugees. The interviews were conducted in the respondents' native languages, audiotaped, and then transcribed verbatim and translated into English. We emphasize the fact that all our primary respondents and most of our elder subjects were women, because gender is a critical variable in understanding the lives of refugees both in the past and in the present. Among the key issues for future research is the impact of gender differences on the experiences of refugees in old age.

The interview schedule included both open-ended and close-ended questions. Because the interviews were audiotaped we also caught the extended comments around close-ended answers (such as occupation, etc.). While the primary focus of the research was on current health status and needs, the respondents often referred to events in the past in order to help explain current circumstances. Because of the importance of their historical experience to understanding their current situations, we provide a short review of that historical background before moving on to the results of our data analysis.

Historical Background[4]

The history of the two Soviet refugee groups is complex. Members of each group were among those who contributed to the building and maintenance of the Soviet state, and at the same time others in each of the two ethnic groups were persecuted for attempting to maintain separate cultural, religious, and national identities. Our older Jewish respondents told two, parallel stories. On the one hand, they were given access to educational and employment opportunities never enjoyed before by Jews living under Russian rule. In fact, older Soviet Jewish immigrants in Philadelphia are on the whole better educated than their American-born counterparts. Jews were able to seek opportunities and live their lives as they never had been able to under Tsarist rule. V.I. Lenin, the first ruler of the Soviet Union, had outlawed physical anti-Semitism, a constant threat under the old regime. Most importantly, Jews were allowed and even encouraged to participate in the majority, that is, Russian, culture.

On the other hand, all formal attempts to maintain their Jewish religious expression or Jewish nationalism were suppressed. Further, even though the Yiddish language continued to be accepted in the Soviet Union, it was not encouraged. Beyond the issues specific to the Jewish community, there were the challenges of living within the Soviet Union itself, with the famines and political terror that were part of everyday life for its citizens. By the 1940s and 1950s Stalin had embarked on a program of murdering Jewish authors and intellectuals. However, it was not until the 1960s that systematic persecution of all Jews began. It should be remembered, however, that Jews were also among the perpetrators of state terror, serving in the Soviet secret police, the NKVD, and other parts of the state apparatus. (However, the number of Jews accepted in these agencies was limited because of anti-Semitism, and eventually forbidden altogether except for a few who served to inform on other Jews). Stalin's "right hand man," and one of the three people most responsible for the artificial famines of the 1930s that killed millions, was a Jew, Lazar Kaganovich. This is important because the roles that Soviet Jews played in the Soviet regime are also an issue for the elderly immigrants, as we shall see.

Although migration of Jews from the Soviet Union to the United States began in the 1970s, it continued and even grew after the collapse of the Soviet government. The reasons for this migration are complex, and include insecurities about the political stability of the new regimes, prejudice, desire for economic mobility, and fear of environmental disasters in the former Soviet Union exemplified by the Chornobyl[5] nuclear disaster in 1986.

The Jews who arrived from the Soviet Union during the 1990s were in many ways very different from the Jews who had arrived in the early and middle decades of the century. These new arrivals had for the most part adapted to Soviet realities and had become not only Russian-speaking, but devotees of Russian culture. There was little left of the traditional Jewish civilization that had flourished in Eastern Europe for centuries. Only a few older persons knew the daily language of East European Jewry, Yiddish, and almost none of the immigrants had any understanding of Jewish identity, either through religion or ethnic/national activities. Further, using the Soviet definition, these Jews defined themselves as a nationality, roughly equivalent to an ethnic group in the United States. However, there was no cultural content to this nationality, only a mark on the internal identity card all citizens had to carry. Many Soviet Jews came in three generation families. Members of the older generation migrated with their children and grandchildren because their only child was leaving the country and without that child they would be without a caregiver in their old age. Therefore, many older refugees left their homes because they had no choice, not from a desire to migrate in old age.[6]

The Ukrainians who had arrived in the United States in the early and middle part of the century were often from the Western part of the country, where there was easier access to routes for migrating to the United States. Many were members of the Ukrainian Greek Catholic Church, Orthodox in rite but in communion with Rome. This church was prominent in Western Ukraine, which had to find a compromise between the Orthodox East and Catholic Poland. After the Second World War there was a significant Ukrainian immigration, especially of intellectuals and others fleeing the Soviet regime, again mostly from the Western part of the country. The generation that migrated after the war was on the whole both religious and nationalistic. Many of the most prominent Ukrainian institutions in the United States were either founded by or strengthened by this generation of migrants.[7] As with the Jews, there were Ukrainians who were prominent in the Soviet hierarchy. There was also an initial interest in building some sort of pro-Soviet Ukrainian national identity. However, the Soviet Union rigorously suppressed any attempt to create an independent Ukraine, and after the Second World War made the Ukraine Greek Catholic Church illegal. Most infamously, during the 1930s Joseph Stalin engineered an artificial famine in Ukraine that murdered millions. Very few ethnic Ukrainians were allowed to migrate to the United States before the fall of the former Soviet Union.

When we began the project we expected to find Ukrainian respondents to be like their Jewish counterparts, Russian-speaking and disconnected from their own religious and ethnic roots. Our initial research, while preparing the grant proposal, showed that there were Ukrainians coming in two and three generation households to the United States, so there would be enough respondents for our study. However, once we began serious recruitment, we learned that most of the Ukrainians arriving were coming from the large cities such as Kyiv and Lviv and were like most immigrants, a young single person coming here to seek their fortune. Where then did we find the bulk of the two and three generation families among the Ukrainians? In a very unlikely place.

Before beginning this research, none of the members of the research team was familiar with the presence in the United States of communities of Baptist, Pentecostal, and other Protestant immigrants from Ukraine. Mennonites and other Protestant groups arriving in the Tsarist Empire generations before had evangelized the ancestors of these immigrants. These Ukrainian Protestants were rural, steeped in their faith, and were in continuous conflict with the Soviet regime. They experienced constant persecution in every part of Soviet society. Children attending school were required to view films on the evils of being a Baptist. They were unable to enter university because they would not take the oath of atheism required for membership in the Komsomol, the party youth movement that was a prerequisite for college. There was also suspicion that because they were originally evangelized by Germans, they were accomplices to the German invasions of 1914 and 1941. Because these Protestants were persecuted by the Soviet regime for their faith, the American government assigned them special status as a persecuted minority, like the Jews, thus making entry to the United States of three-generation families much easier.

Findings

How does this history affect the ability of older refugees in these two communities to express their feelings of generativity? The Ukrainian Baptist elders share many of the same problems that face the Jewish refugees. They do not understand the culture of their new land, and cannot provide all the assistance that was possible for them to do in Ukraine. But that is not the whole story. A long excerpt from a single interview speaks for the group as a whole.

I(interviewer)**: Would you describe yourself as generally happy or sad?* ***R(respondent)**: I am happy because I have discovered God. I have been serving him all my life and he takes care of me...* (Crying)... (Long pause)... ***I**: In general, are you optimistic about your future?* ***R**: Well, of course. I think that the way I have lived my life I am going to have an eternal life...because I have served Him all my life. I was baptized in 1937.* ***I**: Describe the types of things you do with or for your grandchildren and other children in your household.* ***R**: What can I do? I stay with them. They are afraid to be alone in the house. "We are scared, grandmom," they say. So I stay with them...* ***I**: Do you read together?* ***R**: My younger granddaughter—she tells me everything about the world, how it all started, about Adam...about everything... I listen and I correct her sometimes...and so...* ***I**: You talk about the history of religion...* ***R**: She loves it and if you ask her she will tell you everything just like a preacher. She knows it well. Their mother talks to them a lot about it so they know everything well.* ***I**: Do you teach them how to sew?* ***R**: How can I teach them if I can barely see myself? The glasses that I brought from Ukraine don't work for me anymore. I have been asking for a new pair of glasses so I could at least read sometimes. I can't see!* ***I**: Describe the types of things your grandchildren or other children in your household do with or for you.* ***R**: What can they do for me?* ***I**: Do they help you in any way?* ***R**: No...* ***I**: Besides going to the meetings, do you do anything else as a religious person?* **R**: (Smiling) *I pray...* ***I**: What role does religion play in your life? How important is that role?* ***R**: It is the most important part of my life.* ***I**: Could you tell me more about that?* ***R**: Well, what can I tell you? It is the most important...* ***I**: But why? What do you mean when you say that?* ***R**: We can't live without our religion—because God helps us... You look around and see how difficult life is and you say, God, help us!* ***I**: What is your nationality?* ***R**: I am a Ukrainian.* ***I**: Could you describe your cultural background?* ***R**: As I said, my parents were very religious people, they were serving God and they raised us that way.... And so we raised our children. Our parents taught us and we taught our children.* ***I**: What were your parents' occupations?* ***R**: Well, they had land...they had a field. They were peasants. They worked on the land.* ***I**: So, they were peasants...* ***R**: Yes.* ***I**: How would you describe your spouse's cultural and national backgrounds?* ***R**: He was also a very religious man, a Ukrainian Pentecostalist. He was a religious* *person since he was very young.* ***I: *Do you belong to any churches?* ***R:*** *I do. I don't know either its name or where it is located. They take me and I sit and listen to the pastor. How can I tell you where the church is?* ***I:*** *Would you describe yourself as generally happy or sad?* ***R:*** *I am happy in my faith, in God. And I am happy that I have my children.* ***I:*** *In general, are you optimistic about your future?* ***R:*** *As long as I have my health.* ***I:*** *So you are optimistic, right?* ***R:*** *Yes, as long as God gives me life, health, I think I am not going to be like this all the time....*

The issues raised here—poor health and unfamiliarity with the local environment and culture—appear in many of the transcripts of interviews with the Soviet Ukrainians as well as with the Soviet Jews. But for this group generativity is not a problem. In spite of persecution, the continuity of the faith of these Ukrainians provides a link between generations. Even if grandmother's eyesight is so poor that she cannot sew any more, she can still listen to her grandchild's recitation of the story of Genesis and correct any errors in the telling. Even with poor health and lack of knowledge of American culture or even the way to get to church, her status within her own family and her role there is secure. The experiences of persecution, then refugee status, and now living as a "stranger in a strange land," do not prevent these elders from expressing their own sense of generativity, secure in the belief that the faith of their parents and grandparents will also be the faith of their children and grandchildren.

The experience of the Soviet Jewish elders is very different. Let us allow the Soviet Jews to speak for themselves, beginning with how they describe the hardships of living in Stalin's Soviet Union.

I: *How does a person know if she is getting old? What does it mean to be an older person?* ***R:*** *Well, the opportunities to socialize and to attend events go down. In my opinion age affects the general condition of a person. I have permanent pain either in my legs or in my back. Besides, you have to know what my generation of Soviets has lived through. I survived three famines. I don't remember the first one. My parents told me later about it because it happened in 1921. The second famine was in the 30s... The last one maybe was not so awful, but it was during the war, during our evacuation. We had a hard life at that time.*

We can begin to see that the experience of living through the Second World War and the Holocaust existed within a larger framework of the hardships of Soviet life. The Second World War was not even the worst that this respondent experienced. There were other difficult aspects to life in the former Soviet Union.

I: *Your husband died...* ***R:*** *No, he was executed by a firing squad...* ***I:*** *What was the reason he was executed for? What was the sentence?* ***R:*** *He was accused in participating in a military plot... I am not a writer or journalist, but in the last few years I have written my life's history, typed it on ninety pages. It has been printed in a print shop. I have dedicated it to my grandchildren and great-grandchildren for them to know their roots* (showed the manuscript). *I wrote this in 1993. Before that I had written memoirs about my husband...*

As this statement indicates, not everything the older generation wishes to pass on to younger generations is either happy or optimistic. In some cases, the older person simply desires that her children and grandchildren know their own roots and where they come from.

The older Jewish respondents also talk about the decline in Jewish culture. The reference to being unable to vote is because they were considered petite bourgeoisie, a status that in some cases could lead to arrest and possible execution. Also notice the reference to physical anti-Semitism in the Tsarist regime.

I: *Were you raised in a particular religious tradition? If so, please tell me about it.* ***R:*** *Yes. Until I was sixteen and lived with my parents. My mother was a very religious woman. We ate only kosher food. We celebrated all Jewish holidays. We have suffered from the persecutions there for being Jewish. I remember I was beaten by a police dog* (under the Tsarist government)*, and when my mother went to ask him if the dog was sick, he simply threw her out and did not want to even talk to her... Like that. And so, until the time that I left that little town in Byelorussia, I practiced... My mother went to a synagogue on Yom Kippur... I went with her...* ***R:*** *I was taught Yiddish, how to read and write. I don't remember any of that, though. Later, when I left for Leningrad, I lived with my sister. Our older sisters took us in. And there, until the arrival of my parents in '29, I had left in '23, for those six years I had no one to talk with. I never taught my children* (the language). *When my mother came, everything has come back. My parents were denied the vote because my mother had at one point bought and sold goods. They had left everything behind, their house, the store, and came to Leningrad. And here again, mother was religious, and again, up until '40, until her death, I spoke Yiddish with* *her.* Another Respondent: *My father died earlier, in '35. And after that, Yiddish has disappeared from my life. Completely.*

These quotes show that the essence of Jewish culture in Eastern Europe, both religious and linguistic, was disappearing from the landscape within a couple of decades of the Bolshevik Revolution. The great spiritual trauma for many of these Jews was not the physical hardship of the war. It came later when the Soviet Union decided on an anti-Semitic policy. When the Soviet government restricted the number of Jews in the universities and took other actions to limit the economic and social activities of the Jews, many who had felt a strong loyalty to the Soviet system and Russian culture were left without the belief system that had sustained them throughout the worst of times, including the war.

***R**: I love Leningrad. And I love my native country too. That's where my childhood has been, my youth years, my marriage, the birth of my children, all of that is understandable. But I left there without a single regret. It was more of a stepmother to me than a mother, unfortunately. Because my husband was executed, my son perished, and I mean it, although he died of a heart attack, but the endless anonymous letters during the Andropov period* (the early 1980s) *terrorized him, when it mattered.*

The image of Russia being a stepmother rather than the traditional "Mother Russia" is both poignant and revealing. Without that cultural and spiritual link, what can this woman pass on to her descendants? The culture of their youth is the only culture they know. As one older woman said:

***I**: How would you describe your cultural and national background? **R**: I am Russian by culture and Jewish by nationality.*

Another older woman seemed to believe that she should not think of Russian culture as her own, even though she still does.

***I**: How would you describe your cultural and national background? **R**: You see, I consider myself to be Jewish by nationality, but culturally I am Russian because I was raised in Russian culture. I adore Russian culture, Russian opera, Russian ballet, Russian theatre, Russian actors. I adore all those. I adore Russian literature, and I can't help it.*

Another respondent talked about the continuities in her life:

R**: As far as the senior club...I like it there, very much so. It is very pleasant. But, you understand, the women come there only to show* *off their jewels, their clothes. I am sorry, but I tell you what I feel.* ***I*: I am interested in your opinion.* ***R****: Perhaps, that's how it should be done. Life does not stop. Perhaps, it's because my age is different. But I have never worn anything like that in my life. It was not the norm when I was part of Komsomol. And on the whole I have never been interested in trinkets. You see. But nevertheless, I am still very glad I am there because...there are interesting lectures... I presented a lecture myself there twice which was received very well. It was dedicated to the 49th anniversary of World War II... It's very interesting, of course. I enjoy going there very much. But as far as friends...I had tried to be with a few there, even gave them my phone number. But no one has called, and I don't either. I have not found people with similar outlook on life.*

Even though the Soviet system betrayed her, and even though the system and the Komsomol are no more, this woman has nothing else to use as a moral and spiritual base in her old age. But even if the world view she learned as a young girl can still serve as a moral compass for her world, how can it be made part of a legacy for those who come after her? The shock of losing their belief system was only one of three traumas that this cohort of older survivors had experienced since the war. The second was the nuclear disaster at Chornobyl. For some, the evacuation from Kyiv after the Chornobyl disaster brought back memories of the flight from the Nazis as they approached Kyiv in 1941. The third trauma was the collapse of the Soviet Union itself.

I*: What were the reasons you left your native country? How did you feel about leaving?* ***R****: The most important reason was radiation, to which the city was exposed and my grandchildren and my children through the Chornobyl disaster. So we were very nervous because of my children and especially my grandchildren. I didn't think about myself. I thought about my children and my grandchildren. When they offered me to emigrate, I had doubts because I thought that I could stay there. However, I would have stayed alone in (hometown) because my other son lived in Petersburg, and my sister and brother lived in Moscow. So, they talked me into emigrating with them, and I went with them. Generally it was very difficult for me to leave my homeland.*

Many of the elders said that they would have stayed there if not for the fact that their only child was leaving for a new country.

***I**: What were the reasons you left your native country? **R**: Because my children... My granddaughter with her husband left. **I**: Was it the only reason? **R**: Yes, of course. It was the most important reason. **I**: No other reasons? **R**: No. I mean it was getting hard to live there, and our nationality started being a problem, but the main reason was our children. If we stayed there together we might not leave. We would continue suffering as other people do.*

Sacrificing their own lives and future for their children and grandchildren was part of their experience. But how could that be communicated in a way that provided a link to the future for these older persons? In the New World they do not know the language or culture. Even what they considered their greatest accomplishment, military service in the Second World War, is not acknowledged in the United States.

***I**: Could you tell me what organizations you belong to and what kinds of activities you are involved in? **R**: My husband is a member of World War II veterans club. **I**: Is this an immigrants' club or an American club? **R**: This is immigrants' club. Americans don't care. I mean we don't have contacts because we don't understand them, and they don't understand us.*

Another older survivor summed up her misery:

***R**: There is no one else. I am very lonely. Very much so. There are no bounds for my loneliness. I love people and everything, but I am always alone.*

However, the same respondent also described happier times in the United States.

***I**: Please tell me how you spend your time* (leisure, work, family, helping out, organizational activity, etc.) ***R**: We spend time together during any family celebration. We always get together during the family celebrations. All the relatives get together to celebrate. And I am together with them. It's nowhere without me. I am at Bar Mitzvah, or a wedding, I am everywhere, I even give speeches. I always have the first toast.*

The first toast at a celebration goes to the most honored guest. So it is still possible for these older survivors to retain some of the status they had within their families in the Old Country. Some of the survivors also spend time talking to others of their own age and experience. For example:

***I**: What do you talk about? **R**: We often talk about the past, about* *our youth, about the children. About the sickness we are now experiencing. They are hard for us to live with.*

At the same time, much of American culture and society remains a mystery to them. For example, funds from SSI, the Supplementary Security Income program for the very poor, are provided to refugees. However, not all the refugees understand why they are receiving these funds.

***I.** But what is this money? **R:** It's my pension. **I:** Is it SSI? **R:** Yes, SSI, it's my pension. Whatever I had received in Russia, they transferred here. **I:** You think that you are receiving the money from Russia? **R:** Of course, all senior citizens do. The money has been transferred here. I don't know how they do that. But it the fact that we are receiving the pension here. This is lucky.*

***I:** Is your pension a part of the household income? **R:** Of course it is. No doubts about it. See, I feel myself very confident because I can give them something. I can make a gift. So, I am proud of this.*

The SSI check becomes not a sign of being poor but another way of contributing to the family welfare. Of course, the Russian pension is not transferred, and if it was it would probably be worthless after currency conversion. But the desire to be generative, to participate and to contribute to the life of the family, is critical to the sense of self-esteem and self-worth for these older refugees. For some Soviet families, the SSI check is the difference between being able to pay the rent and being evicted from their apartments.

But what can they pass on? One older woman spoke about teaching her granddaughter the writings of the Russian poet, Pushkin. She felt that by doing so she could make a connection between her own cultural heritage and that of her granddaughter. Pushkin represents the best of Russian culture, unsullied by Soviet betrayal or anti-Semitism. But the response of this woman is not the response of many of the other older women we spoke with. As one middle-aged woman said of her older mother's relationship with the grandchildren:

***I:** Describe the types of things your children do with or for your mother. **R:** They like to discuss political news with her, a newspaper article. They like to ask her about her childhood, her life. She tells them about it with pleasure, about the hard years during the war. They try to learn about her life in the past, about her family and relatives.*

What these older women have to pass on, the heritage they can bequeath to their children and grandchildren, is not cultural or national or religious: it is the story of their own family, usually focused on the women in the family, and their own legacy of determination, strength, and hope in the face of adversity. Even the Second World War, which threatened the destruction of all the Jewish people, is something that can be discussed "with pleasure," because it becomes a symbol of the ability of their family, and especially of the women in their family, to overcome even the greatest hardships. These stories are a gift that can be given to young people who cannot imagine the hardships of their grandparents. In the process the elders can contribute to the ability of the family to face new struggles in their adopted homeland.

Conclusions

The desire for generativity—something to leave as a legacy for future generations—seems to be part of the human condition. The ability to express that desire can, as it does in the case of the Ukrainian elders in our study, provide a role in the family and a source of meaning when health conditions and migration have taken other important roles from them. The Ukrainian elders can continue as contributing members of their families, giving them a sense not only of love but of respect, and most importantly knowledge that despite their infirmities and ignorance of their new cultural surroundings, they are needed. For the Soviet Jews, who came with little of a formal heritage that they could pass on to their family, a creative replacement was found that allows the elders to proudly teach a very personal family tradition. In both cases, the human desire for a family legacy for the future and for a family role in the present found its expression.

Notes

1. The author would like to thank Neville Strumpf, Renée C. Fox, Tanya Koropeckyj-Cox, Svetlana Shevchenko, Marina Mistetsky, Leanna Kantarovich, Olena Mitnik, and Robin Goldberg-Glen for allowing me the opportunity to gain an understanding of these two, fascinating refugee communities.
2. In 1992 the National Institute on Aging and the National Institute of Nursing Research published a Request For Proposals asking for studies of barriers to long-term care services for older persons who are members of minority groups. In response, two investigators at the University of Pennsylvania and the author of this

paper submitted a proposal to compare access and barriers to community-based long-term care for older minority and non-minority refugees. Neville Strumpf of the School of Nursing and Robin Goldberg-Glen of the School of Social Work served as principal investigator and as a co-principal investigator respectively. Goldberg-Glen supervised data collection among the two Asian populations. The author of this paper, trained as a sociologist and working at the time at the Polisher Research Institute of the Philadelphia Geriatric Center, served as the other co-principal investigator and was responsible for data collection among the Soviet populations. Renée C. Fox served as ethnographic and sociological consultant on the project. Tanya Koropeckyj-Cox served as project manager for the portion of the project that dealt with the Soviet-born populations. Leanna Kantarovich, Elena Mitnik, Marina Mistetsky, and Svetlana Shevchenko, all native speakers of Russian and Ukrainian, served as interviewers on the Soviet portion of the study. These four interviewers became part of the research team, contributing their own insights and comments on all aspects of the study, from instrument construction to data analysis.

3. For a fuller description of the project, see Strumpf, et al. 2001.
4. For an extensive discussion of Jewish life in the former Soviet Union, see Ro'i 1995. For more information on Ukraine under Soviet rule, see Subtelny 1988.
5. In the article the current Ukrainian names for locations in Ukraine, rather than the more familiar Russian names, are used. So Chornobyl rather than Chernobyl, Kyiv rather than Kiev, and Lviv rather than Lvov.
6. For extensive discussions of the experience of Soviet Jewish immigrants to the United States, see Gold 1994, and to Philadelphia see Levin 1986.
7. The experience of these immigrants is well described in Kuropas (1991).

References

Erikson, Erik. 1980. *Identity and The Life Cycle.* New York: Norton.

Gold, Steven J. 1994. "Soviet Jews in the United States," pp. 3-57 in *American Jewish Yearbook*, New York: American Jewish Committee.

Kuropas, Myron B. 1991. *The Ukrainian Americans: Roots and Aspirations 1884-1954.* Toronto, Buffalo: University of Toronto Press.

Levin, Nora. 1986. "Home and Haven: Soviet Immigration to Philadelphia, 1972-1982," pp. 201-222 in *Philadelphia Jewish Life: 1940-1985*, edited by Murray Friedman. Ardmore, PA: Seth Press.

Ro'i, Yaacov, ed. 1995. *Jews and Jewish Life in Russia and the Soviet Union.* Portland, Oregon: Frank Cass.

Subtelny, Orest. 1988. *Ukraine: A History.* Toronto and Buffalo: Published by the University of Toronto Press in association with the Canadian Institute of Ukrainian Studies.

Strumpf, Neville, Allen Glicksman, Robin Goldberg-Glen, Renée C. Fox, and Elizabeth H. Logue. 2001. "Caregiver and Elder Experiences of Cambodian, Vietnamese, Soviet Jewish, and Ukrainian Refugees." *International Journal of Aging and Human Development.* 53(3): 233-252.

4

It Couldn't Hurt: An Ethnographic Study of a Ritual for Healing

Gail G. Glicksman

Introduction

Those investigating the intersection of religion and medicine devote considerable attention to the ways that religious involvement or beliefs shape response to illness, or even health outcomes. One of the most popular research questions today is the role of prayer in promoting healing.[1] To explore my interest in the ways that the awareness of illness affects a religious community, I did field work using participant observation and analyzed the results from a symbolic interactionist perspective. This approach proved to be an effective way to collect data about sensitive issues such as illness and death and religious beliefs.[2]

During the first few months of my rabbinic internship, I discovered that there was something distinctive about the synagogue Makom Tikvah. (I have selected fictitious names for all proper names in this paper, in order to preserve confidentiality.) At the time, the 200-member congregation, composed primarily of immigrants and first-generation Americans in the 70+ age range, became focused on a brief prayer for the restoration of health, the *Mi she-Berakh le-Holeh* prayer. Since the chair of the congregation's ritual committee, and not the rabbi, recited this prayer, elaborations of the ritual surrounding its recitation reveal the congregants' strategies for coping with illness, and provide insight into the social dynamics of the congregation.

What is the *Mi she-Berakh le-Holeh*, the Prayer for the Sick?

Mi she-Berakh prayers are benedictions offered when a person is called to the public reading of the Torah during a prayer service.[3] This class of prayers was introduced early in the development of the Torah service, perhaps as a way to fill the time while the Torah scroll was rewound to the proper position. During medieval times this class of prayers became associated with efforts to raise funds for the community. Many traditionally observant Orthodox Jewish communities use a version of the text which mentions that the person requesting the prayer pledged funds or is planning to perform good deeds for the community.[4] These prayers are recited for various occasions, varying from a standard offering for the individual's well-being to a commemoration of a joyous occasion. Their name is derived from the first few words of the prayer, "*Mi she-Berakh*"—He who blessed.

In Hebrew, *le-Holeh* means "for the sick." The *Mi she-Berakh le-Holeh* prayers—the *Mi she-Berakh* prayers that focus on the wish for the recovery of the sick—differ in the ways that they are published in various prayer books and rabbis' manuals. As early as medieval times, the prayer caught the popular imagination and the number of blessings multiplied greatly, overshadowing other parts of the service. Over the generations, some prayer book editors have intentionally omitted the *Mi She'Berakh Le'Holeh* prayer for logistical reasons, because they found that it prolonged the service, or for ideological reasons, because they worried that it encouraged congregants to think of prayer as fostering specific, concrete responses.[5] The version that is recited in the Makom Tikvah congregation is found in the *Weekday Prayer Book of the Conservative Movement* (Rabbinical Assembly 1965: 85). It is based on quotations from Biblical and Talmudic sources. In Makom Tikvah it was recited only in Hebrew. At first, the congregation followed the traditional custom, reciting two versions of the prayer—one for all men and one for all women who are ill, including the individual names within each gender group. As congregants felt moved to add special attention to the prayer, they decided to recite an individual prayer for *each* person. They devoted considerable attention to the prayer, and developed a ritual surrounding it, taking pride in the time and devotion they lavished on it, and, by extension, on those who were ill. After a number of years, however, they decided that they could not bear to acknowledge the scope of the suffering by listening to so many individual prayers, so they returned to the traditional approach. The version they currently use is a combined version of the male and female prayers. The English translation found in the prayer book is:

> May He who blessed our fathers, Abraham, Isaac, and Jacob, Moses and Aaron, David and Solomon, bless . . . ., [son/daughter of (name of the mother of the *holeh*, person who is ill)]. May the Holy One, praised be He, mercifully restore him/her to health and strength. May He grant him/her, and all who are ill, health of body and health of mind. Let us say: *Amen.* (Rabbinical Assembly, 1965:85)

One unusual aspect of the *Mi she-Berakh le-Holeh*, which distinguishes it from other varieties of *Mi she-Berakh* prayers, is that the *holeh* (the person who is ill) is identified with the mother's name, not with the father's name as in all other arenas in traditional Jewish communities. There are several common explanations. On the elite level, scholars of Jewish liturgy have explained that "in this way there could be no question as to the identity of the [person] prayed for." (Marcus 1947: 221) On the folk, or "lived religion" level, the traditional interpretation has stressed the symbolic association of mothers with healing and "tender loving care."[6] In addition, some hypothesize that mothers would have a closer, more intimate, relationship with their offspring than fathers so they would be expected to intervene more ardently on behalf of their afflicted children. (Donin 1980: 53, 251-252)

"How Could It Hurt?!"

During the first few months of my tenure as rabbi of Makom Tikvah, Bertha Pappenheim discovered that she had breast cancer and had a radical mastectomy. The prognosis was not promising. The cancer spread rapidly through her body. At her bedside, when I asked whether she wanted me to recite a *Mi she-Berakh* prayer, she replied candidly: "How could it hurt?!"

After conducting numerous services at Makom Tikvah and spending countless hours with congregants, I learned that even the innocent musing, "How could a *Mi she-Berakh* prayer hurt?" would not be accepted by all congregants. Indeed, some believed that a *Mi she-Berakh* prayer *could* hurt. The congregation's ritual director received a message from a neighbor of Eli and Anna Bernays: "Stop reciting *Mi she-Berakh* prayers for Eli. You're only hurting him. You are keeping him alive and prolonging his suffering. He's only being '*tse-mitchert*,' (tortured). You're cruel if you continue to recite the prayers!" How else could a *Mi she-Berakh* "hurt" a *holeh*, a person who is ill? Some congregants believed "hurt" was ensured by reciting the prayer incorrectly, "mispronouncing" the name of the *holeh*, thereby confusing God, or by reciting the prayer and keeping alive a person who was suffering, without hope of recovery.

Social Roles of the *Mi she-Berakh le-Holeh*—Announcing Illness

Since the *Mi she-Berakh le-Holeh* prayer is recited with individual names of the sick, it announces illnesses, recoveries, and deaths. Makom Tikvah is a small congregation, which has a strong social network. Most of the congregants who are actively involved live in the same neighborhood and see each other during the week. The Saturday morning prayer sessions, which include the *Mi she-Berakh le-Holeh*, bolster the congregants' own system of communications. Although most of them do not understand all of the Hebrew words, they listen for the names of those who are ill. Often, one can hear murmurs as names are added. Individuals ask about a person's identity. Is he or she a relative, a friend, a neighbor?

During the week or on Shabbat (the Sabbath) before the service, congregants present the ritual director with slips of paper on which they have written the name of the *holeh*, the person who is ill. Others wait until all the prayers have been recited to request that we add a prayer. Some of the most poignant interactions occur at these times. Some congregants become impatient while others ask for additional *Mi she-Berakh* prayers, especially if they take a long time remembering the complete name of the *holeh*, or if they describe the person and his problem at length.

Setting The Agenda: Social Control and the Recognition of Social Status

The recitation of *Mi she-Berakh* prayers is a structured event. Individuals do not offer these prayers spontaneously, at least not aloud. At Makom Tikvah, the ritual director (the chair of the ritual committee) recites the *Mi she-Berakh* prayers. The person reciting these prayers sets the agenda, determining whose names will be recited and setting the order in which they will be offered. That person maintains a list of the names of those for whom we regularly offer prayers. The list reflects a hierarchy. For several months, Rakhel bas Leah

Bayla (Rose Pappenheim), who was battling metastatic cancer and the effects of several strokes, remained in first place. At times, the ritual director recited a prayer first for Sarah Breuer, Makom Tikvah's Sisterhood president and the wife of the congregation president. Although Sarah—who has struggled against very serious cardiac problems—traditionally occupies the first place on the list, and returns to that position when she experiences a crisis, she became second on the list when Rose's health declined.

The *Mi she-Berakh* Prayer as a Gift to the Sick Person and His/Her Family

The *Mi she-Berakh le-Holeh* serves as a gift—an offering the congregation can provide to comfort those who are ill and their families. Many, many times, when there is little else that congregants can say, they have assured sick individuals or their families that they will recite *Mi she-Berakh le-Holeh* prayers as often as needed. Likewise, when they have felt so helpless trying to comfort those facing catastrophic illnesses, they have perceived a sense of relief and comfort when informing them that, as a group, Makom Tikvah will think of and offer prayers for the *holeh.* In this manner, the *Mi she-Berakh* forges group identity by linking those enduring the stress of illness with others in the congregation.

Personal Roles: Facilitating the Expression of Congregants' Feelings

The *Mi she-Berakh* prayer facilitates the expression of a full range of emotions. During these prayers, I notice relatives of the *holeh* expressing sighs of relief or comfort, fidgets, and signs of anxiety, frustration, and desperation. There are also murmurs, hushed conversations, and even comments uttered aloud, to be shared with the entire group.

One Shabbat morning while Schoenberg, the ritual director, was reciting the *Mi she-Berakh* prayers, he fumbled on the words. He could not pass a certain point, despite the prompting that all the men on the *bimah* were eager to offer. Schoenberg started the prayer over again several times, to no avail. Finally, he managed to recite all the words of the *Mi she-Berakh* from beginning to end. During the fumbling, Schoenberg exclaimed: "I'm getting '*oyver a buttle*!' (going senile) I'm forgetting things." Most chimed in, rebutting

Schoenberg's assertion. Schoenberg, buoyed by the words of support, added that he must have a mental block, a "simple" mental block. I added that the great number of *Mi she-Berakh* prayers recited that Shabbat must be daunting. "There's too much illness," I observed. Schoenberg agreed, as did most of the congregants, who nodded in affirmation.

Fear of senility is pervasive among Makom Tikvah congregants. They, like many older adults, are frightfully concerned about the acuity of their mental functions. As the public awareness of and attention to Alzheimer's Disease increases, Makom Tikvah congregants have become exquisitely sensitive about their mental skills. The slightest slip, a memory lapse, even a slip of the tongue, provokes tenuous quips about dementia.

In the vignette, we also perceive despair over the great number of *Mi she-Berakh* prayers, disgust with the pervasiveness of illness. Often, the despair is channeled as "anger at God" and "anger at physicians." The persistence of illness despite the many *Mi she-Berakh* prayers they have offered is met with expressions of "gallows humor" and by the anxious exploration of the possibility that the *Mi she-Berakh* prayers are not efficacious.

Most congregants feel uncomfortable about expressing anger at God. For the most part, they were socialized to believe in a supernatural equation, in which one portion of good deeds should be rewarded with one portion of good fortune. When they suffer, they try to identify concrete ways in which they might have failed to meet God's expectations, ways they might have angered God. Sacred rage represents a socially appropriate way to express anger without blasphemy. It also reveals that these congregants identify with God in an individual way. If they didn't expect anything from their relationship with God, they would not feel so disappointed and so bitter. One phrase typically invoked on such occasions is: "Man plans and God laughs." It expresses frustration, the feeling that they are working so very hard, trying to be good people, working to reach goals, but they cannot realize their dreams. They blame God for thwarting those dreams.

Anger at physicians is also expressed when many *Mi she-Berakh le-Holeh* prayers are recited. At times, individuals blame physicians for suffering even if they have not increased the misery as a result of invasive procedures and even if they could not have done anything to alleviate it. Confronted with a bewildering amount of affliction, many individuals try to contrive a way to make sense of it. Physicians are particularly vulnerable as targets for such explanations and for such anger. Breuer, Makom Tikvah's president, has a favorite phrase: "Physicians aren't sure about anything. They're merely 'practicing' medicine."

Gallows humor is often expressed during the *Mi she-Berakh* prayers. On one particular Shabbat morning, it seemed that everyone was coughing or sneezing, particularly toward the end of the service, as we were waiting for the final announcements and an invitation to recess to the small chapel for *Kiddush* (the formal proclamation of the sanctity of the day, usually recited over wine and accompanied by refreshments). One congregant's response to the chorus of coughs evoked many laughs: "We'll have to serve Robitussin rather than sacramental grape wine." Another congregant retorted: "*Oy vey!* We must have goofed on the *Mi she-Berakh le-Holeh*, because it seems that we're all sick."

On some level, many congregants expect God to answer their prayers in a direct and concrete way. Thus, the pervasiveness of illness calls into question the efficacy of the *Mi she-Berakh le-Holeh* prayers. Other expressions are common among congregants confronted with the pervasiveness of illness. As mentioned above, they typically sigh, and say in Yiddish that "Man tries, and God laughs." The other common expression is: "Everyone has his own *pekele* or *bintele* (package) of *tzurres* (troubles)." Usually, this is accompanied by some variant of a folk story about individuals who become consumed with self-pity, but finally realize that if they had the choice of selecting their problems, "no one would really want to trade his *tzurres* (problems) for someone else's *tzurres*."

Fear of Confusing God with Mistakes in the *Mi she-Berakh le-Holeh* Prayer

Congregants express intense concern about the pronunciation of the prayer. They worry that God will not recognize the name of the *holeh*. In part, they are projecting their self-concepts onto God. As I noted earlier, they also project onto God their fears about losing their mental acuity. In addition, when they complain about the pronunciation of a name, they are also adopting a cultural pattern of approaching illness. In expressing concern about the accuracy of prayers, they are perpetuating an age-old tradition of concern for precision in offering prayers or in reading the Torah. In attributing the capacity to become confused to a supernatural power, they also are expressing an ancient tradition. Many folk customs and superstitions have developed about attempts to confuse the "Angel of Death." Through personal experience, many congregants are aware of the custom of changing one's name in time of grave illness, in order to confuse the "Angel of Death." (Marcus 1947: 224) For example, when Ignaz Schoenberg was seriously ill as a child, his mother went to a rabbi and begged him to change Ignaz's Hebrew name. They added a name, which he has continued to use.

Conclusion

Through this examination of the role of the *Mi she-Berakh le-Holeh*, we have learned about the role of religion in the health of a group of older adults. This prayer generates ambivalent reactions, focusing on two seemingly contradictory perceptions about the prayer. On one hand, the prayer is perceived as innocuous—pleasant, but not particularly efficacious. On the other hand, it is perceived to have powerful and possibly magical qualities.

Despite congregants' ambivalence about the *Mi she-Berakh* prayer, they persist in demanding it. First, they are not certain about its effectiveness. If they felt sure that it couldn't help, they wouldn't experience conflict about it. Second, the prayer serves a variety of social functions. On some level, congregants are aware of the role of the *Mi she-Berakh* prayer in promoting feelings of solidarity within the congregation. Third, the *Mi she-Berakh le-Holeh* provides individual benefits. It offers support and solace and enables them to express feelings about illness.

Significantly, the experiences of the congregants, either as immigrants or first-generation Americans, have rendered them transitional figures and forged a creative tension between tradition and modernity. Some of the group's coping strategies are original, developed to respond to the peculiarities of the group. Others are age-old, derived from the chain of Jewish tradition. Those coping strategies that are based on tradition seem to generate the most intense comfort, for they inspire a sense of security and highlight the solidness of the chain that links one generation to another. This sense of permanence in the face of stress enables individuals to realize that they can "live on" through their affiliation with a larger group. In a synagogue without this particular blend of traditional and modern members, we might not find such ambivalent feelings about the *Mi she-Berakh, and* these prayers might not serve the same purposes. In this congregation, though, the *Mi she-Berakh* prayer is indispensable, and it serves a variety of particularly significant roles.

This ethnographic description highlights the creative potential of elders and lay members of congregations to contribute creative changes to the traditional liturgical practices. It also shows the potential of elders when they are allowed to express their full range of interests, including those explorations of illness and death that might be troublesome to some listeners. This group, rather than become morose or paralyzed when they realized that a bewildering percentage of their members were becoming ill or were dying, appropriated an age-old tradition and forged a new way to try to express their concerns and fears.

Notes

1. For further reading on religion and health, and the role of prayer in promoting health outcomes, see Sloan, Bagiella, VandeCreek, et al. 2000; 342 (25): 1913-1916; Sloan and Bagiella 2000; Stannard 2000.
2. This paper emerged from a University of Pennsylvania course, "Medicine and Religion in Society," co-taught by Renée C. Fox and Willy De Craemer. The author expresses appreciation to the Memorial Foundation for Jewish Culture for the Dissertation Scholarship that supported this research.
3. In this case, *Torah* is used in the narrow sense, as the reading of the portion from the Five Books of Moses during the service. "Mi She-Berakh," in *Encyclopaedia Judaica,* 1972.
4. See Elbogen (1993); Rosenberg (1997: 122-123); Hertz (1965, notes on pp. 488-490 and 492). For an example of a contemporary prayer book with a *Mi she-Berakh le-Holeh* that includes a pledge of charitable works or contributions, see Scherman (1984: 442-443): "May he bless and heal the sick person, son/daughter of ___, because the supplicant (to be named) will contribute to charity on his/her behalf."
5. See Elbogen (1993: 150). Examples of prayer books that omit the *Mi she-Berakh le-Holeh* include Silverman (1946) *Sabbath and Festival Prayer Book*; Jewish Reconstructionist Foundation (1945) *Sabbath Prayer Book;* Stern (1994) *Gates of Prayer for Sabbath and Weekdays, A Gender Sensitive Prayerbook*; and Union of Liberal and Progressive Synagogues (1995) *Siddur Lev Chadash.*
6. Notes, Dr. David Jacobson, Modern Hebrew Literature, Reconstructionist Rabbinical College, Spring, 1985.

References

Donin, Hayim Halevy. 1980. *To Pray As A Jew*. New York: Basic Books.

Elbogen, Ismar. 1993. *Jewish Liturgy: A Comprehensive History*, Trans. Raymond P. Scheindlin, Philadelphia: Jewish Publication Society.

Hertz, Joseph Herman. [1948] 1965. *Authorized Daily Prayer Book*. Twelfth Printing. New York: Bloch Publishing Company.

Jewish Reconstructionist Foundation. [1945] 1979. *Sabbath Prayer Book*. Ninth Printing. New York: Jewish Reconstructionist Foundation.

Marcus, Jacob R. 1947. *Communal Sick-Care in the German Ghetto*. Cincinnati: The Hebrew Union College Press.

"Mi She-Berakh." 1972. *Encyclopaedia Judaica*. Volume 12, Columns 86-87. Jerusalem: Keter Publishing Company.

Rabbinical Assembly Prayer Book Committee. [1961] 1965. *Weekday Prayer Book*. Third Edition. New York: The Rabbinical Assembly of America.

Rosenberg, Arnold. 1997. *Jewish Liturgy as a Spiritual System: A Prayer-by-Prayer Exploration of the Nature and Meaning of Jewish Worship*. Northvale, New Jersey: Jason Aronson.

Scherman, Nosson. Editor. 1984. *The Complete ArtScroll Siddur—Nusach Ashkenaz*. Brooklyn, New York: Artscroll Mesorah Press.

Silverman, Morris. Editor. [1946] 1973. *Sabbath and Festival Prayer Book*. New York: The Rabbinical Assembly of America and the United Synagogue of America.

Sloan, Richard P., Emilia Bagiella. 2000. "Data Without a Prayer," [Editor's Correspondence], *Archives of Internal Medicine* 160 (12): 1870.

Sloan, Richard P., Emilia Bagiella, Larry VandeCreek, Margot Hover, Carlo Casalone, Trudi Jinpu Hirsch, Yusuf Hasan, Ralph Kreger, and Peter Poulos. 2000. "Should Physicians Prescribe Religious Activities?" [Sounding Board] *The New England Journal of Medicine* 342 (25): 1913-1916.

Stannard, Russell. January, 2000. "The Prayer Experiment." *Second Opinion* No.2, pp. 26-38.

Stern, Chaim, Editor. 1994. *Gates of Prayer for Sabbath and Weekdays, A Gender Sensitive Prayerbook*. New York City: CCAR Press.

Union of Liberal and Progressive Synagogues. 1995. *Siddur Lev Chadash, Services and Prayers for Weekdays and Sabbaths, Festivals and Various Occasions*. London: Union of Liberal and Progressive Synagogues.

5

Overused and Underappreciated: Culture in an Academic Medicine Merger

Carla M. Messikomer and Judith P. Swazey

In 1987, a little-known, Pittsburgh-based health care organization, the Allegheny Health, Education and Research Foundation (Allegheny), came to Philadelphia to become the parent of an historic and financially struggling medical school. The Medical College of Pennsylvania (MCP), founded in 1850 as the first medical school for women in the United States (Peitzman 2000), balked at the idea of mixing business with medicine, but eventually settled into an uneasy working relationship with its non-profit corporate parent. Securing the residency programs of its elite flagship community hospital in Pittsburgh initially brought Allegheny east, but once there, it dreamed of becoming the first statewide health care system in the country. Four years later the vision seemed more within reach when Allegheny bought the United Hospitals group in Philadelphia, adding four more hospitals to its growing holdings. Then, in 1993, in its most daring and unusual move to date, it acquired a health science university, Hahnemann University (HU),[1] and with it a second medical school, which had an unusual and important history of its own as the first homeopathic medical school in the United States (Rogers 1998). With that acquisition, Allegheny began the process of merging its two schools, an event unseen since the beginning of the twentieth century (Ludmerer 1985).

This paper draws on qualitative data gathered as part of a five year study[2] of the unfolding merger of the two medical schools, which is one of the few, if not the only, long-term and continuous sociological examinations of an organization, private or public. Our study began in spring 1994, a few months after the merger was announced, and ended in 1998 when the Allegheny corporation and the university filed for bankruptcy. During this period we conducted more than 500 interviews and observations and collected over 1500 primary source documents. Respondents included corporate and university officials, faculty, staff, board members, students, and alumnae/i leadership. Observations included meetings of the university and hospital boards of directors, senior management, faculty governance bodies, and students groups.

Our work documented the ways in which a merger is a structurally complex, multidimensional phenomenon, both in terms of its formal organization and social life. It contains a number of identifiable and overlapping phases of development, each of which, in turn, has several dimensions along which activity and movement occur. In this paper we focus on aspects of the "initial consolidation" phase, when the organization put into place processes and undertook activities intended to reconfigure the structure and combine the function of the two schools. The patterns we identified illuminate some of the hidden risks, both human and organizational, that academic medical centers confront as they attempt to re-fashion themselves at the beginning of the new century (Ludmerer 1999).

Once the merger was announced, change came so fast and furiously, without pause, that it became institutionalized, preventing the medical school and its teaching hospitals, as well as the other units of the health sciences university, from achieving any real stability. It created a climate of ambiguity and tension, particularly on the part of the medical school faculty and staff, about what lay ahead. The secrecy surrounding the 1993 consolidation negotiations, the uncertainty created by the scope and pace of organizational change, the lowered levels of trust among members of the organization, the intended and unintended deterioration in communication, the under-appreciation of symbols, and the cultural strains between both the corporation and the academy and the two academic institutions were patterns of behavior that were apparent in this early phase and persisted, at various levels of intensity, as the legal and structural merger evolved. They were not only evident, but prominent once again when the parent organization plunged into bankruptcy in 1998, dragging the medical school, and the health sciences university of which it was a part, along with it (Burns, Cacciamani, Clement, Acquino 2000).

Context of the Merger

The twelve multi-billion dollar mergers that were disclosed in the press in August 1995, as our first work-in-progress report was being written, cross-cut a number of industries and included giant and seasoned corporations with familiar names such as Walt Disney, Westinghouse, ABC, and Chase Manhattan. Partially because of their celebrity and stock market influence, news of radical change in these organizations was not confined to the business section of newspapers but frequently warranted front-page coverage. The acquisition of Hahnemann by Allegheny and the subsequent merger of MCP with Hahnemann's School of Medicine were part of this larger economic and social phenomenon, one that began in the 1980s and wildly accelerated in the next decade. In addition, the context of the merger we studied was, and continues to be, dominated by sea changes in the organization, financing, and practice of medicine, and the merger mania that has gripped other parts of the health care industry. Health care institutions in general, and academic medical centers in particular, anticipated grim times ahead, and scrambled to devise strategies to insure their own survival (Blumenthal, Weissman, Griner 1999; Fuchs 1997).[3] One of these, pursued not only by Allegheny, but also by a number of health systems in Pennsylvania and elsewhere, was the acquisition of hospitals that in one strategic way or another were seen to fit the long-term survival plan of the acquirer.

With the requisite accreditation approvals granted by the Liaison Committee on Medical Education in 1994 for the consolidation of the two medical schools; its legal identity formalized on January 1, 1995, less than fourteen months after the merger agreement was announced; and the arrival of the inaugural class of the newly formed school of medicine in August 1995, many at Allegheny—executives, academic administrators, and several high ranking faculty—were already privately and, even on occasion, publicly describing the merger of the schools of medicine as "a done deal." Although the specific event they considered to be constitutive of the merger varied, they defined the "legal" creation of the organization and the educational approvals required to carry out its mission as tantamount to the merger itself. The merger was viewed as a static event that could be tied to a specific action and date, a view that gave the executives a sense of control over the consolidation process.

During the initial consolidation phase, the corporation directed its energy to the structural fusion of the two schools and to a range of financial problems that demanded attention. Neither HU nor MCP were fiscally strong at the time of merger, and HU, in particular, had incurred substantial deficits. Moreover, when the medical schools were combined, budget projections showed a sizeable excess of expenditures over revenues. The shortfalls were due to several factors, two of which were mounting problems for most other medical schools as well: the teaching hospitals' declining clinical revenues, translating into a decrease in the so-called "dean's tax" for operating the medical school, and the fact that many areas of basic and clinical research had become cost rather than income centers. While tackling the financial problems and the many structural reorganization tasks were essential, there was not, however, a concomitant emphasis on identifying and dealing with the functional aspects that also were vital to the successful joining of organizations. Thus, as we observed, to the lasting detriment of the consolidation process, there was a striking inattention to the cultural complexities that lay above and beneath the surface of the merger enterprise. That was indeed the case, despite our respondents' trendy overuse of the term "culture" when discussing Allegheny and the medical schools and their teaching hospitals. More generally, we also found that persons involved in other mergers in business and academic medicine arenas, at least as reported in the press and in some scholarly literature, made frequent and cavalier references to "clashes of cultures" as reasons for serious problems, including the demise of merger negotiations or of a merger itself. Not unlike the academic administrators or corporate officials whom we interviewed, the print media's glib, almost perfunctory use of the term "culture clash," and its reductionist conception of culture, were evident across reports of mergers in a number of industries—ranging from communications to petroleum.[4] Both our study and accounts of other mergers suggest that far too little, if any, attention has been given to organizational cultures, if indeed the principals fully comprehended the meaning of the term and scope of what constitutes culture in the first place.

Although legal and regulatory authorizations allow an organization to exist, they do not breathe life into it. Its precise nature, shape, and form, and its meaning to insiders and outsiders must be negotiated through multiple and ongoing interactions among and between members of the organizations: in this case, managers, educational administrators, faculty, staff, students, and alumnae/i. In this sense it matters very much what people do, what the meaning of their work is, and what the anticipated and unanticipated consequences of their actions and inaction turn out to be.

Accounts of corporate mergers suggest that some features of the MCP-Hahnemann venture are inherent to mergers more generally. Others, we believe, are distinctive, deriving their singularity either from the union of these two academic institutions[5] or from the organizational peculiarities and characteristics of the parent corporation. Examples of the ways in which this merger was similar to corporate mergers include the secrecy surrounding the 1993 negotiations, the subsequent lowered levels of trust among members of the organization, and the deterioration in communication within and between organizational units, particularly from the top down. As we will see, culture is particularly important at this stage of a merger because it entails an early groping for a new, fused social identity. When the culture of two or more formerly independent organizations with distinctive histories and styles of managing and operating bump up against one another, what occurs, at the very least, is subliminal tension that in some cases may evolve into ritualized disagreement, and in others may erupt into open conflict. The risk is inherent in the phenomenon of mergers (Buono and Bowditch 1989, Pritchett 1985). However, from a theoretical perspective as well as from empirical observation, the critical issue of social system identity was one of a first order magnitude to the well being of Allegheny and its medical school.

One of the most distinctive features of this merger involved the complex layering of diverse organizational cultures, which included the mingling of corporate, academic, and teaching hospital cultures. The necessary interfaces between the multiple units of the organization—including the school of medicine, other professional schools, the hospitals, and the managing corporation[6]—created an atmosphere in which the tensions arising from their cultural differences became more likely, more difficult to manage, and more important to accommodate.

Culture Wars: The Corporation versus The Academy

The conflict between the corporate and the academic cultures was foreshadowed by the formal, public announcement of the merger on November 17, 1993 made by the presidents of Allegheny and Hahnemann University shortly after their respective boards had approved the Resolution of Consolidation. At that meeting Iqbal Paroo, the president of Hahnemann, told those assembled that "the news I have to share is exciting and historic...and will ensure Hahnemann University's future in becoming a new...stronger, growth-oriented configuration that survives long into the next century." He went on to outline where Hahnemann would fit into the expanding Allegheny structure, and obliquely raised but did not address important faculty concerns and several hospital issues (Hahnemann Consolidates 1993). Paroo was followed by the CEO of Allegheny, Sherif Abdelhak. Responding to a faculty member's question, the CEO's closing remark, "Remember, don't cross me," set the tone for the troubled, sometimes rancorous relationship between management and faculty which, in that first year of the merger, reached a high pitch and did not significantly change over time, except among pockets of faculty members. In what became the corporate equivalent of the political sound bite, the admonition "don't cross me" was recalled, quoted, and used by many respondents in our study as a point of entry into a discussion of the innate tensions between the ethos of the corporation and that of the academy. As one department chair put it:

> Abdelhak...is not interested in winning the minds of the faculty. That distasteful comment...was instructive of his approach to understanding the academic culture—manage it from on high.

The wedding of these cultures continued to be questioned by organizational members as the initial consolidation processes and activities unfolded, and indeed throughout the course of our study and the life of the Allegheny corporation and its eastern Pennsylvania health care system. It was raised most vocally around what at the time was the relatively unique development and implementation of faculty goals and objectives. The administration publicly held[7] that the goals and objectives were a tool for faculty development, but faculty, from the outset, viewed them as tied to decisions about matters such as retention, compensation, and a threat to the tenure system, despite vehement and vocal denials from administration. The furor over the use of goals and objectives erupted soon after the merger agreement, when Allegheny realized that the consolidated medical school had an unusually large number of tenured faculty, partly due to Hahnemann's history of the almost automatic awarding of tenure to all basic science faculty with the rank of associate professor or above. In summer 1994, as part of cost control measures, Allegheny developed provisions to dismiss a number of tenured faculty, and then sought to do so. A group of tenured and nontenured Hahnemann faculty filed a grievance about the attempted dismissals, charging the university administration with violating tenure agreements and academic freedom by setting goals and objectives concerning matters such as the amount of salary to be raised through external funding, areas of research, and types of publications. The grievance was settled out of court in December 1994 (American Association of University Professors 2000).

Many faculty and administrators at the medical school believed that the organization's approach to goals and objectives, and the faculty's reaction to the events surrounding their use, had to do with the "clash of cultures." "Chairs don't approve of the [assessment] process and are embarrassed by being part of it..." a faculty member told us, echoing the view held by many. "If we don't go back to the academic process, the institution will not be taken seriously." The culture of the corporation, however, was clearly winning. One feature of Allegheny's corporate culture that was particularly salient for the way its leadership dealt with faculty, and other aspects of its management of the medical school, was the fact that it had originated and developed as a hospital management organization. The system's executives were grounded in hierarchical and centralized hospital management practices, and although Allegheny had acquired MCP in 1987, they had little training or direct experience with managing an academic institution. Nor, despite having had a medical school as part of their organization for several years, did they seem to understand—or if they did, were impatient with—the nature of academic norms and governance and the ways that it differed from their management culture.[8]

The conflict between the corporate and the academic cultures was anticipated and often recognized, to varying degrees, by people at every level of the organization. Perhaps the most compelling and revelatory in this regard was the fact that for many at MCP, Allegheny's acquisition of Hahnemann revived dormant apprehensions and insecurities that had lingered since the time of MCP's own takeover in 1987. "There is just as much angst among the MCP faculty as the Hahnemann faculty," said one member of the MCP administration.

Supporting this view, a full professor told us that "it became apparent...quickly after the AHERF-MCP merger" that they had what he called "an oil and water problem," one which, seven years later, had not resolved. "The corporate versus academic culture and mentality," our respondent concluded, "seems to be a long-term problem." When the scope, content, and nuances of culture in its varied forms are comprehended, it is not surprising that the process of change is met with resistance, fraught with difficulty, and glacially slow in its movement.

Historical and Cultural Traditions of Hahnemann and MCP

Most people who raised the issue of culture tended to emphasize the divisions between the corporate and academic ethos, assigning less weight to the substantial cultural strains that the fusion of two academic institutions inevitably created. In that first year of our study, a contrasting picture of the broad outlines of these cultures emerged. MCP's was an expressively verbal and material one, one that could be and was convincingly articulated by every person we interviewed, and which was imbued with a proselytizing quality. Faculty came on board, we were told "because of the atmosphere, the intimacy, the small size [of the school]...the ability to make a difference...the friendly feeling, the family feeling." The family metaphor was universally present in every characterization of MCP—those of administrators, faculty, and students. Its ethos was also gender-centered, a product of its rich and proud history as a women's medical college. That "gender sensitive" and "women's issues" were in every definition of MCP while class, race, and ethnicity were not suggest that MCP was exclusionary in its inclusiveness.

In contrast to MCP's self-confident presentation, Hahnemann's culture was subdued, almost silent, and at a gross level, invisible. Because of these characteristics, people could, and often did, mistakenly believe that Hahnemann had no culture—or at least none worth preserving. What was described as a "lack of confidence" by Hahnemann faculty in the school's administration prior to the merger translated into a lack of confidence in a collective sense. While gender-centeredness was a hallmark of MCP's culture, class-centeredness was a critical definitional characteristic of Hahnemann, evidenced by its center-city location and strong community orientation, its history of recruiting working class students, and its belief in the strength of ethnic diversity. Hahnemann's culture was articulated in action rather than words.

Allegheny forged ahead with the process of incorporating Hahnemann into its system and with plans to begin the inaugural year of the new School of Medicine. Among other things, departments and programs were consolidated, chairs were appointed by the provost and Allegheny's president, information systems were modified, personnel policies were drafted, and the physical location of the medical school at MCP's suburban-like campus was designated. What occurred, unequivocally, was that the policies, processes, and structural arrangements adopted for the new school were modeled, in almost every instance, after those of MCP. This was a source of widespread acrimony among former Hahnemann respondents. The Hahnemann community was told, as one administrator put it, "that the best [of each school] would be chosen," but despite that promise and what was regarded as Hahnemann's clear superiority in certain areas, "MCP's [way of doing things] took precedence." The bitter antagonism that we witnessed among Hahnemann faculty and staff stemmed from what they viewed as a kind of organizational arrogance on the part of Allegheny, whose decisions, in several instances, were based on the assumption rather than the evaluation that the MCP paradigm should prevail in every aspect of the organization.

The wholesale disregard of Hahnemann's material and symbolic culture was expressed most thoroughly and most poignantly by an Allegheny executive who spoke with unexpected candor. The failure to assess whatever strengths Hahnemann might have brought to the newly consolidated organization occurred, in his view, "more out of an unwillingness to consult...to engage...and to recognize that maybe things at Hahnemann were worth preserving—systems, procedures, processes.... That kind of analysis wasn't done and I think the organization is suffering now because of it." The remarks of another colleague supported the view that "Allegheny-MCP has the attitude that whatever they have is better than anything else and they also have a reluctance to let go of something that they have invested time and money in."

Symbols: The 19th Floor

Symbols, material and non-material, are constitutive elements of every culture and are embedded with meaning. As such, symbolic meaning is necessary to maintain human groups in a variety of organizational arrangements, including universities and corporations. This fact was implicitly recognized by the members of the Hahnemann and MCP communities who rallied active and vocal support against renaming the consolidated university in the summer of 1994. When Allegheny capitulated to the schools' demand to retain the names of the two schools, the decision was framed in ideological and philosophical terms. "It is important," an Allegheny spokesman said, "to carry on the names of both institutions." But, months later, he confided that had Allegheny chosen "to deal with the name" at that time, it "could not have [dealt] with anything else." The strength of the attachment to name and the social identity it reflects, if not comprehended at the highest level of the organization were, at least, viewed as insurmountable obstacles in the earliest phase of the merger.

As the consolidation process continued to unfold, the inattention paid to the symbolic meaning of name and place was supplanted by the failure of corporate and academic leaders to recognize and appreciate the importance of other symbols, exemplified by the reactions to "the 19th floor." "There is anger everywhere," an MCP administrator conceded in a conspiratorial tone "about the fact that the executive offices [on the 19th floor] at Hahnemann have been so elegantly renovated...[at the same time] that faculty layoffs [are occurring] and departments are being denied budget for this year..." In its most concrete form, the "19th floor" was the physical space where authority and power were concentrated. What this comment and many others in the same vein revealed was an acute but controlled resentment of all that the "19th floor" symbolically represented. In a system that many described as "fiscally driven," and at a time when budget cutting measures were instituted affecting entire departments and the people within them, the executive offices of the university were undergoing a corporate facelift. Viewed by many as hypocritical, the renovation gave tangible expression to the "us versus them" mentality that was used to characterize the uneasy relationship between the corporation and the academy.

Timetables and the Organization of Work

Another corporate pattern that frequently met resistance was a steadfast focus on timetables within which specific dates were firmly established for accomplishing particular tasks related to academic life. This approach was used, in part, to reduce ambiguity and uncertainty in a changing environment. "Timetables," one executive explained, "...force people to communicate quickly." Indeed, such timetables, in the case of developing a consolidated curriculum, for example, forced Hahnemann and MCP faculty to work together at a time when many were demoralized and their futures uncertain. Despite their coming together on a joint project as important as the new medical school curriculum, however, members of the Curriculum Committee were apprehensive about the time constraints under which they were working, raising doubts about the quality of their product. The pace of work was "too fast" a committee member confided, noting that "...curricula take years to evolve and develop. But according to the dean, this is our opportunity to be innovative and unique...as if that could come out of a pressure can.... The faculty have spent a lot of time working on this...but everyone realizes what a charade it is..."

In a few instances, the imposition of corporate-style timetables was viewed constructively, giving people a context within which to interact and an impetus to do so. For the most part, however, the timetables were regarded negatively by the faculty and many administrators not so much for the burden of work they exacted, but the lack of appreciation for the sociological calendar of academia that they reflected and for the disruption to it. Many of the deadlines were set based on the corporation's fiscal calendar, which also undergirds the operation of academic institutions. But the day-to-day life of the academy is organized and governed by a less structured and more leisurely system of time that both shapes the organization of academic work and is shaped by it.

Where the fiscal realities of the corporate calendar collided most powerfully with the realities of academic life and the calendar that organizes its work was the adoption of the goals and objectives used for the faculty assessment process. The "behind-the-scenes" activity that preceded its implementation gave an unexpected picture of unpreparedness that contradicted the notion of corporate efficiency. As one administrator put it:

> Two days before we were going to eliminate faculty...we were still drafting letters...and we were establishing goals and objectives for seventy or so faculty members a week before we were going to tell them that they either met these [goals]...or rightfully could

> lose their positions.... And it was all done hurry, hurry, hurry instead of through a very deliberative process.... And, what was driving the timing? Clearly, dollars...

Many faculty members had the impression that Allegheny was primarily "driven by dates," by an urgent sense that they had to accomplish certain tasks by certain dates, for legal and financial reasons, among others. Indeed, that was sometimes the case, forcing necessary movement on the legal and financial dimensions of the merger. However, the timetables simultaneously obstructed some aspects of organizational function and set back the pace of development along other dimensions. Many, like the administrator quoted here, worried about the errors that haste and enslavement to the corporate calendar generated:

> At the very top levels we're losing creativity that we need, and errors are being made that we're spending a lot of time reworking. [On the one hand] we don't have time to plan and implement something optimally but [on the other] we make time to rework the mistakes...if we took the time we'd have less rework because we're taking the time anyway.

Communication as Social Control

In hindsight, some of the major patterns characterizing the nature of the communications within and between various layers of the Allegheny corporation and its schools were evident in the acquisition of Hahnemann. The merger negotiations between Allegheny and Hahnemann were tightly controlled, secretly conducted, and done within a short time frame. The rationale for this process, the university's provost later explained, was that a prior merger attempt in 1990 (Knox 1990) had shown "how the democratic process, sadly, can be counter-productive in a time of rapid and dramatic change.... Discussions were held in an open and democratic forum, but a groundswell of opposition from the constituencies caused leadership to abort the discussions." Consequently, the 1993 attempt "was engaged in a 'surgical' manner, with all discussions and negotiations conducted behind closed doors. Only the required management representing the institutions was involved. When announced, the consolidation was presented as 'a fait accompli'" (Ross 1996:270). The negotiations, indeed, were kept so quiet that several people described the merger as "a startling thing" when it was revealed. In the words of one full professor, the acquisition was "one of the best kept secrets in an institution where secrets are seldom kept." With the consolidation agreement in hand, Hahnemann faculty were invited to a meeting with the university's president, who was slated to "speak on the steps being taken to insure that Hahnemann remains strong and relevant as health care reform moves forward." The cryptic language of the announcement reflected the same "close to the vest" approach that characterized the merger negotiations, giving no hint of the direction of change or the participants in it. The merger negotiations and public disclosure of the agreement were orchestrated in such a way that secrecy began to be used and viewed as an institutionalized mode of organizational communication. In fact, as time passed, it became clear that what we termed a "frozen pattern of communication" typified the Allegheny culture, and its restrictive style of communication was foreign to the academic setting and those who worked in it.

Historically, the academy operates on a "right to know" basis which is, for the most part, viewed as an entitlement. Corporations, on the other hand, apply a "need to know" strategy, which Allegheny did in many instances, including the repositioning of senior personnel that came in the wake of the merger. At some critical junctures, however, the corporation grossly miscalculated the correct timing of the "need to know." In two important cases during the first year, for example, members of the university who held positions of authority and responsibility found themselves in the humiliating position of receiving news of their promotion in one case, and their removal as a sitting chair in another, from outside sources. What the faculty viewed as egregious violations of the norms of professional ethics was also remarkable from an organizational management perspective. In one instance, the person in question had not been officially informed of the change more than two months after it occurred and had been publicly discussed. Similar, too, in these cases as in others, were the not-so-subtle overtones of a modern day form of corporate paternalism, in which the chief executive officer determines not only what is best for the organization, but what is in the best interests of individuals as well. In both instances, it was reported that the corporation had stripped the faculty members of their standing titles and positions and reassigned them, without consultation and without their knowledge. And, again illustrating the issue of corporate timetables, these cases were viewed by faculty as further instances of management's not taking the time "to do it right."

Concluding Thoughts

The lack of appreciation for cultural differences within any newly merged organization—public or private—slows the process of integration and diverts attention from collective goals to individual or sub-group concerns. Moreover, disregard for a culture that has developed its own routinized way of doing things can sometimes, and in this case did, cause efficiency—which many organizations pride themselves on—to suffer. An organization such as Allegheny that has become both an "academic corporation" on the one hand, and a "corporate academy" on the other, will require not only the "corporate socialization of the academy" but also, to a lesser but important extent, the "academic socialization of the corporation." To succeed in its acquisition of and integration or alliance with academic institutions, corporations ideally need to internalize the critical ideas and values that are distinctly academic in nature, but more importantly and more urgently, they need to develop an institutionalized respect for the traditions and modes of conduct that characterize the academic world. The same is true for the other side of the partnership, although greater energy and resolve are needed on the part of the corporation because it is operating from a position of strength and power, with less incentive to change.

The style of communication that characterized most interactions between administration, faculty, and staff also has a moral message worth noting. The reality of the merger, as a Hahnemann administrator reflected on it, was that "expectations have just not been borne out." In announcing the consolidation, he recalled, Hahnemann's president, who briefly was president of the merged institution, "said optimistic things," many of which "turned out to be false." The subsequent sudden appointment of Allegheny's CEO as president of the new university, for instance, was not what Hahnemann expected. They had been led to believe that its incumbent president would remain in office, either "because we were lied to or because our president thought that [would] be the case." And in either scenario, they reasoned, honesty had been compromised.

This view, to a greater or lesser extent, represented the collective sentiments of the Hahnemann community. But what is more remarkable about it was the fact that many of those in the upper echelons of MCP's administration and Allegheny's management agreed with that interpretation—and felt compelled to tell us so. It was clearly stated this way by one high-ranking MCP administrator: "Allegheny didn't deal with change...they didn't deal with people honestly.... What they said to us at MCP was...'don't worry—your dean and CEO are in charge.' But, what they said *there*, at Hahnemann, was a lie: 'Don't worry—your leaders are in charge.' Hahnemann has been so royally lied to that they don't trust nobody no how."

Secrecy has a time and place in the life and activities of organizations, particularly when mergers and other forms of restructuring are being contemplated or negotiated. But Allegheny's style of communication and its images—of both groups and individuals—became "frozen" so that secrecy prevailed and duplicity followed. In the end, the organization suffered for it—faculty morale plummeted with each new revelation of untruthfulness, misleading statements, and secret executive negotiations and decisions that violated the norms of academic governance. And when we left the field, five years after our study began, the hoped-for melding of the cultures of Hahnemann, MCP, and Allegheny had not taken place in any palpable and meaningful way.

Looking at what occurred in the very early phase of this historic merger can help us better understand what happened when Allegheny filed for bankruptcy four years later. The same patterns we witnessed in that very first year of the merger were visible throughout the short life of Allegheny University of the Health Sciences and its medical school, but erupted with great force in the months preceding Allegheny's demise. And, many people whom we came to know, who spoke to us in confidence and with courage, suffered enormously—on both professional and personal levels. That is, perhaps, the most important moral message of all.

Notes

1. Allegheny's acquisition of Hahnemann University was not driven by a desire to have a second medical school in Philadelphia. Rather, the corporation wanted the major center-city teaching hospital location provided by Hahnemann Hospital and market strength in several clinical programs including cardiac surgery and cardiology, as well as the university's degree programs in allied health fields and nursing that, it hoped, would provide staff for its hospitals.
2. Funding for the study was provided by the Acadia Institute, the Charles E. Culpeper Foundation, The Greenwall Foundation, The Henry J. Kaiser Family Foundation, Menlo Park, CA, and the Office of the Provost of the former Allegheny University of the Health Sciences.
3. For a detailed account of the economic forces leading to, and the outcomes of, the mergers of six prominent teaching hospitals—the Brigham and Women's and Mas-

sachusetts General in Boston, New York and Presbyterian in New York City, and the University of California, San Francisco and Stanford University Hospital in California—see Kastor 2001.

4. See, for example, Truell 1998; Harmon 1998; Quinones 1998.
5. The merger of academic institutions has been a relatively rare event, and has occurred primarily among two-year colleges. In contrast to the conventions governing most corporate mergers, however, higher education professionals have emphasized that conventions of open dialogue among stakeholders and shared decision-making are important elements for a successful merger or other actions (Martin and Samels 1994).
6. As of 1994, the organizational units consisted of the Allegheny Foundation, which included for-profit subsidiaries; Allegheny General Hospital and its Allegheny-Singer Research Institute in Pittsburgh; and MCP-Hahnemann University (later renamed Allegheny University of the Health Sciences). The university included several schools, adult hospitals, and a children's hospital. The schools were medicine; health sciences and humanities, which had a nursing program that gained separate school status in 1995; the graduate school; and a proposed school of public health. Adult hospitals were Hahnemann and MCP, with the latter including the Eastern PA Psychiatric Institute and two suburban hospitals.
7. In private discussions with us, senior medical school administrators acknowledged that the goals and objects were, as the faculty believed, intended to be used as a means for determining compensation and retention.
8. It is important to note that the imprint of a hospital-based management orientation was not unique to the MCP-HU School of Medicine, despite its being the only corporately-owned academic medical center. A 1999 AAUP statement on Academic Freedom in Medical Schools, for example, observed that "The modern medical school has many of the attributes of a complex, market-driven health care system with professors often acting as entrepreneurs in research and patient care. It is marked by conflicting roles and responsibilities, both academic and nonacademic, for faculty members and administrators alike.... Further affecting the academic freedom of medical school faculty is the hospital pattern of hierarchical organization, with deans and department chairs—and often professional administrators who lack medical training or academic experience—making decisions that elsewhere in the university would be made collegially or left to individuals professors" (American Association of University Professors 1999).

References

American Association of University Professors. 1999. "Academic Freedom in Medical Schools. Statement Endorsed by Committee A on Academic Freedom and Tenure on June 6, 1999." *Professional Ethics Report* (Spring):4.

American Association of University Professors. 2000. "Report. Academic Freedom and Tenure. Termination of Tenured Appointments: MCP Hahnemann School of Medicine (Pennsylvania)." *Academe* (May-June): 42-58.

Blumenthal, D., J. S. Weissman, and P. F. Griner. 1999. "Academic Health Centers on the Front Line: Survival Strategies in Highly Competitive Markets. *Academic Medicine* 74: 1037-1049.

Buono, A. F. and J. L. Bowditch. 1989. *The Human Side of Mergers and Acquisitions: Managing Collisions between People, Cultures, and Organizations.* San Francisco: Jossey Bass.

Burns, L. R., J. Cacciamani, J. Clement, and W. Acquino. 2000. "The Fall of the House of AHERF: The Allegheny Bankruptcy." *Health Affairs* 19: 7-41.

Fuchs, Victor R. 1997. "Managed care and merger mania." *JAMA* 227: 920-921.

"Hahnemann Consolidates with Allegheny Health, Education and Research Foundation." 1993. *Degrees and Stitches* (Hahnemann University Newsletter) 17 (Nov. 24) 1-3.

Harmon, Amy. 1998. "Culture clash seen in merger of companies: Gap between Netscape and America Online." *The New York Times* (24 Nov.): C-1, 4.

Kastor, John A. 2001. *Mergers of Teaching Hospitals.* Ann Arbor, MI: The University of Michigan Press.

Knox, A. 1990. "No merger deal for Hahnemann and med school." *Philadelphia Inquirer* (21 Feb.):F1.

Ludmerer, Kenneth M. 1985. *Learning to Heal: The Development of American Medical Education.* New York: Basic Books.

Ludmerer, Kenneth M. 1999. *Time to Heal: American Medical Education from the Turn of the Century to the Era of Managed Care.* New York: Oxford University Press.

Martin, James, James E. Samels and Associates. 1994. *Merging Colleges for Mutual Growth. A New Strategy for Academic Managers.* Baltimore: Johns Hopkins University Press.

Peitzman, Steven. 2000. *A New and Untried Course. Woman's Medical College and Medical College of Pennsylvania, 1850-1998.* New Brunswick, NJ: Rutgers University Press.

Pritchett, P. 1985. *After the Merger: Managing the Shockwaves.* Homewood, IL: Dow Jones-Irwin.

Quinones, Eric R. 1998. "Culture clash could undermine big oil merger: Mobil and its boss are seen as more freewheeling, Exxon and its chairman as stodgy." *The Philadelphia Inquirer* (3 Dec.): C-1, 2.

Rogers, Naomi. 1998. *An Alternative Path. The Making and Remaking of Hahnemann Medical College and Hospital of Philadelphia.* New Brunswick, NJ: Rutgers University Press.

Ross, Leonard. 1996. "Health Workforce Policy and Planning in a University: A New Approach," pp. 263-273 in *The U.S. Health Workforce: Power, Politics, and Policy.* Edited by M. Osterweis, C. J. McLaughlin, H. R. Manasse et al. Washington, DC: Association of Academic Health Centers.

Truell, Peter. 1998. "The potential clash: The corporate culture gap at 2 securities subsidiaries." *The New York Times* (14 Apr.): D-11.

6

Transplanting the Transplant: Japanese Sensitivity to American Medicine as an American Mission

William R. LaFleur

"I believe the impression [left on the Japanese] was that I was a butcher as well as a doctor..."
—*Dr. William Willis in Kagoshima in 1870*[1]

Carry-over and Carry-back

Many books get translated. Usually the process calls no attention to itself and that is the way publishers prefer things. After all, a translation can be judged successful when the persons reading the book in the "recipient" language are unaware that they are reading a text that had been taken out of one language and put into another.

When, however, the topic of what could be called the "donor" book is the medical practice of moving internal organs out of one body and into another, certain formal similarities between "transplantation" and "translation" will, at least to the alert publisher, invite attention. In that case the one mode of carry-over can be itself carried over into some kind of explicit or implicit relation with the second type of carry-over. And this is apparently what happened when *Spare Parts: Organ Replacement in American Society* by Renée Fox and Judith Swazey was released in 1999 in an excellent Japanese translation by Naoki Morishita and three colleagues.

I hope to demonstrate that in this case the linguistic "play" with this matter went considerably beyond being a clever but otherwise insignificant detail of the publishing process. Instead, it deserves to be seen as having its own role in bringing to the Japanese readership's consciousness the profound and extensive cultural and religious ramifications of something that occurred in Japan during 1999—the date of the first legal cadaveric organ transplantation. Translating *Spare Parts* for a Japanese readership was intended, according to Morishita, as a "telescope" for looking, via America, back at Japan and what would soon be happening there (Morishita 1999a:425).[2]

Here I try to turn that telescope around. That is, I examine how things that were part of the process of introducing *Spare Parts* to a Japanese readership can have significance for North Americans. I also explore reasons why this has relevance for more generalized thinking about medicine and how it features in the interactions between cultures. This exercise in what might be called "carry-back" will be done through select translations from Japanese and a comparative analysis.

We are in debt to Margaret Lock for pioneering, data-rich, and insightful work in English on the Japanese public struggle over brain death and organ transplants (Lock 1996, 1997). Her work does much to fill in the huge gap in the West's knowledge of how a society such as Japan reacts to the introduction and promotion of a medical procedure such as transplantation. The Anglophone world, at least in comparison with the Japanese, is still relatively ignorant of the comparative issues. The volume of our writing about both medicine and bioethical issues that gets translated into Japanese is vast, and, by contrast, that in Japanese conveyed into English is minuscule—especially in terms of critical reaction to our perspectives and methods.

Arthur Kleinman (1995) has impressively brought materials and perspectives from China into direct comparison with those of North America so as to demonstrate the contingency of the latter, and Fox and Swazey (1984) have made explicit some of the problems of assuming that American bioethics is easily transferable into Chinese society. Yet, in some ways the Japanese materials may potentially be the richest resource of all. For Japan is so technologically advanced that many of their concerns about biotechnology arise because in at least some things an attitude of prudence results from having already tasted much of that technology and having seen some of its deeply problematic aspects—social, political, philosophical, and religious. Awareness of horrible medical experiments carried out in China during Japan's own imperial period also contributes to a greater readiness to exercise caution.

However, as long as these concerns are locked up in writings still virtually unknown in the West, our own ignorance of them contributes to the misperception here that our technologies and presuppositions are universalizable. Thus, the Japanese debates about transplantation can tell us much. My contention is that the Japanese reaction to cadaveric transplants could serve *us*, in its own way, as a well-equipped laboratory. It can be a ready-made means for testing an entire spectrum of our own culture's procedures and assumptions—not only technical but also cultural, philosophical, and religious.

One index to the importance seen in the publication of *Spare Parts* in Japanese is the fact that it was speedily reviewed in a wide range of national weeklies, the equivalents of *Time* or *The New Yorker.* This contrasts with the fact that most reviews of books on "specialized" topics are placed in journals and professional newsletters (Personal communication, Naoki Morishita, April 27, 2000). Morishita, a bioethicist in the School of Medicine of Hamamatsu University, and himself the author of philosophically sophisticated analyses of changing conceptions of death (Morishita 1999b), appended to his translation an interesting and important "comment," one he wrote also on behalf of his co-translators. In it he described the longer trajectory of the Fox/Swazey research project; explained why the conclusions of *Spare Parts*—as in the now oft-cited paragraphs about "leaving the field"—are of great importance to a Japanese society still apprehensive about doing transplants from putative cadavers; told why—as a precise rendering of "spare parts" as a title would have left Japanese readers mistaking it for a book about mechanical engineering or production control—another title was chosen; introduced the individual strengths of his co-translators;[3] and selected from *Spare Parts* an array of things constituting the "dark side" of transplants—items overlooked by those Japanese who might tend to be overly impressed with the public promotion there of this technology as a sign of "progress."

To me, one of the salient phrases in the ten pages of Morishita's commentary is the phrase *burêki o kakeru*, literally "applying the brakes." To Morishita, the message of *Spare Parts* to the Japanese is one concerning both the difficulty and the necessity of halting medical research programs even though they may be ethically compromised. He sees America as having difficulty doing this. Therefore, Morishita applauds the authors of *Spare Parts* for their readiness to face head-on various internal contradictions in American society—as shown by the report that, although some can get exorbitantly expensive multiple organ transplants, perhaps as many as 43 million other persons in the United States receive inadequate medical care (Morishita 1999a: 428). From my own reading of Japanese writings, this is a commonly expressed point and one often made by Japanese physicians who trained and practiced in America and then returned to Japan. Although their instructors and colleagues on our side of the Pacific may not realize it, these persons often tell of how it came about that, while in America, they first began to entertain doubts about the juggernaut character of high-tech medicine. The point they stress is that their skepticism arose out of hospital and laboratory-based experiences in the United States, not out of ignorance of it. Notable among these are the writings by Teruo Hirose, one of which could, if translated, be rendered as "Warnings Concerning Modern Medicine: What is Taking Place Ethically in the Most Advanced Medicine Today?" (Hirose 1992). Dr. Hirose, a cardiovascular surgeon who did some groundbreaking surgery, had, if my calculations are correct, spent approximately three decades doing medical research in Chicago, Philadelphia, and New York.

Supply-Side Children

As of spring 2000, the Japanese version of *Spare Parts* had been reviewed—and in every case praised or commended—in at least eleven publications. Among the reasons for this favorable reception is the fact that this book documented in detail certain things that some Japanese writers on the topic had already guessed to be the case. Fox and Swazey, that is, are seen as providing independent and objective data on things already surmised in Japan to be the case in American transplantations procedures. Chief among these, at least in the reviews, is that once cadaveric transplantation is regarded as ethically acceptable in society, the great demand for organs results in a shortage and this, in turn, leads to a sequence of ethically compromised measures to fill the gap.

Among the developments regarded as shocking is one—perhaps because not known or fully grasped in Japan before the publication of *Spare Parts*—that strikes the reviewers as especially egregious. It is that some Americans would actually decide to conceive a child with the intention that the newborn might then serve as a "resource" for tissues or organs needed by an older sibling. Morishita puts this practice within a longer list of items he sees as having gotten oddly reversed in Americans' consciousness and practice. He writes:

> Another problem given close attention in *Spare Parts* is the shortage of organs (chapters 3 and 4). That such *shortage* is a fact is very clear from the outset. Although it had been hoped that traffic accidents might provide a sufficient means for coping with the shortfall problem, there turned out to be a statistical decline in the number of young people who could be declared "brain dead." In spite of this, the attitude seems to be that, precisely because of this shortage, such organs are even more deeply desired and then even more unusual measures can then be employed to get them. Does this not strike us as upside-down reasoning? Yet in America such twisted logic goes virtually uncontested. And then all kinds of measures are taken to fill in for the lack of organs. It starts with taking organs from persons who may still in fact be alive. Next comes the use of parts of an anencephalic infant. From there it is the xeno-transplant. And this extends even to the practice of conceiving and giving birth to new children just so that their organs, through transplantation, may save the lives of existing ones. Anything and everything will get to be brought forward for use once things start going in this direction. Matters which had initially been thought of as purely voluntary acts of goodness turn soon enough into ones conceived of in terms of "obligation" and from there degenerate all the way into commercialized procedures. What you get, then, is the buying and selling of body parts (Morishita 1999a: 428).

Although it is this entire downward trajectory that Morishita wishes to bring to his readers' attention, that with which he ends the list—in other words, what seem to be its *most* reprehensible practices—are two in number. They are the production of a child for the use of its organs and, second, any and all sales of organs.[4] These two comprise the moral nadir.

It is noteworthy that child-production for donor sourcing is also singled out for reference or comment in some of the reviews of Fox/Swazey. The fact that it is given space even within relatively short reviews indicates that it strikes the Japanese as showing how far—including misconstruals of human relationships—some Americans will go to procure tissue and organs. In his review in *Shûkan Gendai,* a major weekly, Yasuichi Abe writes:

> Chapter 3 takes up the topic of organ shortage. In the process of organ procurement how are ethical concerns to be preserved? What is extremely shocking among things presented in *Spare Parts* is the case of parents of a daughter with leukemia who "produced" another child, a younger daughter, so that the latter might be the donor of bone marrow. Would the older child not feel an immense debt to the younger in this kind of situation? And would the younger one not be filled with great questions concerning just why she had even been brought into the world? And is it necessary [for the medical community] to comply with any level of demand made by parents for the sake of saving their child? (Abe 1999)

The reference here is to what Fox and Swazey detail under the rubric of "Making a Live Donor: Bone Marrow Transplants," and specifically the case of Mr. and Mrs. Ayala, who conceived Marissa so that this child could, if there proved to be a tissue match, provide bone marrow needed by her older sister, nineteen-year-old Anissa. This action drew criticism from within the American bioethical milieu, and the sources and points of this criticism are referenced in both the English and Japanese versions of *Spare Parts*. Yet what probably amazed and appalled Japanese readers was that between 1984 and 1989 there were forty cases in America of infants conceived for this purpose, that the physicians in charge suggested or at least sanctioned this, and that a *Time* poll in 1991 indicated a 47 percent approval and only a 37 percent disapproval of this practice in the United States (Fox and Swazey 1992: 55-56; Morishita 1999a: 114-116).

The greater degree to which the Japanese were shocked by these cases calls attention to our need for a comparative bioethics that attends closely to what at first may seem to be small but ultimately unimportant nuances among cultures in such matters. The details may be the locus not only of the devil but also of some of the more important heuristic data. A "comparative bioethics" that glides over these will rightly be charged with being implicitly imperialistic. This principle is illustrated by the reasons for which producing children for their organs is likely to seem much *more* egregiously wrong in Japan than it will in the contemporary United States.

Cultural difference often gets evidenced in language. And large issues can at times be at stake when a translator faces a snag. For instance, although in their account Fox and Swazey had written that "Marissa...at age 14 months was old enough to have the bone marrow withdrawn and infused into her sister," Morishita's team had no alternative but to render this as a transfer from a "younger sister" to an "older sister." They had at their linguistic disposal no term for "sister" that was not pre-loaded with information as to birth-order. Those of us who translate Chinese and Japanese texts into English know the exact same problem...but from the opposite direction. When we come upon Sino-Japanese ideographs that have birth-order built into them, we can anticipate that many readers of our translations into English will find the references to "elder brother" or "younger sister," if not labored, then at least quaint, culture-heavy, and probably "Confucian." It is not insignificant that *our ears* find the birth-order modifiers to be gratuitous and, by comparison, our own unmodified references to "sister" or "brother" wholly *natural.* This, I suggest, is because our culture has probably come to think of birth-order as having virtually nothing to do with ethics.

The East Asian locution, however, has its own impressive logic. Since "sister" and "brother" are, in fact, words that do not make sense unless at least one other sibling exists, in the East Asian language contexts it seems completely natural, logical, ethical, and even economical to have written and spoken forms into which the notions of "elder" and "younger" have already been built. An only-child *with* a sibling is an impossibility both in nature and in logic. In the case of siblings, being born in order is a *biological* and natural necessity—even in the case of twins. And so sisters such as Anissa and Marissa could not do other than comprise the pair "older sister and younger sister" [姉妹 *shi-mai* in Japanese].

In East Asia, to be aware of one's place in such a temporal sequence is to be cognizant not so much of some kind of social construct as of something dictated by something intrinsic to being born—that is, a sequencing in which "culture" can play no role. Conversely, to fashion language so as to "free it" from reference to such a fact of nature is to court illusion. And it is, then, to prepare the ground for denying that at least in some domains *nature constrains us ethically.* This is something refracted both through how Morishita and his colleagues were forced to translate the terms for the Ayala siblings and through the higher level of disgust registered in Japan concerning the production of "supply-side" children for the sake of transplantation. My point is that, however much we in our own specific cultural context may wish to read the differences here as just variations in the construction of culture itself, the persons on the other side of this specific "cultural" difference are apt—and not without a powerful logic in their point of view—to see our practices, both in language and in bioethics, as not just strange or even self-deceived but, in fact, as running contrary *to nature.*

The assumption that nature in some ways entails specific forms of ethical behavior is demonstrated by the greater disgust felt in Japan vis-á-vis parental production of children who, sometime after being so born, will be expected to "give" organs to their seniors. This goes directly contrary to what is seen as the natural pattern of inter-sibling obligation. Chronological seniority automatically gives an earlier mastery of language and social norms, and thus it seems almost too obvious to need stating that it will be the older siblings who transmit these things and are the nature-determined "givers." The younger ones are recipients and will never be able to reciprocate for what they have received. This is the way things *are*—that is, how the irreversible structure of temporal sequence articulates into normal expectations and how these, in turn, take on the character of normative values. And it is why the very idea of giving birth to a younger sibling so that he or she may "give" an organ or tissue to its senior sibling—itself a gift never capable of being reciprocated—seems to be putting something dictated by nature, not just culture, askew.

In his own review of the translation of *Spare Parts* in a prominent weekly, Tsutomu Wada sees this practice as ominous, not easily palliated by euphemistic language:

> There is also the problem, one which surfaces especially in the case of kidney transplants, of turning the transplantation of organs from parents to children and among siblings into something implying a sense of obligation. But being the recipient of such a gift imposes a tremendous psychological burden. And the kinds of lamentable complications that this injects into the human relationships of the persons involved are not likely to be palliated by language about "the gift of love." [In America] there have been more than forty instances of parents intentionally conceiving and giving birth to a child solely so that it might possibly provide bone marrow to an older child facing death. In the situation where there is a shortage of organs, things are bound to move in the direction of the buying and selling of them, etc. This book provides us with empirical proof of the kinds of "burdens" which come into existence with the carrying out of organ transplants (Wada 1999).

The point here is that on a deep level the surface language about "love" and "giving" will not remove the likelihood that something is going wrong, not just superficially but seriously, within a society so ready to take such radical measures to make organs procurable.

Therefore, although I very much respect her work, I disagree on this point with Margaret Lock when, in an essay entitled "The Unnatural as Ideology: Contesting Brain Death in Japan," she readily reads Japanese concerns about "the natural" as little more than nation-serving rhetoric (Lock 1997). This is not to deny that a disturbing chauvinism can be found in a number of statements about the Japanese as being "closer" to nature than other peoples. Nor is it to gainsay the importance of calling attention to the fact that in many, perhaps most, societies the use of language about "natural" and "unnatural" behaviors, perhaps especially in matters having to do with gender and sexual practices, can be politically loaded, conformity-demanding, and oppressive.

My concern is different. It is that in the domain of bioethics, especially if we want it to be truly comparative, we must refrain from prematurely closing down an important trajectory of potential inquiry via a quick dismissal of all references to "the natural" as only cultural constructs at best and political ideology at worst. The problem with a knee-jerk and unreflective employment of the notion of "cultural construct" is that, when universalized as *the* important feature to note about human behavior, it reduces all reference to "the natural" as laughably naive, whereas, in fact, many of them may not be so at all. And one outcome of disallowing the category of "nature" to function as at least one means for registering concern and caution is to make our bioethics the mirror-image and companion piece to an increasingly common assumption about the human body—that it is being proven to be an almost infinitely flexible, malleable, and interchangeable concatenation of separable parts. That is, we move towards a "spare parts bioethics" to fit our "spare parts" practices in medicine.

The Barbarian Frontier

One cannot read very far in the vast Japanese literature concerning the social and moral ramifications of introducing organ transplant technologies without gaining the impression that it is quite commonly seen there as a Trojan Horse. That is, however innocent in appearance, it is loaded with cultural, even philosophical and religious, presuppositions and values. Persons thinking you can skim off and use only the technology are naive. The surgical suite where organs are given new bodily loci cannot escape also being a context wherein cultural assumptions, including those of religion, get carried along as well.

The Japanese title for the Fox/Swazey book and the design of its jacket make this point overwhelmingly clear. The book's Japanese title, if translated back into English, is "Organ Transfer Societies: America's True Present Condition and Japan's Imminent Future."[5] This title says that the book describes the way things *really* are in America; the words chosen to render the phrase "true present condition" imply a contrast between it and idealized representations or illusions. But the Japanese title also suggests that Fox/Swazey can be read as predicting the shape soon to be taken by Japanese society itself if organ transplantation is accepted and promoted within it. That is, to the descriptive modality of the original book concerning America has been added a predictive one concerning Japan.

Not just organs alone, but through them whole systems—or at least sub-systems—of cultural assumptions get transplanted. The design of the cover for Morishita's translation makes that point very skillfully. It divides that space into upper and lower halves, with one reclining body silhouette just above the dividing line and another just below it. These paralleled images, while representing any two bodies involved in an actual transplantation of organs, also function synecdochically. They represent the much larger "body" of intellectual, religious, and cultural assumptions that are bound to get carried along. Organ transplants transplant much more than organs.

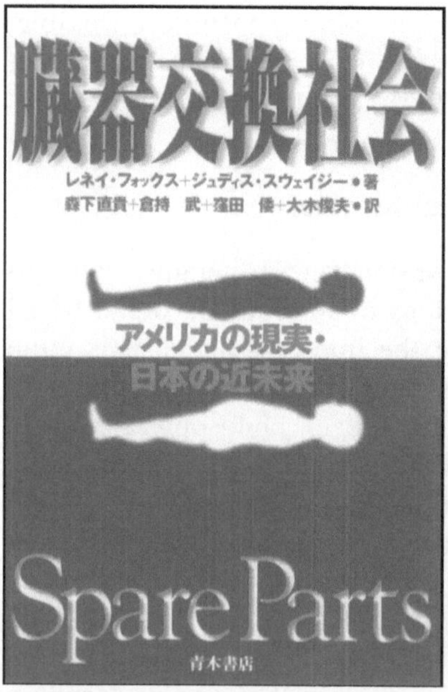

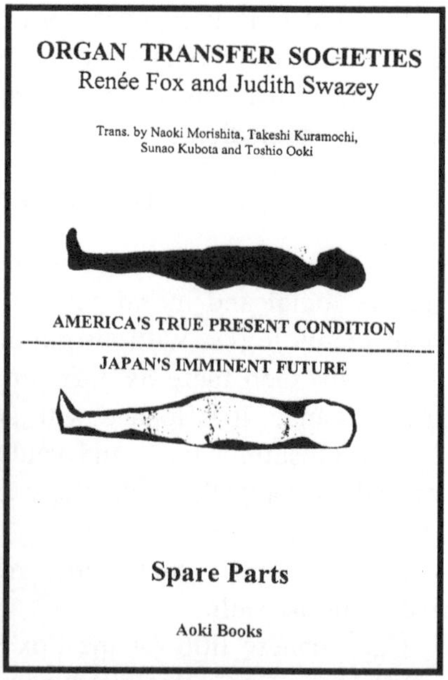

The cover seems clearly designed to raise the following questions: Is Japan really ready for this? Is this technology not, in fact, a total cultural package? And is it not likely that we Japanese, once informed by the data provided by Fox and Swazey concerning America, will emphatically want to reject it?

The appended "commentary" by Morishita also suggests the questions to be asked. In a passage that strikes me as especially interesting, Morishita calls attention to what in *Spare Parts* is an astute recognition of the "courage to fail" value system role within the ethos of America. In the original, Fox and Swazey had written:

> This ethos includes a classically American frontier outlook: heroic, pioneering, adventurous, optimistic, and determined. It also involves, however, a bellicose, 'death is the enemy' perspective; a rescue-oriented and often zealous determination to maintain life at any cost; and a relentless, hubris-ridden refusal to accept limits (Fox and Swazey 1992: 199).

Morishita reiterates that the notion of "frontier" encapsulates much of the American ethos. However, in a fascinating spin on the text he expands on this notion. Having just recapitulated Fox and Swazey's depiction of medical researchers "with such courage to move forward that they were unafraid to make mistakes," Morishita, in parentheses, suggests a pair of synonyms. In Japanese he writes "*furonteia seishin = banyû*" (Morishita 1999a: 425). What is significant in the interpolated equation is that, while its first half consists of a straight transliteration of "frontier" [*furonteia*] plus an old word for "spirit" [*seishin*], the term on the other side of the equalizer, *ban'yû*, is an old Sino-Japanese compound that denotes "savage valor" or "barbarian courage."

It is a term with a history. The ideograph translatable as "savage" or "barbarian" had long usage in East Asia. In China it had early on been employed to designate persons or groups of people somewhere beyond the edge of the civilized world—that is, outside the circumference of the "middle kingdom," its culture, and its values. The Chinese graph, originally pejorative beyond a doubt, includes a component meaning "insect" and the implication that people so designated may not only be living in "buggy" habitations but also themselves be somewhat less than human.

When used to designate peoples to the south of China—those of Southeast Asia—the term "southern barbarian" [南蛮人] had been commonly used. The Japanese later adopted this compound as their own and found special value in an extension of the reference. "Southern barbarian" [read *nanbanjin* in Japanese] came to denote those Portuguese and Spaniards, Christian missionaries for the most part, who initially arrived in Japan in the sixteenth century from points which were, at least to a Japanese geographical perspective, "south"—that is, Macao or the Philippines. Because they were being totally literal about the direction from which this religion entered their archipelago, the Japanese of that epoch took Christianity to be a "southern" rather than "western" religion. In fact, a Jesuit church built in Kyoto in 1576 was called the Nanban-ji or "Southern Barbarian Temple" (*Kodansha Encyc. of Japan* 1983, vol. 5: 321-323).

Over time this term lost much of what we might identify as its original racist and dehumanizing implications.[6] (In fact, an entire sub-genre of sixteenth- and seventeenth-century painting in Japan done in what later came to be called the "Western" style is today officially referred to, without any derogation, in the international art-world as *nanban-e* or "southern barbarian art.") Therefore, Morishita's use of a term for "barbarian" should not be judged to be racist. But it continues to suggest something coming in from "outside" Japan and likely be rather "alien" to the indigenous culture. Moreover, given the fact that most Japanese reading Morishita's account would be aware of this term's historical association with the early Christian enterprise in East Asia, linkage between it and religion, especially *religion in a missionizing modality*, would likely be present on some level.

This makes, I suggest, the equation fashioned by Morishita especially interesting. It places within a longer and wider historical context that which Fox and Swazey had referred to as the "American frontier outlook" expressed in our organ transplanters' "courage to fail" ethos. That is, while undoubtedly "American" in many ways, the "frontier outlook" had antecedents in world history—most especially in the history of European Christianity during its most aggressively expansionist phase. The Jesuits and Franciscans of the sixteenth century saw East Asia as new territory and they had adopted their own "frontier outlook" in dealing with it. Then too the mindset had been "heroic, pioneering, adventurous, optimistic, and determined." With an almost "barbarian courage" these missionaries had striven to transplant their religion onto Japanese soil

Medicine as Mission

In today's Japan the Christian missionary presence is rather different than it once had been. Today it is largely institutionalized in colleges, universities, and service organizations. Both physically and culturally, the missionary from the "West" is not as *conspicuous* there as would have been his or her counterpart in the sixteenth century. Moreover, the need for physical courage is largely gone and too overt a "pioneering" spirit would be socially and psychologically out of place. And much of the advanced "know-how" that earlier had been a privileged possession of the Catholic and Protestant missions in Japan has by now passed into the general society as commonly held intellectual and technical property. The hospital with Christian origins in today's Japan will have no advantage in terms of being able to dispense medical therapies more "advanced" than any other.

Yet there is at least one interesting exception to this decline in the general conspicuousness of the Christian missionary. Significantly for this discussion, the exception is both uniquely "American" and one that *Spare Parts* shows to have had, at least in terms of religious valorizations, its own tight connection to certain developments in transplantation technology. That to which I refer is the missionary work in Japan carried on by members of the Church of the Latter Day Saints, known more widely in both countries as "the Mormons."

It did not escape the attention of their Japanese readers that Fox and Swazey had interesting things to say about subtle connections among the Mormon interpretation of Christianity, the religious ambience of the "frontier spirit," and the explicit way in which some figures in the developing transplant technologies, themselves Mormons, prized what they saw as research explicitly expressive of their religious commitment. Morishita, for instance, writes: "The sixth chapter of *Spare Parts* makes for extraordinarily interesting reading, especially because of the way in which it pictures the American value system as embodied in Mormonism" (Morishita 1999a: 429). And Masaaki Sakamoto, who himself did research in the United States in preparation for a book titled *Amerika no kagaku gijutsu saizensen* [America's Most Advanced Scientific Technology], in reviewing Fox and Swazey in the journal *Saiasu*—a review titled "On being Astounded by How the American 'Frontier Spirit,' for the Sake of Medicine, 'Runs Roughshod over the Corpse'"—writes:

> Both Dr. William DeVries, a surgeon regularly doing transplants, and Barney Clark, the person [who had the Jarvik heart implanted by DeVries], were members of Mormon families. And the "dream of progress" that had been a symbol in the development of the mechanical heart meshed neatly with the value perspective of Mormonism. What is especially fascinating, then, about *Spare Parts* is that it provides an analysis by cultural anthropologists of the surprising degree of connectedness between high-tech medicine and religion (Sakamoto 1999).

These interpreters show a clear interest in the underlying connections among the Mormon church, the degree to which it embodies what is most "American" about religion here, the value placed on "high risk" projects on the Western frontier, and the development of organ transplant technologies in their most risk-assuming phases.

I suspect, however, that for a number of Japanese readers of *Spare Parts*, something else will come to mind, because they will be aware that Mormons have been missionizing in Japan with a zeal and conspicuousness now hard to find among Catholics or Protestants there. Probably to a degree surprising to most Americans, Mormons have had a proselytizing street presence in Japan and a fairly conspicuous one at that. Something mentioned in *Spare Parts*, but not known to most Americans, is that virtually all Mormons in their twenties have a religious obligation to serve a two-year stint as either domestic or foreign missionaries (Fox and Swazey 1992: 163). And especially during the 1970s and 1980s, it appears, a favored location for bright young Mormons to spend these two years of service was Japan. This is why they then showed up on the streets and corners of big cities such as Tokyo, Osaka, and Kyoto, and why not a few Americans, myself among them, had their first interaction with Mormon missionizing not in some American context, but in the cities of Japan.

The Mormons were missionaries but they were also, because of an "accident" of sartorial history, especially conspicuous in Japan. They did not look like the average American living or touring there in those days—a time when Americans abroad often adopted a *very* casual manner of dress. According to a somewhat inverted sense of what might be de rigueur, most American males during the '70s and '80s went tieless and jacketless, dressed in shorts even in the heart of foreign cities, and frequently wore on their feet the kind of rubber "flipflop" sandal (deemed "Oriental") that Japanese themselves never wear except in bathrooms or at the beach. It was a time when Americans often had long and abundant hair and, unlike today, had virtually no Japanese counterparts in this.

In such a context the male Mormon missionaries were conspicuously different. Their short haircuts, polished shoes, pressed business suits, conservative neckties, and white shirts (even in hot or humid weather) made them stand out and be objects of public curiosity. They were Americans, but unusual ones. Their mode of attire was one that many Japanese, then having similar sartorial tastes or so constrained by social pressure, openly praised.[7]

For these reasons they were hard to overlook when they took up positions on the public sidewalks of major Japanese cities—although the fact that they *were* missionaries was often not made very clear. Their pattern was to issue written and oral invitations to classes of English conversation with themselves as "native" speakers—then a very "hot" and sought after commodity. Persons who accepted the invitations and attended the classes often reported that they only later recognized that these teachers of English were, in fact, missionaries and their *real* project was religious conversion. Not a few Japanese came to regard the classes as having been a kind of bait. A hidden agenda had been part of things.

Thus, in the minds of such persons, "Mormon" is related to impressions of an America in *its most missionizing* mode. Even today Japan is still something of a "frontier" for some Christians. And the pioneer spirit—whether exercised in religion, medical research, or some *combination of these two*—is alive and valued. Therefore, one of the most interesting features of *Spare Parts* may be what it reveals about how these things came together in Mormon-connected research on transplants in general and the Jarvik artificial heart in particular (Fox and Swazey 1992: 106-109, 162-169). Sakamoto, in the citation above, wrote of having learned from *Spare Parts* of "the surprising degree of connectedness between high-tech medicine and religion" in America. That within medicine, in spite of pronouncements about it being strictly secular, there may be semi-hidden religious agendas—in ways not entirely unlike those of missionaries proffering classes in English—is, it seems, one of the important features of the Fox/Swazey book for Japanese readers. It confirms for them an earlier suspicion.

To persons eager to retain their own culture's religious integrity, the perception of such agendas means that there are substantial risks involved. The technology of organ transplantion comes from an America where "zeal," whether in religion or in medicine, sometimes seems not very different from recklessness. The cultural embodiment of the "frontier spirit" means so great an orientation toward the future that serious ethical blind-spots come to be tolerated in the present. And the fact that these things carry over into medical research is not then surprising. In his review of *Spare Parts* Sakamoto tells how he himself had once been told by Dr. Robert Jarvik, the inventor of a mechanical heart, that he had been very fearful that his experimental patient, Barney Clark, might die during the surgery. And Sakamoto expresses his own shock. "Why," he asks, "is it that experiments posing *this* level of risk to human subjects are permitted?" (Sakamoto 1999). The posing of this question is immediately followed by Sakamoto's reference, as quoted above, to Mormons and the deep "connectedness between high-tech medicine and religion" in America.

The point of such reviews in Japanese is not that a Mormon influence *per se* is pervasive in America. Nor is it that it has had a great impact on how bioethical issues are debated and decided here. Rather it is that the Mormons make overt the *covert role of zeal* in America, one that sometimes carries over easily from the domain of religion to that of medicine and medical research. The old-style "medical missionary" may have long been absent from Japan, but the sense of mission, one largely Christian, may not yet be out of the mind of some Americans in the medical field. Japanese experience with how cadaveric organ transplantation has been pushed there will tend to reinforce that point.

As I have shown elsewhere, the history of the acceptance and promotion of cadaveric transplants in America occurred at what was, at least for its promoters, a uniquely opportune historical moment. The late 1960s and early 1970s was a period when theological discussions, especially among Protestants, had fastened upon love in the *agapé* mode as not only distinctly expressive of Christianity's essence but in need of being articulated into societal forms. Documents of the time show how quickly and eagerly explicit connections were seen as existing between that epoch's most "advanced" theological positions and its newest, most awesome, developments in medical technology. *Agapé* and the transplant seemed to have been made for one another (LaFleur 2001).

It should not be surprising, therefore, that at least some Americans hold that the Japanese resistance to cadaveric transplants is evidence that Japan still is not a society sufficiently open to the Christian perspective in these matters. I have been personally told by a self-identified American Christian, who travels to Japan in medical contexts, that at bottom their ignorance of Christianity is the *real* reason many Japanese resist the use of cadaveric organ transplants. It was also suggested to me that, if I were to check on the matter, I would find a high percentage of Christians among those physicians in Japan active in promoting organ transplantation. I have had no way to verify or disprove such a claim. It may, however, be significant that in a recent essay in one of Japan's premier intellectual journals, Kenji Doi, a Japanese theologian skilled both in the interpretation of the Greek New Testament and in theoretical analysis, forcefully contends that being a Christian can, in fact, be *totally compatible* with being opposed to the societal acceptance of the cadaveric transplant (Doi 2000). The fact that Doi, as a Japanese Christian, even felt the need to present such a case may indicate the extent to which, although he himself resists such, a significant number of individuals and groups in Japan assume that the Japanese public's acceptance of transplants will serve—for better or for worse depending on how one views the result—as a step either in Japan's adoption of Christianity, or at least a deeper level of congruence between Japanese society and the values of the "Judeo-Christian" West.

Another level of the American "mission" is not nearly so visible—or even recognizable—as such by persons engaged in it. It exists simply through the procedures of internationalized medical education, physician travel, and international conferences on medicine or bioethics. It is based on the assumption that the latest procedure is likely to be the best and, because whatever is best will also probably save the most lives, its export for use in societies other than our own is an unambiguous moral imperative. The universality of the basic human anatomy and responses to treatment is taken to mean that the particularity of culture is a matter of little or no consequence. Pleas for sensitivity to what might be prudence-based concerns within a given society—that is, concern that the "new" may *not* be the "best"—will seem both unnecessarily abstract or even too ensconced in another society's "traditional" religion to merit caution or even much attention. The "traditional religion" is judged from the outset to be stagnant and an impediment to the very societal changes that will be a moral advance.

Although certainly not the only American so engaged, Dr. Thomas E. Starzl, among the most eminent of transplant surgeons, tells in his autobiography how and why he was active in assisting his Japanese colleagues who wanted to have the "brain death" definition of death legalized there and, through that, the possibility in Japan of doing cadaveric transplants. In his writings we can see that the all-too convenient assumption that the transfer of medical technology is a strictly secular affair supports the pioneering spirit and prevents it from being recognized as also a religiously missionizing one. Starzl writes of Japan in 1990 as a "hotbed of industry and technology where social and legal inertia had frozen the conditions of organ donation into the mold that the Western world had shattered two decades before." Using the colonialist's caricature of the Other's culture as stagnant, he continues: "Brain death was [still] not accepted, and public debate over what defined this condition remained at the same level as when I visited Japan for the first time in 1968" (Starzl 1992: 311).

Perhaps it is part of the pioneering spirit to assume that the possession of one type of technological skill obviates the need to acquire another one when doing diagnoses in a totally different domain. Somehow Starzl assumed that, even without the ability to read Japanese, and thus without the skills requisite to handle the massive amount of data involved, he could easily judge that it was nothing but "inertia" that blocked cadaveric transplants in Japan and that in 1990 "the public debate in Japan...remained at the same level" as it had been in 1968. He could not know that things far more intellectually interesting than inertia had been blocking an easy acceptance in Japan. Nor did he possess the tools to be able even to consider the possibility that Japan's debate on this issue might have been, in fact, more extensive, informed, and vigorous than that of any other nation in the twentieth century. What is telling is that he not only lacked the evidence for his judgment, but also appears to have assumed that the ability to access *evidence,* commonly considered the highest desideratum in any science, simply was not requisite for him to make his own diagnosis of what was ailing Japan.[8]

All missions and missionaries know the value of the political route, often the quickest one, to their objectives. On December 4, 1991 Dr. Starzl wrote a letter to Barbara Bush, wife of the American president, just prior to the latter's departure for an official visit to Japan. In that letter Starzl noted that "because of controversy in Japan about brain death, organ transplantation has been slow to develop in that country...." He requested Mrs. Bush to ask her husband to meet with Japanese members of TRIO [Transplant Recipients International Organization]. Such a meeting with the American president, Starzl predicted, "would be widely reported in the [Japanese] media and would help to expedite transplant acceptance and development" (Torio Jyapan, 1993: 249).

I assume that Dr. Starzl's impulse to "help out" in overcoming resistance elsewhere to the technologies taken as "normal" in our own culture is not uncommon. It appears to have been characteristic of those persons and nations with "advanced" medical technologies to assume they have an obligation to help these gain universal acceptance. Yet it is fairly clear that the American physician in this instance viewed the cultural and intellectual *reasons* for the "controversy in Japan about brain-death" as dismissable and he wanted the American president to help overcome them. The fact that there was—and still is today—scientific doubt about the definition of brain death as personal death, something extensively reported upon and analyzed in Japan, was simply overridden in the effort to see to it that the American practice be adopted and universalized. The problem here is that, especially when taken as "secular," such practices are thought to not interfere with anything—at least not anything of real *value*—in the "Other," the resistant society. But this attitude, however dressed in the language of the strictly secular, cannot do other than turn medicine into something operating in a missionizing mode. And this is why it remains deeply problematic—to a degree pithily articulated by Eike-Henner W. Kluge:

> There is little that can be done about a refusal to donate [organs] which finds its basis in religious conviction, short of changing the tenets of the relevant religion or prohibiting adherence to the religion itself. Neither of these is morally acceptable (Kluge 1999: 388).

Notes

1. Quoted in Cortezzi 1985: 179.
2. Although Fox and Swazey are the authors of both the English and Japanese versions referred to here, for the sake of differentiating the two I refer to the latter as "Morishita," its principal translator, in citations.
3. Morishita notes that one of the team, Sunao Kubota, had when younger been planning a career as an organ transplant surgeon but abandoned this plan when realizing what it involved.
4. It has not gone unnoticed in Japan that in America there now are small measures and larger proposals to "compensate" the surviving kin of donors and that this introduces the "sale of organs" in an indirect way. This has been a live issue in Japan in part because individuals are known to have gone abroad from there and paid to receive a kidney from an indigent person.
5. The force of the "mechanization" image connoted by the phrase "spare parts" is not entirely lost in the Japanese. Although in Japan the average automobile driver, compared to his American counterpart, is less likely to know junk-yards as reservoirs for auto parts, the word chosen to render "transfer" in the Japanese title, *kôkan,*

is one most commonly used when a vehicle undergoes an "oil change" or "tire change."

6. Modern linguistics, contesting a somewhat notorious error made by Ezra Pound and Ernest Fenollosa, holds that the original components within Chinese graphs are, through habituated usage, often not items of which their users are conscious. Just as in English we can use the word "cynic" without intending, in spite of etymology still latent in the term, to animalize another as a "dog" [Greek: *kynikos*], so too the Chinese graph for "barbarian" can be written without any intention of referring to another as "bug." That is, the "insect" can remain in the graph without being in the mind of the person writing it.
7. A number of these Mormons, having received excellent training in Japanese, later went on to receive higher degrees and to become American scholars with expertise on Japan.
8. Other ways in which transplantation promoters at times simply disregard negative data are examined in LaFleur 2002.

References

Abe, Yasuichi. 1999. "Seizonritsu, tôjishi no shinri, chôtatsu no rinri nado iryôgenba no uchigawa kara ishoku no honshitsu o tou" [Examining the Realities about Transplants from Inside the Medical Facility—in Terms of Survival Rates, the Psychology of those Involved, and the Ethics of Procurement]. *Gendai shûkan* June 19.

Cortezzi, Hugh. 1985. *Dr Willis in Japan: British Medical Pioneer 1862-1877.* London: The Athlone Press.

Doi, Kenji. 2000. "Rinjinai no bimei no moto ni—nôshi ishoku ni taisuru kirisutokyôteki shiten kara no mondai teiki," pp. 242-263 in *Gendai shisô* 28:10, Sept.

Fox, Renée C. and Judith P. Swazey. 1984. "Medical Morality is not Bioethics—Medical Ethics in China and the United States," pp. 336-360 in *Perspectives in Biology and Medicine* 27:3.

Fox, Renée C. and Judith P. Swazey. 1992. *Spare Parts: Organ Replacement in American Society.* New York and Oxford: Oxford University Press.

Hirose, Teruo. 1992. *Kindai iryô e no keikoku: Ima iryô rinri no saizensen de nani ga okite iru no ka.* Tokyo: Kanehara shuppan.

Kleinman, Arthur. 1995. *Writing at the Margin: Discourse between Anthropology and Medicine.* Berkeley: University of California Press.

Kluge, Eike-Henner W. 1991. "Organ Donation and Retrieval: Whose Body is it Anyway?" pp. 387-389 in *Bioethics: An Anthology*, edited by Helga Kuhse and Peter Singer. Oxford : Blackwell Publishers Ltd.

Kodansha Encyclopedia of Japan. 1983. Tokyo: Kodansha International, 9 vols.

LaFleur, William R. 2001. "From *Agapé* to Organs: Religious Difference between Japan and America in Judging the Ethics of the Transplant," pp.271-290 in *Ethics in the World Religions*, edited by Joseph Runzo and Nancy M. Martin. Oxford: One World.

LaFleur, William R. 2002 [in press]. "Philosophy and Fear: Hans Jonas and the Japanese Debate About the Ethics of Organ Transplantation," in *Technology and Cultural Values: On the Edge of the Third Millennium*, edited by Peter Hershock, Marietta Stepaniants, and Roger T. Ames. Honolulu: University of Hawaii Press.

Lock, Margaret. 1996. "Deadly Disputes: Ideologies and Brain Death in Japan," pp. 142-167 in *Organ Transplantation: Meanings and Realities*, edited by Stuart J. Youngner, Renée C. Fox, and Laurence J. O'Connell. Madison: University of Wisconsin Press.

Lock, Margaret. 1997. "The Unnatural as Ideology: Contesting Brain Death in Japan," pp. 120-144 in *Japanese Images of Nature: Cultural Perspectives*, edited by Pamela J. Asquith and Arne Kalland. Surrey: Curzon Press.

Morishita, Naoki with Takeshi Kuramochi, Sunao Kubota, and Toshio Ooki. 1999a. Trans. *Zôki kôkan shakai: Amerika no genjitsu, Nihon no kinmirai* by Renée C. Fox and Judith P. Swazey. Tokyo: Aoki shoten.

Morishita, Naoki. 1999b. *Shi no sentaku: Inochi no genba kara kangaeru.* Tokyo: Madosha.

Sakamoto, Masaaki. 1999. "Iryô made ga 'Shikabane o norikoe' susumu Beikoku no 'furonteia seishin' ni odoroki" [On being Astounded at How the American 'Frontier Spirit,' for the Sake of Medicine, 'Runs Roughshod over the Corpse']. *Saiasu,* July.

Starzl, Thomas E. 1992. *The Puzzle People: Memoirs of a Transplant Surgeon.* Pittsburgh: University of Pittsburgh Press.

Torio Jyapan 1993. *Korekara no ishoku iryô: Ishokushatachi kara no hasshin.* Tokyo: Haru shobô.

Wada, Tsutomu. 1999. Review, *Zôki kôkan shakai. Shûkan posuto*, June 4.

7

Forty Years of Fieldwork: Renée Fox and Belgium/Belgium and Renée Fox

Yves Winkin

In June 1959, Renée Fox took the ocean liner *Niew Amsterdam* to come to Belgium for the summer. "Why Belgium?" to use the title of one of her best known papers (1978). It was because she wanted to know more about a society that was able to call back home young and brilliant physicians after their training in the United States. They had no promise of a career in Belgium, and yet most of them decided to return home. Renée came to know quite a few Belgian physicians while working on her study of Ward F2 at Boston's Peter Bent Brigham Hospital, which became her now classic book, *Experiment Perilous* (1959). During that summer, she refined the focus of her sociological inquiry to learn "how social, cultural and historical factors affected clinical medical research and research careers in a contemporary European society" (Fox 1994:4).

When she settled in Louvain that summer, Renée had no idea that she was going to return to Belgium almost every year for the next four decades. Over the course of those visits her perspective changed: "What began as a study of Belgian medical research, and its social and cultural framework, was rapidly transformed into a study of Belgium through the windows of its medical laboratories"(Fox 1994: 5).

Her "Belgian work," which culminated in her 1994 book, *In The Belgian Château: The Spirit and Culture of a European Society in an Age of Change*, is probably better known in Belgium, where it was published in a French translation in 1997, than in the United States. This is not the place, however, to present it in any systematic way. My focus will be on the ways her Belgian work was received in

Belgium over the years. My argument is that she played an important healing role in Belgium at a time, 1997, when the country sank into a deep collective moral crisis. Today she also could play an important role in exemplifying the way social scientific work might be conducted in Belgium on Belgium.

In 1962 Fox published a paper in *Science*, titled "Medical Scientists in a Château" (1962), which focused on a colloquium on cardiac surgery held in the Royal Castle in honor of three foreign medical scientists. To her, this was a "symbolic gathering": the "Château" was emblematic of the ways medical research was carried on in Belgium. The many political, cultural, and religious bodies of Belgium were present at the gathering; to move around easily in such a complex maze of relationships required many years of social science training. No wonder building a medical research career was so slow and difficult.

The paper triggered a wave of reactions. In Belgian newspapers they were predominantly negative. Although the paper was focused on the organization of medical research, it was derided as an all too subjective analysis of the ways the country "worked" (or rather, did not work). As the weekly *Pourquoi Pas?* editorialized on June 15, 1962: "Are We a Ridiculous Country?" Renée Fox was seen as a young American *blanc bec* (arrogant know-it-all). In more private circles, however, her paper was seen as the work of a courageous young writer who gave a voice to people who could not speak up for fear of losing the possibility of a career. But such appreciative comments were obliterated by defensive replies.

Thirty-five years later, the French translation of the *Belgian Château* appeared in Belgium (Fox 1997). This time, the positive reactions were overwhelming. About fifteen reviews appeared in the French-speaking Belgian press, but there were also reviews in the Flemish-speaking and the German-speaking Belgian newspapers. They were not short reviews. The book made first-page headlines of *Le Soir* and *La Libre Belgique*, the two most widely circulated Belgian, French-speaking newspapers. There were many interviews, from popular women's magazines (*Femmes d'Aujourd'hui*) to sophisticated radio programs (*Arguments*). The book ranked fourth or fifth for several weeks on the list of best-selling books in Belgium.

The dominant theme of the reviews, comments, and questions to the book's author can be summarized as: "So, really, you think that

Belgium does exist as a whole?" From the United States, it may sound like a weird question. But the Belgian media and the Belgian political and intellectual circles have been filled for many years with debates about the existence or non-existence of a country that was "artificially created" in 1830 as a buffer zone between France, Holland, Germany, and Great Britain, and which has always been marred by the "linguistic question." In recent years, the question became "*when* do we split up ?" The example of Czechoslovakia was offered systematically in the mid-90s.

Then the country was very badly shaken up by a horror story: in 1995, a sadist kidnapped, raped, and let die two young girls in a hidden cell. Two other young girls were saved almost by chance. All over the country, spontaneous meetings of protest took place: parents were afraid for their children, and people could not believe the police had acted so poorly. It all culminated in a huge "White Walk" in Brussels in late 1996, in which the linguistic divide was transcended. In a new epilogue to the French edition of the *Belgian Château* Renée stressed that the meeting was very important symbolically (1997: 341-364). The subtitle of the book, "Un Peuple se Retrouve" (A people rediscovers itself) aptly captured her vision of the event.

As I systematically combed the press clippings, I was struck by the repetitiveness of the questions asked by the journalists. It was as if they wanted to say: "Please, tell us again we are not so bad after all"—as if an outsider could offer some redemption and comfort. One leading journalist, Jacques de Decker of *Le Soir*, completed his review of the book with the following lines: "One is caught looking at oneself from a different eye and, in a way, one realizes that some new self confidence is building up. In order to learn again how to like oneself, isn't it sufficient sometimes to know that someone loves you?" (1997:13).

What is remarkable about these lines is that they are full of emotions. It perfectly illustrates what Renée had written when she analyzed the reaction to King Baudouin's sudden death in 1993: "... the tendency of Belgians to be highly sensitive to the sphere of their individual and collective existence where emotions and beliefs, values, and symbols reside, while verbally denying their importance in daily life and systematically excluding them from their intellectual and scientific work" (1994: 321).

Le Château des Belges helped Belgians express publicly their emotions at a time of crisis. Through her interviews and public addresses in Belgium in the spring of 1997, Renée found herself in the role of a public healer. She did not say anything more than she had written for many years, but the context was such that her analysis reached broad audiences and was accepted with gratefulness. The collective attitude was a symmetrical inversion of the 1962 reaction, except in one segment of Belgian society: the academic social scientific "community."

The few negative reviews of *Le Château des Belges* were written by sociologists or "intellectuals" who considered the analysis anecdotal, superficial, and outdated. I vividly remember one incident that illustrates this attitude. I attended a talk Renée gave in the basement of a bookshop in Brussels in April 1997. The room was packed. Just behind me was a group of people exchanging facial signs and hushed comments on Renée's dialogue with the audience. I later found out they were members of the editorial staff of *La Revue Nouvelle*, a left-of-center, "Christian democrat" intellectual review which played a significant role in the atmosphere of doom that prevailed for years in Belgium. They could not accept her views—and yet they came to the lecture. But they did not address her publicly, although they later published the harshest review of the book (Halen 1997). They reminded me of the attitude of several colleagues at the University of Liège, who thought I had wasted my time editing the French version of *In the Belgian Château*. "Sociologie de château," as one of them wrote to me: castle sociology—implying that Renée only pictured a rosy tableau of the country, closer to *Paris-Match* style journalism than to sociology.

To account for such negative framing, one may return to her remarks, quoted above, regarding the exclusion of "emotions and beliefs, values and symbols" in Belgian intellectual and scientific work. In a nutshell, her writings on Belgium are considered too mawkish by traditional Belgian social scientists. Belgian sociology was partly founded by professors first trained as law scholars (Fox 1982: 30-32). Only manifest structures of Belgium could be studied scientifically: libraries are full of monographs on economic, political, and historical aspects of Belgian society. But latent cultural and symbolic dimensions of Belgian life were left to writers and painters. Such a positivistic attitude long prevailed in Belgian social sciences, which never accepted anthropology as a full–fledged discipline. Belgian anthropologists of Renée's generation were trained and taught abroad (Jacques Maquet and Jan Vansina, to give two American examples). The situation is getting better today but there is no tradition to build upon.

The lack of an anthropological tradition in Belgium explains why Fox's ethnographic work was never quite understood by her Belgian colleagues. Fieldwork for her is not only based on long interviews with many kinds of people. It is also a kinæsthesic mode of participant observation in the ambiance of a culture: the staccato noise of the footsteps on a sidewalk, the perfume of roses, the colors of the sky. Fieldwork is thus as much an inner experience as a collection of "data." She lets her own "inner landscape" resonate with her observations. She incorporates them and later renders them through a very delicate prose. All this is foreign to the methodological traditions of Belgian social sciences. Not that the literature on Belgium by Belgian social scientists is filled with statistics—but again, "you don't speak about your dreams" when you do research, as I was once told by a colleague.

Fox's approach to Belgian society could thus lead to the development of a new interdisciplinary field: Belgian Studies (preferable to "belgiumology"). In a few universities spread around the world, from Canada to Romania, there are departments or at least professors and seminars devoted to Belgian arts and literature. But such creative productions are rarely considered to be manifestations of cultural patterns that should be incorporated into social scientific investigations on Belgium as a whole. This is even more so since the federalization of Belgian administrative structures led people to think that the "Flemish community" culturally belongs to the Low Countries (and Low Countries Studies), while the "French community" is ready to join France (and French Studies). This is not a superficial foreign reading of the complex situation of Belgium: as a matter of fact, it is even more prevalent within Belgian universities, which were "communitarized" a few years ago. Their sense of belongingness is anchored in a linguistic community or an economic region, not into a country as a whole. There is no way they are going to consider Belgium as an integrated field of study, except possibly in history.

Renée Fox's role could thus be extremely important in the redefinition of the frames within which Belgium could be studied, both abroad and at home. Both conceptually and methodologically, her work on Belgium opens new vistas. It may well be that a new generation of scholars, less enmeshed in the academic traditions of their elders, will dare explore them systematically.

References

De Decker, Jacques. 1997. "Une Américaine en Belgique." *Le Soir,* March 28: 1, 13.

Fox, Renée. 1959. *Experiment Perilous: Physicians and Patients Facing the Unknown.* Glencoe, IL: Free Press.

Fox, Renée. 1962. "Medical Scientists in a Château." *Science* 136: 476-483.

Fox, Renée. 1978. "Why Belgium ?" *Archives Européennes de Sociologie* 19:224-26.

Fox, Renée. 1982. "Is Religion Important in Belgium?" *Archives Européennes de Sociologie* 23:5-37.

Fox, Renée. 1994. *In the Belgian Château. The Spirit and Culture of a European Society in an Age of Change.* Chicago: Ivan Dee.

Fox, Renée. 1997. *Le Château des Belges. Un Peuple se Retrouve.* Bruxelles: Duculot.

Halen, Pierre. 1997. Review, *Le Château des Belges. La Revue Nouvelle*, October: 93-95.

II

Becoming and Being a Physician

8

Responding to a Poor Evaluation: What Constitutes an "Honest" Response in the Eyes of Residency Program Directors[1]

Virginia Adams O'Connell and *Charles L. Bosk*[2]

Introduction

During a study of attrition in surgical residency programs,[3] we found that program directors designated honesty the most important trait that a resident could possess, yet complained that honesty was the hardest trait to assess and measure. Table 1 shows how program directors ranked honesty against a host of other traits, aptitudes, and characteristics. As the table shows, 94 percent ranked honesty as very important, whereas no other trait, aptitude, or characteristic was ranked very important by more than 55 percent of program directors.

Table 1

Trait, Aptitude or Characteristic	Percent of Program Directors who ranked as "very important"	95% Confidence Interval for the Mean
Honesty	94%	4.901047-4.952336
Patient Relationships	55%	4.399189-4.516383
Maturity	54%	4.390859-4.502199
Personality	49%	4.263576-4.390559
Ability to Handle Stress	49%	4.298845-4.421606
Staff Relationships	42%	4.235678-4.353441
Clinical Judgement	41%	4.171312-4.299498
Cognitive Knowledge	39%	4.170986-4.290552
Manual Dexterity	19%	3.559386-3.709917

1=unimportant, 5=very important

We all share a cultural understanding of what we mean when we say someone is honest, but how do we measure that quality in a person? What does an honest person do that a dishonest person does not do? And how do we assess and reassess our understanding of an individual's honesty over time? Honesty is not a static quality, but a trait that can change with the setting. It is assessed over time through repeated interactions with individuals. We usually assume that the person we are dealing with is "honest" until they prove us wrong. Once labeled dishonest, the tainted individual must work hard to regain trust.

A person is supposed to be honest with others, to tell the truth. We also have a concept of what it means to be honest with oneself. Individuals are often judged as being "honest with themselves" when their self-perceptions match the perceptions that others, especially those people with authority over them, have about them. When there is a discrepancy, those in subordinate positions are thought by superiors to be "kidding themselves" or "out-of-touch." Shared perceptions create a shared reality, a stable context in which interactions can occur.

When surgical program directors use the term, they mean both types of honesty. Residents should be truthful when they say that they have seen Patient X and completed the work up. But honesty also means sharing the attending faculty's perception of the proper role of the surgeon and, more broadly, of the culture of surgery. This broad perception includes everything from having the proper demeanor to sharing the faculty's view of the surgeon as the head of the medical team. It means assuming responsibility for your own as well as others' actions or misdeeds. It means demonstrating that you are a team player who recognizes the hierarchical structure of surgical work. These are some of the qualities that a good surgeon displays, so to fill the role honestly, the resident must display the proper attitude, demonstrating that he or she accepts and validates the many different aspects of the culture of surgery.

Honesty in this latter sense translates to a complete acceptance of responsibility. To accept the responsibility for a patient's life on the operating table but to fail to make sure that pre-op and post-op care has been managed well is considered dishonest. To not get along with some members of the medical staff may be very human, but it is considered dishonest. To challenge a faculty member's negative evaluation means that you are denying personal responsibility, which is considered dishonest. By looking at the culture of surgery, we will see why these infractions are such grave ones.

Since the central focus of our study was on attrition, we gathered information about residents who resigned, were terminated, or who problematically completed their residency training.[4,5] We asked specifically for information on the resident's response to faculty criticisms of performance for two of our groups—terminations and problematic completers. No resident gets through a residency program without some criticism at one time or another or without some correction from a superior. So the question follows, how does the individual respond to criticism? In the context of the interaction between teacher and student, much information is relayed. The teacher asserts authority by identifying an area that needs improvement. The manner and content of the student's response conveys whether or not the trainee recognizes the authority of the teacher, and indicates the student's willingness to make the necessary changes: i.e., the acceptance of some personal responsibility. And finally, it reflects the degree to which the student believes that the teacher's perspective on the situation is correct. From the teacher's perspective, there are correct and incorrect responses which, in these residency programs, are defined as "honest" and "dishonest." Focusing on this phenomenon, we will show that the nature of the response has a significant effect on a resident's experience in a residency program. In short, a good response signals an honest resident and can save a poor performer from termination.

For the interaction to be successful, both student and teacher need to know the rules of the game. What should be the tone of the response, how should it be worded? What should be the student's demeanor? Passive? Aggressive? A bit of both? How about the teacher's demeanor? How will the behavior and response be interpreted? How well will a man interpret the response of a woman, and vice-versa? How well will an American interpret the intonations and body language of a foreign national? Such questions illustrate that a great deal of cultural knowledge and cultural mastery is involved in all human interactions. We found that female and racial minority residents are at a disadvantage in the culture that still dominates the world of surgical practice today. Female and racial minority residents differ from white males in the quantity and quality of interactions with faculty members, and attending faculty show a greater intolerance for their responses to criticism.

The Culture of Surgery

As is characteristic of professions in general, physicians believe that their work is special and worthy of note and esteem, and laymen also accord it prestige. Doctors are given special privileges because of the special nature of their work (Glantz 1985:63). Given the patient's state of vulnerability and the intimacy of physician-patient contact, the fiduciary role of the physician is central (Parsons 1951). Patients sometimes literally put their lives in the doctor's hands. The amount of faith that this act requires is substantial. The patient must "trust" that the doctor has his or her best interests in mind; that the doctor will do his or her best; and that he or she will not take advantage of the patient's vulnerability. For these reasons among others, honesty is a vital trait for physicians.

Surgery has been defined as the most hands-on of the medical specialties, and surgeons are held to be the epitome of medical competence (Good 1995:66). They sit at the top of the medical hierarchy. Surgeons recognize that with work involving such direct intervention in the body comes a more direct and visible line of responsibility. When something goes wrong during an operation, it is hard for the surgeon to claim that he or she had no hand in the outcome, even if the surgeon was not directly responsible for the bad turn of events (Bosk 1979). As one resident stated, "you feel like if there is one false move, it's like leaving a trail of blood on the water" (R27). But the trail is not just physical; it is moral, evidence of a failure to fulfill the surgeon's fiduciary role (Parmer 1982:2). Shoddy surgical work risks far greater damage to the integrity of the patient's body than other less invasive medical procedures.

Surgery occurs in a surgical theater, and it is not a one-person show. Although the surgeon is the head of the operating team, he or she relies on other team members—the anesthesiologist, the scrub nurse, the residents, etc.—to perform successfully. This team aspect necessitates that the members work together and cooperate. The ideal is that harmony and cooperation prevail.

Ideally, there also must be harmony and cooperation among all staff members in a hospital department. Sharing patients, call coverage, and covering for each other during sicknesses and other personal crises, the medical staff must trust that the care given by any member of the team is comparable to the care given by any other member. Each team member, including the nurses, should be replaceable (Zerubavel 1979:44). Each member must have faith in other members' technical proficiency as well as in their "honesty, compulsion" (R23), and commitment to providing good medical care. Some quotes from our respondents illustrate this point:

> In my program, I want someone who is going to blend with the rest of my people, I don't want a totally independent soul (A14).

> The most important thing, no question...is the ability for the residents and the attending staff to work well together...I think the ability for the residents and the attending staff to communicate, particularly when they have disagreements in taking care of patients (R35).

White males have historically staffed surgical residency programs. Despite their growing representation among the medical school graduates, women and racial minorities are still underrepresented among the surgical residents. Although women comprised 43 percent of 1997 medical school graduates, only about 17 percent of new surgical residents were women and only one-tenth of one percent were in surgical subspecialties (Steinhauer 1999). The homogeneity of surgical programs has facilitated the harmonious functioning of the resident staff and the engendering of trust. The shared context for social and professional interaction is already well in place when a group is as alike as possible (Kanter 1977). With growing diversity comes a change in the rules governing those interactions. There is some question, however, whether women and racial minorities have entered the field in significant enough numbers to challenge the white male idiom of surgical work (Cassell 1998, Conley 1998).

A price for being different for both women and racial minorities appears to be fewer and poorer resident/faculty interactions. Among our survey population we found many significant differences between these interactions for white males and all other race and gender groups. Program directors and attendings were significantly less likely to speak with women and non-whites than with white males about their performance. They were also significantly less likely to help non-white residents secure posts after their residency training.

However, a harmonious department group is an ideal that is rarely achieved, even in departments that are comprised exclusively of white males. The reality is that people have trouble getting along:

> ...a guy who is a bit of a loner...who isn't one of the crowd, but yet may be a really great guy. Guys like that tend to have more trouble. They don't become 'one of the boys'...they (the other residents) may use this guy as the fall guy, faulting him, and they can make his life miserable...that's one unfortunate situation where a guy falls by virtue of some circumstance beyond which he really didn't have a lot of control, but in essence he has to take ultimate responsibility because it was his own makeup which resulted in antagonizing some people...who just won't tolerate a guy who just doesn't fit in (A27).

Irrespective of race and gender, the medical faculty and the residents also acknowledge that attendings can be petty and arbitrary when evaluating residents. Personal conflicts do exist between some teachers and students:

> Ten different attendings... All of them have different superficial expectations and I am always interested in the extent to which a resident lives up to my major expectations for responsibility, maturity, things like that. They get tripped up trying to meet superficial expectations (A32).

> Then he [program director] always finds the one he can pick on. Resident X is his new one that he can pick on now. So no matter what goes wrong, it's X's fault. I mean the poor man could be on vacation and it would still be his fault (N18).

But even in an imperfect world, patients and the medical staff have to decide if they trust the medical resident. The patient must trust that he or she will have the very best care. The members of the medical staff must believe that the resident can be trusted to fulfill the doctor's fiduciary role whenever necessary. As these interview quotes illustrate, owning up to a mistake is the mark of honesty and trustworthiness in the setting of the residency program.

> I think the worst residents are dishonest... Each incident in and of itself perhaps has a plausible explanation, but it is the monotonous litany, repetition of never being on target, never quite doing what he is supposed to do, always getting a different story. I think the biggest problem with being dishonest, not only with others but with themselves, is not admitting there is stuff they don't know (A29).

> The most important thing was that you work hard, that you are honest with what you do. If you make a mistake you are honest with it. You are in a position now where you have to be honest. You're learning. I think what attendings hate the most is someone who isn't honest about their mistakes. When they're not honest about their mistakes when they are learning, they're never going to be honest about what they do. That's what scares attendings the most. (R35).

Honesty is taking full responsibility. No one expects a surgeon-in-training not to make mistakes. What is expected is the acceptance of responsibility for the mistake, and an expressed effort to learn from it. The medical staff fears that if residents do not recognize their hand in an error, they will be unable to avoid repeating it.

Do problem residents really have difficulty engendering trust, getting along with others, and accepting responsibility? Although a certain amount of cognitive intelligence and physical skill is necessary to be a surgeon, these talents were not lacking among the problem residents in our study. Less than a quarter of the residents left or were released because of a technical error or technical incompetence. Social and behavioral problems were the impetus behind three-quarters of terminations and problematic performances.

With this definition of honesty in hand, we will first look at the overall risk of attrition in surgical residency programs. Then we will explore what effect a good response to criticism, an honest owning up to mistakes, has on a resident's risk of attrition and on his or her ranking on honesty.

Risk of Attrition

From Part I of our survey, we calculated attrition rates for residents based on four race and gender categories: white males, white females, non-white males, and non-white females. Since surgery remains a professional arena dominated by white males, we had to combine both non-white foreigners and American-born racial minorities into a non-white category to make any statistical analyses meaningful. Table 2 shows the attrition risks for these groups.

Table 2:
Probability of being terminated or labeled a problematic completer by race and gender

Race/Gender		Termination	Problematic Completer
White Male	(n=682)	0.023	0.020
White Female	(n=152)	0.049	0.040
Non-white Male	(n=138)	0.201	0.095
Non-white Female	(n=43)	0.227	0.053
Total:	(n=1015)	0.034	0.023

We can see from this table that white males have the lowest risk for both termination and problematic completion. White females are 2.13 times more likely to be terminated than white males, while non-white males are 8.74 times more likely, and non-white females, 9.87 times more likely. White females are 2.48 times more likely than white males to be labeled a problematic completer, while the corresponding figures are 4.75 times for non-white males and 2.65 times for non-white females. These figures certainly suggest that race and gender matter, even if other variables are involved. How race and gender impact the type of reaction a resident gives to criticisms will be analyzed below.

Responding to Criticism

What are the rules that govern how a resident should respond to criticisms about his or her performance?[6] Some attendings we interviewed offered this advice:

> It's a military type of structure, where the guy who does his job says 'yes' but knows how to ask the right questions in a non-defiant, and sounding like a compliant way, gets brownie points. If he's reasonably good with his hands, doesn't get into trouble, treats nurses with respect, he has it made... The guy with good social, interpersonal skills...he can generate trust and have physicians want to refer cases to him (A27).

> A good response is, 'We're sorry. I don't know how that slipped by us, but you're absolutely right,' and then they go schedule a test for the patient immediately. A bad response is, 'Well, we were busy all day. Everyone was in the operating room. There was the clinic and it was such a busy clinic, just couldn't get out to see the patient. Those nurses, they never tell us when something goes wrong with the patients.' Making excuses (A34).

And the poor responders:

> A resident who is defensive is a real problem. Who, when criticized, can't understand that he isn't being attacked, but rather there is an attempt to teach, can be a problem (A19).

> Any time something went wrong, she blamed someone else, even though she was the chief resident (A25).

Our hypothesis was that residents who respond well to criticism, who accept responsibility for their poor performance when confronted by program faculty, are considered more honest than their colleagues who respond poorly. We did find a strong association between the kind of reaction residents had when criticized by their attendings and their ranking on honesty. Program directors ranked the appropriate responders above average on honesty as compared to their peers. The inappropriate responders were ranked below average. Blaming others for poor performance also reduced ranking on honesty even further.

The Benefits of a Good Reaction

Residents who are eventually terminated and those who are labeled as problematic completers are similar in many ways. They share many common perceptions of the stresses and strains of the surgical training programs, but they also differ in some important ways. Problematic completers can be said to have some redeeming qualities that are demonstrated in their response to criticism and in their own identification of the source of their troubles. The terminated resident, on the other hand, is considered unredeemable within the normal work setting. The reason for taking such a drastic measure as termination underscores the faculty's lack of faith in the resident's potential for improving his or her poor performance.

If residents who are terminated and those who problematically complete their training present many of the same problems, what factors predict whether or not a resident who is having trouble will be terminated or allowed to stay in the residency program? Employing probit analysis, we found that a good reaction significantly decreased a resident's chance of being terminated even after controlling for race, reason for poor performance, and ranking on clinical judgment. The right reaction has a redeeming effect separate from these other effects.

Who Reacts Appropriately?

Because the probit model predicting which residents will react appropriately to criticisms must use only exogenous variables, we could only use the demographic traits that the residents came with prior to residency training. This list of variables includes the residents' gender, age, race, marital status, specialty choice, and medical school. For the medical schools, we had information both on whether the resident attended a foreign medical school and a ranking (Gourman 1991) for all American medical schools. Of these, only two variables were significantly associated with the likelihood that a resident will respond appropriately to criticism: being married and being an international medical graduate (IMG).

Why would married residents be more likely to respond appropriately to criticism than unmarried residents? We offer two possible explanations, which, however, do not disentangle cause-and-effect. First, residents who are married may possess greater emotional intelligence (Goleman 1995, 1998). We are defining emotional intelligence very loosely as an ability to read and respond to a social situation in the best and expected way as defined by a particular cultural system. In this line of thinking, being married itself would be a marker of emotional intelligence. For the relationship to work, married people have to be good at getting along with others. They must know how to be in a relationship in which there is a give and take and a need to demonstrate mutual respect.

A second possibility is that married residents respond more favorably to criticism because they are more concerned with keeping their jobs. They may "say the right thing" not because they share the faculty's view of the situation, but because they are concerned about the social and financial impact that losing their post may have on their spouse and children. Married residents may feel less mobile than single residents and therefore they may be less willing to say and do things that could "rock the boat." So, the propensity to respond correctly among the married residents may have been there prior to starting residency training, or it may reflect their obligations to their families.

It also is possible that the faculty may interpret the response of the married resident through a different lens than that which they use for the single resident. If the married resident is frazzled because he or she has been up all night with an ill child, the attending may not like the resident's fatigue, but may tolerate it. The unmarried resident, however, should not come in after his or her night off fatigued and distressed, for they presumably have no other demands on their time. We have some examples from the surveys of how married residents' problems were related to their family obligations or experiences:

> A married, white male problematic completer: His response to criticism was "concerned, would try harder and spend more time... He had eight children to support. He had to moonlight and this kept him from his reading of surgery."

> Another white male problematic completer who had a major personal tragedy: Although the resident "accepted criticisms well," he "excessively assigned duties to junior residents" and "attempt[ed] to show up senior residents." He was described as a "precocious surgical pupil with a personality that tended to be arrogant." But then we quickly learn that he was "devastated by the loss of his wife who died of cancer in his third year of training." The program director "stayed with this resident because of his underlying abilities." He has by all accounts become "a successful, well-regarded practicing neurosurgeon."

These examples indicate that the marriage effect may be about both how the resident responds and the filter through which the information is received. Program directors appear to have some sympathy for residents who have significant family problems like ill children and spouses.

Undoubtedly, though, being married is a double-edged sword for the medical or surgical resident. Being married suggests that the resident has other demands on his or her time that are not part of the training program. The married resident must answer to someone who is not a colleague or patient. This is often looked upon unfavorably by the medical faculty who ideally wants the resident's total devotion, as is illustrated by the following example:

> A white female problematic completer: "Resident had three pregnancies during her training and had interrupted training due to pregnancy leave-of-absences. Her inservice scores lagged behind where she should have been because of *split loyalties* (italics added). She always rated satisfactory in CCC, but didn't meet our expectations especially in the area of didactic knowledge… She is bright and had adequate promise…but she never reached her full potential. Initially I thought she had great potential for an academic career and so did she. Pregnancy altered her career goals and I supported that change."

While being married may cause troubles, it also appears to buffer how those troubles are managed and perceived. If marriage offers some protection against termination, then the white women in our sample would be less likely to reap the benefits since they were significantly less likely to be married than any other race and gender group. We have examples of women and men struggling with troubled pre-marital relationships. Program directors showed much more tolerance for marital hardships than romantic hardships. Since white women were more likely to be in pre-marital relationships, their relationship troubles were viewed disparagingly.

Why might being an IMG be associated with the likelihood of giving an appropriate response? International medical graduates may be more willing than their American-educated colleagues to admit that they are not well prepared for the rigors of residency training. They may be more aware that they are behind in the basics, and this self-awareness may make it easier to accept fuller responsibility for poor performance. Graduates from American medical schools may feel just the opposite—that they are well prepared. Their self-confidence and accomplishments thus far may make it harder for these residents to admit holes in their medical knowledge or training. Being one step behind may have its advantages for the IMG.

The medical faculty admits some IMGs into residency programs fully aware that their training will have been less rigorous and thorough than their American counterparts. This may actually lead the medical faculty to view the problems that the foreign-trained residents have with more forgiveness than they view the same shortcomings displayed by the American graduate. Here again we note that the issue may not only be one of presentation by the resident but also of perception by the program faculty.

There also is a race effect among the IMG population. There was a preponderance of white IMGs among the pool of problematic completers (87 percent) as opposed to among the terminated residents (40 percent). Although attendance at a foreign medical school has a significant effect, being white in a white-dominated profession helps these residents know what constitutes a correct response and give it accordingly.

Although "married" and "IMG" were the only exogenous variables associated with responding appropriately, other associations provide a richer picture of how reactions are related to perceptions of residents as honest or dishonest. Good responders were significantly more likely to cite marital/family pressures as a reason for poor performance. They were also more likely to cite some self-perceived deficiency in cognitive knowledge, manual dexterity, or clinical judgment. They were significantly less likely to blame other residents or cite clashes with some faculty members to account for their poor performance. This association between how the resident responded and the reason he or she gave for poor performance directly relates to the structure and operation of the surgical culture discussed earlier. Residents who cite a self-perceived deficiency are accepting full responsibility for their actions. Those who blame others or who clash with other staff members disrupt the harmony of the program.

Although good responders did not outrank poor responders in cognitive knowledge or manual dexterity, they significantly outranked poor responders on such interpersonal traits as honesty, personality, maturity, staff relationships, and patient relationships. The resident who responds correctly to attendings displays better interpersonal skills.

Tolerating White Males' Poor Responses

In our model predicting termination we did not see a direct gender effect even though, as Table 2 indicates, white males are significantly less likely to be terminated than the other race and gender categories combined. While the race effect is prevalent in the full model, the gender effect appears to work through other variables such as clinical judgment, a trait where men have historically outperformed women (Martin et al. 1988, Good 1995:66).

A review of the reaction variable revealed another significant effect. Among the poor responders, white males were significantly less likely to be terminated. This effect held even after we controlled for overall ranking, as well as ranking on two significant variables: clinical judgment and quality of staff relationships. This finding suggests that the medical faculty members are more likely to tolerate poor responses when made by white males. Among the eighty-nine white males who responded poorly to their evaluations, only 61 percent were eventually terminated. Among the other race and gender groups, 81 percent of poor responders were eventually terminated, a significant difference.

Excerpts from the surveys give more detailed insight into the form this tolerance takes. In some of the cases, program directors appear reluctant to fire some of the white male poor responders basically because the residents were well liked:

> Resident's reaction was one of "denial" but the "academic committee refused to terminate because resident was 'such a nice guy.'
>
> Another white male responded "defensively." He was described as "technically inept, poor fund of knowledge, untruthful, tried to cover incompetence with over subservience." He was not fired because he was a "pleasant fellow but slow on the pick-up and lacked talent."

In some other cases, consensus could not be reached. Program directors also sought help for some of these white males rather than terminate them.

> Resident who reacted "defensively" and who had "poor scores" [on an in-house training exam]: was sent to "an orthopedic review course to try to help him."

Other white males were kept due to manpower shortages, or to a lack of documentation against the resident that left programs susceptible to legal action.

> Resident "did not acknowledge problem." He was "impossible to deal with." He was not terminated because program "needed him to finish, no one else in PGY4 year."

> The resident was "angry" when confronted with poor reviews of his performance. He was always "arguing with attendings, always had an excuse for everything, denied any wrongdoing when he had complications." (Why not terminate?) "All the facts were not clearly documented. Resident threatened to litigate."

Most disturbing are the cases in which the white male appears to "get away" with fairly gross misconduct with little consequence for his misdeed:

> Resident "felt I [program director] was overcritical." Problem was "patient complained of fondling during an exam."

> This resident responded "very defensively" to criticism. "Resident had poor relationship with some attendings. Antagonized other residents from other specialties. Two weeks before completion of program, he was found to have falsified medical records." He was not terminated because "major incident occurred two weeks before the end of residency."

In a few instances, program directors expressed regret for not having fired the problematically performing resident precisely because the resident encountered trouble in the form of malpractice suits or dismissal from hospitals soon after leaving the residency program.

For our female and minority residents, there were no cases where a poor responder was not dismissed because he or she was a "nice person," or cases in which help was sought for the resident in the form of some sort of counseling service. This tolerance is a significant advantage for the white male resident.

Conclusion

As our analysis shows, a good reaction goes a long way in helping the resident with problems to present him or herself as honest and redeemable. An honest resident, when confronted by claims of substandard performance, accepts responsibility for the poor performance, agreeing with the faculty's assessment of the situation. The dishonest resident blames his or her poor performance on interpersonal conflicts or on other staff members, challenging the faculty's perception of the mistake and of the source of the poor performance.

Our data show that the good responder is more likely to be a white international medical graduate, and is more likely to be married. The good responder outranks his or her colleagues on a number of interpersonal traits, including honesty, personality, maturity, and staff and patient relationships. The good responder is more likely to cite marital/family pressures and some self-perceived deficiency in cognitive knowledge, manual dexterity, and clinical judgment as a reason for poor performance, and is less likely to cite interpersonal conflicts as an excuse for poor performance.

As we hypothesized in the beginning of this analysis, knowing what constitutes a "good" response involves knowledge about the culture of surgery and what denotes an acceptable exchange. Our description of a good responder certainly shows a race effect. The white IMG residents appear to know better what constitutes a valid and acceptable explanation for poor performance than their non-white colleagues. This race effect is even stronger for white males, since we also found that poor responses are tolerated more readily when made by white male residents than when they are made by any other race and gender group. Whites in general and white males in particular have an advantage whether they responded appropriately or not.

It is also true that in order to benefit from a good response, the resident has to have some kind of contact with the medical faculty. Women and racial minorities were less likely than their white male counterparts to interact with the medical faculty. If these contacts do not happen, the benefit of a good reaction cannot be reaped.

The race and gender effects we found raise the question of whether the medical faculty's assessment of such an elusive quality as honesty is fair and just. We can agree with program directors that given the tremendous amount of privilege and responsibility that physicians have, a goodly amount of honesty is vital. We can also agree that evaluating honesty is a difficult process. We rely heavily on the quality of our interactions with people to judge their honesty, and diversity undoubtedly makes this process more challenging. The hope of the medical faculty is that if the resident accepts blame for poor performance, he or she will always be able to proactively improve performance. The acceptance of responsibility suggests that the resident will be able, now and after he or she leaves the training program, to work with different staff members, at different institutions, with incomplete medical knowledge, etc., and still find a way to get the job done.

Many of our respondents acknowledged that the ideal residency setting does not exist. Our respondents recognized that interpersonal conflicts do exist, and that negative evaluations may just be wrong. These were not rare insights, but realities recognized by many of those we interviewed. Abuse, arbitrariness, and personality contests are a part of the reality of the world of surgical residency programs. When a resident's race and gender determine the losers of these interpersonal contests, there is something very wrong about the process. Program directors are not effectively weeding out the deficient among their ranks; they are practicing discrimination. Some of the residents captured by our attrition statistics were very likely asked to leave their programs because they responded inappropriately, said the wrong thing at the wrong time, not because they were unqualified to be surgeons.

Notes

1. This paper was developed and written by Virginia Adams O'Connell, under the dissertation supervision of Charles L. Bosk and using survey and interview data collected by Bosk (see Bosk 1992). For further analysis of the theme developed here, see O'Connell 2001.
2. The authors gratefully acknowledge support from the Pew Charitable Trusts (Grant No. SNS-01) and The Committee on Resident Selection and Evaluation of the Society of Neurological Surgeons (Drs. William Collins, Julian Hoff, David Kelley, Edward Laws, Steven Mahaley, Robert Ratcheson, Richard Rovit, William Shucart, and Martin Weiss). We also wish to acknowledge the assistance of Michael Polgar and Deborah Putnam Thomas in data collection.
3. The paper was written while Dr. O'Connell was an AAUW (American Association for University Women) Dissertation Fellow; she thanks the AAUW for their support.
4. Although problematic completers are not true attrition statistics, they are an interesting category. They complete program requirements before program directors believe that these residents can practice without supervision. They represent an interesting category of "problem" physicians.
5. In 1990, a two-part survey was sent to the program directors of 767 accredited U.S. residency programs in five different specialties: anesthesiology, general surgery, neurosurgery, orthopedic surgery, and plastic surgery. Five-hundred and fifty-six (73 percent) surveys were returned. A second survey, sent to the 410 of the 556 who had experienced attrition, collected information on the residents in these programs who had resigned, been terminated, or who had problematically completed training. From this second mailing, 290 (71 percent) of the 410 were returned. In addition to the surveys, interviews were conducted with 75 attendings, residents, and nurses from five different neurosurgery programs. The information reported in this paper draws primarily on these interviews and on the experiences of 287 terminated residents and 209 problematic completers. Citations from interviews are coded in the following fashion: Each respondent's position is designated by a capital letter. A=attending, R=resident, and N=nurse. The numbering following was randomly assigned. All other quotes are drawn from program directors' responses on the surveys.
6. The response program directors gave to the survey question, "How did residents respond to criticism?" were often brief qualitative descriptions that we coded as a dummy variable. Responses were coded as honest/appropriate, or as dishonest/

inappropriate. Examples of appropriate responses included "acknowledged problem," "expressed a desire to do better," and "with efforts to do better and study harder." We categorized statements such as "denied problem," "defensive, hostile," and "always had an excuse," as inappropriate responses. We had information on residents' reactions for 69 percent of our problematic completers and 44 percent of our terminated residents.

References

Bosk, Charles L. 1979. *Forgive and Remember.* Chicago: University of Chicago Press.

Bosk, Charles L. 1992. "Summary of Progress Report to the Pew Charitable Trusts, Grant No. SNS-01 to the Society of Neurological Surgeons."

Cassell, Joan. 1998. *The Woman in the Surgeon's Body*. Cambridge: Harvard University Press.

Conley, Frances K. 1998. *Walking Out on the Boys*. New York: Farrar, Straus and Giroux.

Glantz, Leonard H. 1985. "Becoming a Lawyer: Education and Socialization," in *Social Controls and the Medical Profession*, edited by Judith P. Swazey and Stephen R. Scher. Boston: Oelgeschlager, Gunn and Hain.

Goleman, Daniel. 1995. *Emotional Intelligence*. New York:Bantam Books.

Goleman, Daniel. 1998. *Working with Emotional Intelligence*. New York: Bantam Books.

Good, Mary-Jo DelVecchio. 1995. *American Medicine: The Quest for Competence*. Berkeley: University of California Press.

Gourman, J. 1991. *The Gourman Report: Undergraduate and Professional Programs in America and International Universities*. Princeton, NJ: Princeton Review.

Kanter, R. M. 1977. *Men and Women of the Corporation*. New York: Basic Books.

Martin, S.C., R. M. Arnold and R. M. Parker. 1988. "Gender and Medical Socialization." *Journal of Health and Social Behavior* 29 (December):333-343.

O'Connell, Virginia Adams. 2001. "Attrition in Surgical Residency Programs," Doctoral Dissertation (draft), Department of Sociology, University of Pennsylvania, July.

Parmer, Michael A. 1982. "Ethics of a Professional Surgeon." *American College of Surgeons Bulletin* (July):2-5.

Parsons, T. 1951. *The Social System*. Glencoe, IL: Free Press.

Steinhauer, J. 1999. "For Women in Medicine, A Road to Compromise, Not Perks." *The New York Times* (March 1).

Weitz, Rose. 1996. *The Sociology of Health, Illness and Health Care: A Critical Approach*. Wadsworth Publishing.

Zerubavel, Evitar. 1979. *Patterns of Time in Hospital Life*. Chicago: The University of Chicago Press.

9

On the Sociological Anxiety of Physicians

Nicholas A. Christakis

Physicians do not speak calmly about prognosis.[1] Indeed, they seem quite anxious about the possibility or necessity of both formulating and communicating predictions about or to their patients. This observation about prognostication begs a more general inquiry into the response of individual physicians, and the profession as a whole, regarding potentially unpleasant sides of medical practice, and, more broadly, into the sources of doctors' anxiety. What is the nature and origin of this anxiety and what does it mean for our understanding of medical care?

Part of the reason physicians are anxious when it comes to prognosis is that, when prognosis emerges as a focus of interest in a clinical encounter, there typically are also other elements of the encounter that are anxiety provoking. That is, prognosis often emerges in medical care in a setting in which other potentially noxious and worrisome stimuli are present—such as death or uncertainty. Such co-occurrence strongly suggests that we are dealing with a social pattern of the type that sociologist Renée Fox has so frequently identified in medicine. Moreover, the stylized responses to prognosis in medicine, and the cathexis of prognosis with these other concerns, suggest that the anxiety regarding prognosis (and regarding the other issues we will be considering) is *sociological* rather than *personal* in nature. Psychiatrist Rollo May draws a distinction between fear and anxiety by arguing that "anxiety is a *diffuse* apprehension, and...the central difference between fear and anxiety is that fear is a reaction to a specific danger while anxiety is unspecific, 'vague,' 'objectless.' The special characteristics of anxiety are the feelings of *uncertainty* and *helplessness* in the face of danger. The nature of anxiety can be understood when we ask *what* is threatened in the experience that produces anxiety" (May 1977:205).[2] And he proceeds to define anxiety as "the apprehension cued off by a threat to some value that the individual holds essential to his existence as a personality [and to his security]." In normal, non-pathological anxiety, the threat arises from an attack upon the foundation of one's security, and the threatened individual cannot "stand outside the threat" and objectify it, and therefore cannot marginalize or trivialize or compartmentalize or demarcate the threat. The threat is fundamental and somehow transcendent or thoroughgoing. One is afraid, one knows it is serious, but one may not be aware of exactly what one is afraid of. Most generally, it seems that anxiety can arise from a realization of human contingency, that is, a realization of human vulnerability to the powers of Nature, for example, to illness or to death. These initial—basically psychological—ideas, expressed about fifty years ago, take us a certain distance, but only so far, in understanding physician anxiety—for reasons I will touch on shortly.

A case drawn from my book on prognosis, *Death Foretold*, can serve to illustrate some of the various reasons that doctors might be anxious, and the kind of threat to their sociological existence and security we are considering here. One young pulmonologist described his intense experience caring for a critically ill patient as follows:

* * *

One of the hardest cases I ever took care of was when I was an intern in the CCU [Cardiac Care Unit]. There was this guy who came in because he had some mid-epigastric burning. Turned out he had a gastric carcinoma. This was all as an outpatient. And they wanted to bring him in for a resection for his carcinoma. But he was an elderly guy, and there was a concern that he had angina, so they wanted to perform a cardiac catheterization to make sure that he could survive his gastric resection. So they catheterized his heart. On the cardiac cath table, he had a ventricular tachycardia. He then had a heart attack. They brought him to the CCU. He eventually went to open heart surgery. He had a heart attack after his surgery. He was on a ventilator. Had pneumonia, lung failure, and renal failure. And actually, they had given him a medicine he was allergic to, and so he had bone marrow failure as well!

So here was a very healthy—healthy, really—functional man in his middle seventies who—it's unbelievable isn't it?—who had the most minimal of symptoms which brought him to immediate attention as having a small, even curable, gastric carcinoma. And he goes through these amazing machinations of our medical facility, and ends up with multi-system failure. Now, his gastric carcinoma is the *least* of his worries. He's on a ventilator and has a heart that doesn't work, kidneys that don't work, and he's in bone marrow failure, and his lungs are shot. It's incredible!

So he's got four-system failure. He's going to die. There is no way he can live. And yet, I took care of him really from the first day I came to the CCU to the day I left about a month later. I think he died on the second-to-last day before I left the unit. So the entire time I took care of him, I began to...I began to hate him. This is the only patient I've ever had that I've ever truly hated. And it was because he wanted to live so badly. Every day I had to take blood from him...new arterial lines, new central lines, feverish all the time, everything had to always be changed... He was blowing up like a balloon from poor nutrition. Edema everywhere. I would have to go in with a needle more than an inch just to hit a vein or an artery. You know, he would weep from his wound every time I would do it. I was clearly hurting him with everything I did. And it showed on his face. But he was *alive*. And, despite all these problems, which should have killed anyone else in just a few days, he lived an entire month. And I had to really hurt him day after day after day after day. And I wanted to quit weeks before he died.

But my superiors—who didn't have to go in with him every day and work with him—would not let me. Basically they told me that I "had to go culture him for infection," or "he needs a new [intra-vascular] line." They're not the ones that have to do it. I'm the one that has to do it. And even despite my discussions with the family—and I think I was as capable of telling them his prognosis, even as a beginning physician, as anyone else—clearly he was not going to live. But the family was always optimistic because the attending physician always said every day that he was still alive. And the family hung on to that, like that was it. That was all they knew: that every day he was alive. And "when was he going to be able to come home?" Not "*could* he ever" but "*when*." And I couldn't understand: they couldn't see it. And so I had to hurt this guy every day.

Finally, they all saw that he wasn't getting any better. And they agreed to make him DNR and not to resuscitate him if he should have a final event. And the day they decided that, that very night he died!And the next day, the family came in to see him. He had died early in the morning. And they came in that morning to see him, and they saw me there, and I told them how very sorry I was. And they were furious...with me! And his daughter told me that she hated physicians, that she hated me, and that she had a young boy who wanted to be a physician, and she would *never* let him. Never let him be a doctor—because of what we did to her father.

I think that was the hardest case...you know, I predicted...I knew he would die. It was remarkable that he...I never expected that he would die the day that they decided to make him DNR. And the patient didn't even know that we had made him DNR.

I can't believe that he carried on like this for a whole month. And yet he died the day his family and we made him a DNR. Even though he did not know that they had done that. Here he is, in this very controlled environment, and the attending is telling them, the family, every day that the patient is alive another day. And all of a sudden we decide that it is hopeless, that he's not getting any better, let's just not push on any further—not *withdraw* life support, mind you, just not push any further—and that day he dies. The day that I don't have to put the defibrillator on him and resuscitate him if necessary, he dies. (Christakis 1999:147-148)

* * *

This case offers a number of insights about several aspects of medical practice. It is clearly relevant to the role of prognosis and it involves a considerable amount of iatrogenesis. Moreover, in a self-fulfilling-prophecy-like fashion, there is the feeling at the end of this case that when the physicians ultimately predicted that the patient would die—when they decided that the case was "hopeless"—they somehow contributed to the patient's death. In other words, just as the physicians' therapeutic interventions iatrogenically hastened the patient's death in this case, there is the sense that the physicians' prognostic pronouncements iatrogenically did the same. This case illustrates the frightening and awesome power of medical care to both keep the otherwise dead patient from dying and to make the otherwise well patient nearly dead. In the face of this power of medical care, it is not surprising that the physician is anxious about, and troubled by, the possibility that his prognostic assessments might have similarly untoward and powerful effects, might run amok just like the diagnostic and therapeutic interventions. Moreover, the experience of caring for this patient—including the foreknowledge that he would die (acquired early in the patient's care), the prognostic estimate that the care was "hopeless" (stated late in the patient's care), and the evocation of "hatred" in several parties (a rather strong word and sentiment)—was very profound for this physician. The physician was anxious and troubled by his painful and ineffective therapeutic interventions, by his ominous foreknowledge, by the proximity of death, and by his and the family's feelings.

The objects (in May's sense of the word) that I think make doctors anxious are: 1) death, 2) uncertainty, 3) helplessness, 4) the future (and its prediction), 5) emotions (such as affection for or hatred of patients or by patients), and 6) iatrogenesis (including medical error).

However, when I say that physicians are anxious about these things, I do not mean merely in a *personal* way, the way any human being might be anxious about some of these occurrences or issues, such as death or uncertainty or helplessness. I mean something more, in that the anxiety here is not merely personal, but also social—much in the way that Renée Fox has characterized other aspects of the predicament of health professionals (Fox 1988,b,d,e). That is, when I state that the doctor is anxious about death, I do not so much mean death as it might affect them personally, but rather about death as an object that impinges on their patients or their practice, an event that affects their professional or social role as a physician and to which this role is unavoidably or inescapably oriented.[3]

Technical advances and discoveries in medicine, especially since the turn of the century, have held such promise that society has endowed physicians with the privilege and the duty to eradicate disease.[4] From this perspective, death or uncertainty or iatrogenesis connote failure—not just of the therapeutic armamentarium to achieve its objective, but also of the physician to fulfill his or her social role. Indeed, when physicians speak of the death of their patients, they often use expressions which suggest rectifiability—such as "we lost the patient"—or which suggest a failing on the part of the patient—such as "that patient died on me." Physicians' dispositions and behaviors (such as ritualized prognostic optimism) and institutional practices (such as rapid sequestration of dead bodies in hospitals) serve to protect them from being identified with the failure to fulfill their role.[5]

Beyond the compunction to fulfill one's social role, powerful emotional and intellectual strands within the professional culture of medicine also lie at the core of the anxiety regarding death. Optimism, activism, meliorism, and a hubris-ridden, "against-the-odds," "we-shall-overcome" attitude is endemic in physicians. Describing physicians' attitudes towards death, Fox has observed:

> The Judeo-Christian tradition [in America] emphasizes that, because human life is divinely given, it is inherently sacred and important, has absolute, inestimable worth and meaning, and should be protected and sustained.... [But] in recent years, the unqualified commandment to support and sustain life has become increasingly problematic in American society, particularly in the medical sector. The sanctity of life ethic has helped to push physicians, nurses, and other medical professionals into a pugilistic

> tendency to combat death at any cost, and to define its occurrence as a personal and professional defeat. This heroically aggressive "courage to fail" stance has been reinforced by the development of more powerfully effective forms of medical technology that increase the medical team's ability to save and maintain life. (Fox 1988a:429-430)

In the face of such rising expectations, it seems only natural that the profession would be anxious.

Similarly, the role of physician requires the confrontation not only with death, but also with other possibly anxiety-provoking phenomena, such as uncertainty. Indeed, in the foregoing case as more generally, prognostication instantiates a particularly acute kind of uncertainty that transcends the classic types described by Fox (1988e).[6] A fundamental uncertainty arises in prognostication from the mere fact that knowledge of the future is *irremediably* provisional. Uncertainty about the future results both from a personal ignorance that is unavoidable and from a limitation in medical knowledge that can never be fully remedied. The limitations in ability to predict future events and their timing is a particularly thorny form of uncertainty, especially since, paradoxically, situations in medicine with high unpredictability both demand and subvert efforts by physicians to render prognoses.[7] However, the key observation for present purposes is that uncertainty, whether arising from prognostication or the more customary sources, is an inherent part of medical care that physicians cannot avoid much as they might want to.

In short, physicians have sociological anxiety because they are structurally confronted with danger and threats to their social duty. They cannot escape some of the problems we have discussed since these problems (death, uncertainty, emotions, prediction, etc.) are inherent in their social roles. Yet, these dangers threaten physicians' social roles, and this is what I mean by sociological anxiety. Doctors are supposed to like their patients and be liked by them, they are supposed to know things, be certain, be effective, see into the future, cure disease, and forestall death. Doctors' failure to meet these objectives, or even the risk of failure involved in facing these challenges, threatens to make their practice *meaningless*, by rendering actions harmful, therapy ineffective, the future inscrutable, patients rageful, or experience amoral. To paraphrase sociologist Robert Merton in his discussion of sociological ambivalence: unlike a psychological perspective on anxiety, a sociological one focuses on the ways in which the anxiety comes to be built into the structure of social roles. A sociological perspective draws attention to the processes in the social structure that foster anxiety in particular kinds of role-relations. And a sociological perspective also draws attention to the social consequences of anxiety for the workings of social structures (Merton and Barber 1976:5).

All of these observations, of course, borrow heavily from Renée Fox's path-finding work in medical sociology. She has examined in numerous places the distinctive and socially structured experiences of patients and doctors in the context of illness, as well as the stresses, anxieties, and coping responses that these experiences have engendered. Whether we are thinking of patients on Ward F-2, or medical students in the dissecting room, or physicians being socialized to cope with uncertainty or to manifest "detached concern," or transplant surgeons demonstrating a "courage to fail" ethos, in all of these cases we are confronted with how such socially-situated actors are responding to stressful, anxiety-provoking situations in which they must confront death and attempt something that might well both be impossible and absolutely imperative. Moreover, her work has called attention to the melding of the personal and social and moral experience of such actors, and it sets the framework for finding analogous processes at work at both individual and social levels. The sources of physicians' anxiety have moral overtones because they are connected to a possible failure to fulfill their social role, which, consequently, suggests a possible delict or culpability on the part of the physician and of the profession.

Fox has thus been profoundly concerned with not only the determinants of social processes, but also with their personal, social, and moral consequences. This begs the question of what the beneficial and harmful consequences of this sociological anxiety in physicians might be. But she has had something to say about this too, in her work on how physicians confront death, uncertainty, and the potentially dehumanizing threat of illness.

At an individual level, anxiety can certainly be useful. For example, the anxiety medical students feel about their training and competence can motivate them to study and work harder. The confrontation of their mixed feelings about examining the human body can serve to bolster their ability to deal with its decrepitude, which is such a necessary part of their profession. Like its individual counterpart, sociological anxiety, in moderation, can enhance performance. That is, a certain amount of sociological anxiety may help to keep the medical profession in balance, fulfilling its role adequately. For example, the "courage to fail" ethos that Fox and Judith Swazey identified in the area of organ transplantation can be seen as productive (Fox and Swazey 1978). Similarly, the argument that Fox makes in her classic work on "training for detached concern" is also an institutionalized way that members of the profession are systematically socialized to cope with the structural, anxiety-provoking aspects of their profession. These responses attempt to balance the personal and professional risks and benefits of avoiding anxiety-provoking objects.On the other hand, if the challenges of the circumstances become overwhelming, physicians may avoid the object. This is one of the reasons that physicians avoid prognosis: high expectations for prognosis, coupled with the manifest difficulty in meeting them, make physicians structurally anxious and, consequently, lead away from engagement with this domain. Similar arguments can be made about the other sources of anxiety. In excess, therefore, anxiety can lead to blind spots in a profession and a kind of institutionalized denial that, in the long run, is not merely counterproductive but also intrinsically unstable. A profession that inescapably faces death and so many other threats cannot avoid them completely.

Notes

1. I attempt to get to the root of this anxiety and to understand the thoughts and behaviors that the necessity of prognostication engenders in Christakis 1999. This book grew from a dissertation I did under Renée Fox's supervision at the University of Pennsylvania from 1991 to 1995.
2. Emphasis in original. By "objectless," May does not mean that the anxiety lacks a stimulus or trigger. Similarly, when I argue that physicians are anxious about something, I do not mean that the cue to the anxiety is unknown (e.g., it might be death), but rather that there is an additional aspect to the anxiety-provoking object that threatens the social nature of physicians' existence and that is often, at least initially, not manifest.
3. This is analogous to the difference that sociologist Robert Merton has drawn between a personal, psychological ambivalence on the one hand, and a sociological ambivalence on the other (Merton and Barber 1976, Merton 1976).
4. For more on the status gradually assumed by the medical profession, see Starr 1982.
5. It reflects both irony and arrogance that physicians feel guilt when their patients die—irony because they are not (ordinarily) truly responsible for the patient's death and arrogance because they believe that they are so powerful that they might have prevented it (see Christakis 1996). Regarding the "ritualization of optimism" in prognosis, see Christakis 1999.

6. Uncertainty in medicine has been classically described by Fox as having three principal sources: "The first results from incomplete or imperfect mastery of available knowledge. No one can have at his command all skills and all knowledge of the lore of medicine. The second depends on limitations in current medical knowledge. There are innumerable questions to which no physician, however well trained, can as yet provide answers. A third source...derives from the first two. This consists of difficulty in distinguishing between personal ignorance or ineptitude and the limitations of present medical knowledge" (Fox 1988e:20; see also Fox 1988c).
7. The situation is not so simple, of course, because, as I discuss in *Death Foretold*, formulating a prognosis may be a way for physicians to cope with the uncertainty in medicine. Making a prediction can make physicians feel as if they have some rational understanding, and therefore control, over a patient's disease. The uncertainty associated with serious, life-threatening diseases is both unsettling and threatening to physicians, and they thus welcome situations where they can cope with it through prognostication. The ability to prognosticate can provide reassurance. Similarly, prognostic *certainty* can, paradoxically, also be problematic for physicians. Certain knowledge of an unfavorable future can be perceived as a burden. See also Fox 2000.

References

Christakis, Nicholas A. 1999. *Death Foretold: Prophecy and Prognosis in Medical Care.* Chicago: University of Chicago Press.

Christakis, Nicholas A.1996. "Managing Death: The Growing Acceptance of Euthanasia in Contemporary American Society," pp. 15-44 in *Must We Suffer Our Way to Death? Cultural and Theological Perspectives on Death by Choice*, edited by R. P. Hamel and E. R. DuBose. Dallas, TX: Southern Methodist University Press.

Fox, Renée C. 1988a. "Advanced Medical Technology—Social and Ethical Implications," pp. 413-461 in *Essays in Medical Sociology*, edited by R. C. Fox. New Brunswick, NJ: Transaction Publishers.

Fox, Renée C. 1988b. "The Autopsy: Its Place in the Attitude-Learning of Second-Year Medical Students," pp. 51-77 in *Essays in Medical Sociology: Journeys into the Field*, edited by R. C. Fox. New Brunswick, N.J.: Transaction Publishers.

Fox, Renée C. 1988c. "The Evolution of Medical Uncertainty," pp. 533-571 in *Essays in Medical Sociology: Journeys into the Field*, edited by R. C. Fox. New Brunswick, N.J.: Transaction Publishers.

Fox, Renée C. 1988d. "The Human Condition of Health Professionals," pp. 572-587 in *Essays in Medical Sociology: Journeys into the Field*, edited by R. C. Fox. New Brunswick, N.J.: Transaction Publishers.

Fox, Renée C. 2000. "Medical Uncertainty Revisited," pp. 409-425 in *Handbook of Social Studies in Health and Medicine*, edited by G. L. Albrecht, R. Fitzpatrick, and S. C. Scrimshaw. London: Sage.

Fox, Renée C. 1988e. "Training for Uncertainty," pp. 19-50 in *Essays in Medical Sociology: Journeys into the Field*, edited by R. C. Fox. New Brunswick, N.J.: Transaction Publishers.

Fox, Renée C., and Judith P. Swazey. 1978. *The Courage to Fail. A Social View of Organ Transplants and Dialysis.* 2d ed., rev. Chicago: University of Chicago Press.

May, Rollo. 1977. *The Meaning of Anxiety*. Rev. ed., New York: Norton.

Merton, Robert. K. 1976. "The Ambivalence of Physicians," pp. 65-72 in *Sociological Ambivalence and Other Essays*, edited by R. K. Merton. New York: The Free Press.

Merton, Robert K., and Elinor Barber. 1976. "Sociological Ambivalence," pp. 3-31 in *Sociological Ambivalence and Other Essays*, edited by R. K. Merton. New York: The Free Press.

Starr, Paul. 1982. *The Social Tranformation of American Medicine*, New York: Basic Books.

10

The Transplant Surgeon, the Sociologist, and the Historian: A Conversation with Thomas E. Starzl

Renée C. Fox

It was a conversation that I had hoped to have some day with transplant surgeon Thomas E. Starzl—one that would explore the three decades-long relationship that medical historian Judith P. Swazey and I have developed with him over the course of our collaborative first-hand research on organ transplantation. This unusual triad, formed by a surgeon, a sociologist, and a historian, is integrally connected to our mutual sense of the more-than-biomedical significance of organ transplantation. Based primarily on the intermittent field research visits that Judith and I have made to Thomas Starzl at the University of Colorado and the University of Pittsburgh medical centers—the chief settings where his lifetime of pioneering clinical, technical, and scientific contributions to the field of transplantation have taken place[1]—the dynamic center of the relationship has turned around the questions that we have raised in our interviews with Tom, and in our publications (that he has assiduously read) about the "courage to fail"/"spare parts" ardor with which this form of organ replacement has been pursued, its therapeutic justification, its accomplishments, and its unintended harmful side-effects (Fox and Swazey 1974, 1992). Rather than being alienated by these questions, or defensive about them, he has consistently welcomed the opportunity to candidly discuss them with us. His responsiveness went beyond the intellectual importance that he clearly attached to pondering the social and moral quandaries that the evolution and deployment of transplantation have posed. Despite his sense of mission about organ transplantation—or perhaps because of it—these were matters with which Tom appeared to be continually wrestling, in an acutely personal and often angst-ridden way. His at-once ebullient, thoughtful, and pained reflections, along with the opportunities that he afforded us to observe him in the midst of his daily professional round, and our close, between-the-lines reading of the connotations of his evocative medical writing, have given Judith and myself a view of Thomas Starzl that is more intricate, and also more compelling, than the unbridled picture of him conveyed to us by some members of the transplant community.

The chance that I had sought to make explicit what had long been implicit in this relationship occurred on December 5, 2000, when Tom traveled to Philadelphia expressly to be interviewed by me about it. The trip was both a sequel and a supplement to the symposium that was held to mark my becoming an emeritus professor. Starzl had reluctantly declined an invitation to give a paper at the symposium because of his prior commitment to participate in an international congress on transplantation in Turkey. But he flew from Turkey to Philadelphia, with only a brief stopover in Pittsburgh, to be present at the celebratory symposium dinner. Following this occasion, when he agreed to schedule a conversation about what I termed "the transplant surgeon, the sociologist, and the historian," it was with the understanding that in lieu of a paper, it might contain the ingredients for a contribution to this volume.[2] I anticipated that the talk would reveal lesser-known facets of this illustrious transplant surgeon, with deep relevance to the unifying theme of the colloquium and book: the social, moral, and spiritual dimensions of medicine. In addition, I hoped that it would provide intimate insights into the content and import of a profound, long-term relationship rooted in the kind of ethnographic research underlying many of the colloquium presentations.

Our conversation began with reminiscences about our first meeting in Denver in Starzl's office at the Veterans Administration Hospital where he was then chief of surgery. Judith and I had come to see him, I recalled, because of his renown in the clinical history of kidney transplantation and of immunosuppressive therapy to manage the rejection reaction that transplanted organs trigger in recipients, and because of his path-making role in the surgical and biomedical development of liver transplantation. We had no preconceptions about the kind of man he was, but in studying his publications, we had been struck by the fact that he was an uncommonly good writer—somebody who was not just a wordsmith, but an author with sufficient literary skill to imbue his publications with meaning that was not confined to the narrowly technical aspects of organ transplantation, without undermining their scientific rigor. We did not know at this juncture that he had "ink in his veins," as the son of the editor-owner of a newspaper in his hometown, Le Mars, Iowa, on which Starzl had worked, and the nephew of a general manager of the Associated Press. Our most vivid memories of this meeting were the large photographs of snow-capped mountains that hung on the walls of his otherwise spartan office; his pensive remarks about the city-borne smog that was polluting the vista of Rocky Mountain peaks visible through his office windows; and the visit that he insisted we make with him to see one of his favorite pigs, whose liver graft seemed to be surviving indefinitely without immunosuppressive drugs, and who had consequently become a sort of transplant mascot.

The photographs were taken by one of his sons, Tom said, and the laboratory technician who had accompanied them on the endurance trips they had made in the mountains, and on their 2000-mile bicycle trip above the Arctic Circle down to Helsinki. The environmental pollution in Denver had gotten worse, he lamented—adding that he had truly meant what he said when he told us that he considered dealing with environmental problems to be more crucial than involvement in transplantation. My invocation of our "call" on the prized pig brought forth a colorful initial response from Starzl about the group of randomly matched outbred pigs to which this particular animal belonged, and on whom he and his colleagues had performed experimental orthotopic liver allografts. A few of those pigs who spontaneously accepted their transplants and never required any immunosuppressive therapy "grew to be horrendous in size," he exclaimed. "They started out small, but some of those pigs got to be a couple of thousand pounds!" Despite the clear demonstration in pigs, and subsequently in certain rat and mice strains, of what Starzl termed "the relative immunologic privilege of the liver"—its greater "biological easiness" in this respect than the kidney or the heart—he reminded me that from a technical point of view, the liver was surgically more difficult to transplant than virtually any other solid organ. He did not go on with this train of thought, but I silently recalled that the first five attempts he made between March and October 1963 to perform liver transplants on patients with end-stage liver disease resulted in their rapid deaths after no more than 0 to 23 days. This led him to call a three-and-a-half year-long self-imposed moratorium on further attempts at human liver transplants until he felt that he had made sufficient progress in surgical technique, organ preservation, and metabolism, and that more efficacious immunosuppressive treatment strategies existed.

Tom interrupted our pursuit of this topic by saying that he would like to move "in a different direction," and "try probing the discussions that we've had"—discussions he alleged, with a mixture of seriousness and mischievousness, that he "treasured" because "most of the time...we disagreed.... But never in a way that would arouse the slightest anger [he added]. These were, I thought, very productive exchanges," he continued, because "in a clean way...a hygienic way [that] took away the passion, they allow[ed] some thoughtful consideration of somebody else's point of view...an opposite point of view.... I think that's even more important to me in retrospect than it was at the time...for a very good reason.... I feel that we—but especially I—was very, very lucky in the way that the whole story [of clinical organ transplantation] played out."

Here Starzl proceeded to give what he termed his "assessment of things" at the inception of the clinical history of transplantation:

> At the beginning, it looked as [though] transplantation, if it were going to succeed, had to violate some very hardcore biologic laws, and to erode some qualities of biologic defense that were absolutely essential for people who live in a hostile environment. It had to weaken the immune system. So in order to do that, you had to make your patients subject to tuberculosis, malaria, right across the line. You had to expose them to a much higher incidence of malignancies, but more than anything else, you had to erode their quality of life to the point that if you were in the position of that patient, sitting there with the moon-face and the buffalo hump, and striates as if they had been pregnant nineteen times—if you had to go through that, broken hips and crumbling bone—you probably wouldn't have done it yourself. So the only way you could justify what you were doing at that particular point is the grim determination to never emphasize triumphs, but always to emphasize deficiencies. Then to devote your efforts to improve things. That's what I did, never knowing at the end of the day, or the end of the decade, or the end of the third of the century, whether what you were striving for was actually going to be anything resembling what you'd hoped it would be. And you were that little voice of conscience that would not let anyone forget that....I think in a very real way you were asking, right from the beginning, whether what was being pawned off as treatment might, in a very real sense, be a disease in and of itself. In other words, if the treatment were so morbid, so uncertain, so emotionally destructive, and fundamentally so unbiologic that the game was not worth the candle, that the penalties exceeded the gains.... [T]hat

> questioning was always there, although it was pretty covert in your first book [*The Courage to Fail*], but it was naked in your second book [*Spare Parts*]. And it's a legitimate question because what you were laying out in your writings, actually if it hadn't occurred to *someone* in the darkest moments of night who was doing these things, then they were not exhibiting any insight.

"But," I commented, "although many of your colleagues saw you as being fervently and relentlessly committed to transplantation, you didn't need two social scientists to come along in order to have such questions occur to you in the middle of the night." Tom agreed, but he persisted in affirming that the questions we raised were "important and truthful," and that "the point of our lengthy professional relationship [was that he] understood very well that [our] points were well taken, and that the only thing that could possibly override your concerns was that if at the end of the line things could be made right...the suffering that was being seen in those early cases."

"We always felt that you were deeply attuned to that suffering, and that you suffered, too," I ventured to say. "Absolutely," Starzl responded. "It was life-destroying." "What do you mean by life-destroying?" I asked.

> First of all, it precluded a normal life for me [he replied]. I think I probably would have been almost the prototype of somebody who would have lived a pretty normal middle-class life.... But...after we had done the first kidney, we already realized certain things that hadn't been observed before. First, that you could easily reverse rejection, which had been thought to be one of biology's most inexorable reactions. Secondly, we had a patient, this young African-American boy, who had spent four weeks in the operating room.... That boy was going to go back to school only six or seven weeks post-operative. We already knew that the fat was in the fire.... I went out to dinner—my wife, a senior colleague [who was] chairman of the department out there [Colorado], and his wife—and we agreed that we had, by accident, grabbed a tiger by the tail, and there would be no way to let loose. We would either hang on until we could finally climb up and ride the brute, or else we would be destroyed in the process. [T]hat's an important point. I think that once you do something as bold as what we had done with the kidneys, and then particularly by violating the extra-renal organ barrier with liver transplantation...you either succeed, or you're destroyed by it because it was just too draconian a thing to have done.

"Is it sort of like climbing mountains?" I asked. "Yes, I think it's a little bit like [that]," he answered. "If you climb up so high on a mountain by a pathway that is impossible to retreat on, then the only way to get over is to go all the way to the top and find a way down on the other side." A formidable audacity was involved not only in "figur[ing] out how to transplant organs," and in "taking out an unpaired organ" [the liver] but, above all, in "[breaking] down a barrier that superseded the scientific limits." The impact of liver transplantation, he told me, was listed as the 213th event in a book called *The Thousand Milestones of the Last Millennium*.

Although the Thomas Starzl whom Judith Swazey and I had come to know over time was continually trying to "scale the highest peaks," he struck us as a haunted climber—someone whose seemingly dauntless, public displays of pushing limits were privately accompanied by pensiveness, a sense of tragedy, a fear of failing and harming his gravely ill patients, anxiety about adversely affecting the careers of younger colleagues, and something akin to remorse about all the animals he had injured and "sacrificed" in the laboratory in the course of conducting experiments on them. I broached these matters by alluding to the fact that we had always felt his questing and striving were connected to something larger than personal ambition, and to bigger questions of meaning with which he had struggled throughout his life. This appeared to be borne out, I commented, by *The Puzzle People*, his autobiographical "memoirs of a transplant surgeon" (1992).

Starzl admitted that he had "always felt that if [he] wasn't very careful, there were wolves just outside the campfire, wolves of melancholy that were ready to pounce. I had a lot of sad things happen in my life," he continued, "but I was able to get through them because there was a refuge, and the refuge was simply to work." "Work was more than work, then," I remarked. "It was more than work," he agreed. "It was solace.... It had to be not just small work...not just learning more and more about less and less.... It had to be some big problem.... [G]etting some big vision was what it was all about."

Nonetheless, he insisted, "I wasn't very ambitious actually. Strangely enough, I never wanted to be a chairman. It was imposed on me! In fact, I fought it for a while." "I became chair of the Sociology Department at the University of Pennsylvania at the same time that you assumed the chairmanship of the Department of Surgery at the University of Colorado," I recalled, "and I remember your saying that my heading a small liberal arts department of some thirty faculty members was comparable to the administrative magnitude and complexity of the much larger assignment that you took on. That greatly flattered and also amused me," I said. "But you lasted vastly longer [in the job] than I did!" he laughingly retorted. "I didn't like being a chairman," he stated vehemently. It "has some very bad obligations. You have to make decisions that influence" and can "destroy... a person's life"—for example, in a surgical training program, "the decision that somebody can't do the job.... So, I never was able to fire anybody. I never fired anybody in my whole life!"

"With that kind of sensitivity and dread," I asked him, "how did you ever manage to pick up a surgical instrument and cut into anybody?" "Oh, I didn't really like to operate," he said frankly. Starzl stopped performing active surgery in 1990, when he reached the age of sixty-five. It was not until then, that he was able to discuss openly his "torment[ing] anxieties" about operating, making mistakes, and "failing the patients who had placed their health or life in my hands"—anxieties that were not "relieved by each new layer of skill or experience," as he wrote in *The Puzzle People*, but that "grew worse":

> [I]nstead of blotting out the failures, I remembered them forever. With growing concern, I came to believe that I was not emotionally equipped to be a surgeon or to deal with its brutality. The incongruity was that I did not like doing the one thing for which I had become uniquely qualified. It was as if I had trained all of my life to become a violin virtuoso, only to discover that I loathed giving concerts or even playing privately. (1993:59-60)

If he were starting anew, Tom told me, he was not sure that he would re-become a surgeon. And as for the dogs he used in the laboratory research—"I couldn't do it again! I could *not* do it again! In fact, I haven't been able to do any experimental work on dogs for more than twenty years, because more and more they become dear objects." Ophelia, an abused and abandoned dog that Starzl and his wife rescued from the streets, has become an especially dear part of their lives. "Maybe by being so attached to this dog," he mused, "I was doing some penance for the dogs on which I did laboratory research."

"You not only stopped doing experimental procedures on dogs," I commented, "but in your clinical practice, you called a permanent moratorium on transplanting kidneys from living donors." Yes, "I stopped doing live donors," he confirmed, "and that was something you were not critical of," he remarked. "On the contrary, we were appreciative of it," I said. The possibilities of donor coercion made the concept of living donation seem less acceptable to him as the years went on, Tom explained. "Under [the] Judeo-Christian circumstances that we live in, the whole question of whether you can give informed consent is really an open one.... Where self-sacrifice is such a part of our moral code, [if] you go to somebody and say, 'Here, your brother needs a kidney. Will you give it to him?' how can you say no? And if you do, then you'll be ostracized" [by the family]. "What about the problem of the surgeon deliberately doing harm to live donors and their bodies by removing vital organs from them to help recipients?" I queried. If you could have "complete assurance that you weren't going to cause harm," he answered, along with "complete assurance that you could get [uncoerced] informed consent," it would be "acceptable." "But real harm is done to this extent: about one out of every thousand live donor kidney transplants results in the death of the donor. The official figure UNOS [the United Network for Organ Sharing] puts out is one every 2,200; but that's not really correct. It's just a little over twice that. It's probably about one in a thousand":

> I never had a death, but what did happen was that a young woman who was a professional softball player, a wonderful athlete, was going to give a kidney to a sibling. They put in these catheters to do an angiogram, and when they took them out, a clot came off and went down to her feet. It was done at another hospital, which in a way [was] exculpatory for us. But on the other hand, if it weren't for us, they wouldn't [have been] doing an angiogram at the hospital across town.... So anyway, they shipped the girl over and I spent the whole day in the operating room with that woman, cleaning out clots. Just when I would be ready to let her go back to the room, it would clot again.... Back and forth, back and forth.... After about a day, I realized that we [were] going to lose this woman's life in trying to save her leg. I ended up doing a foot amputation.... It alter[ed] her life. She never played softball again.

"It's very hard to do good without the risk of potentially doing harm," I opined. "The iatrogenic side-effects of medical and surgical interventions seem to me to be an irreducible part of practicing medicine. Yet, experiencing this in the context of the medical humanitarian work in which they are engaged has come as a kind of culture shock to many of the young physicians whom I am observing and interviewing in my current study of Médecins Sans Frontières [Doctors Without Borders]," I informed him. "Their utopian belief that if you have the right motivation as well as the right training you can do harm-free good, has been called into question." "You touched an interesting point," said Starzl, "and that is the motivation":

> It's very tempting to pass yourself off as a saint. But there are all kinds of motivations that go into striving; and trying to perpetuate somebody's life or return them to society is, of course, not an ignoble undertaking. It could be empowered by all the wrong

> reasons, like greed, or pride, or competitiveness like in an athletic contest. I think there is no pure reason.... [Even] being impelled by a sense of creativity is [not] necessarily such a great thing.... [G]reat things could come from it, but it could be creative in a lot of wrong ways.... [It's] an important issue to get into because everything in medicine is justified by this idea of salvaging or perpetuating life. [And] almost anyone who's practicing [medicine] has to be alive to this kind of idolatry.

Judith Swazey and I had never found Starzl inclined to idolatrize the work of a surgeon, in this or other respects. "In fact," I noted at this point, "you always gave me the sense, which quite astonished me, that you thought that being a sociologist or a teacher was just as important as being a surgeon." "Well, I think it *is* just as important," he rejoined. And "it isn't just a matter of sociologists, or of surgeons, or of authors, but [of work] up and down the line." However, he declared, "teaching is the most noble profession.... That's my view of it. It's the most selfless of the professions. It would be nice to be a schoolteacher. I wish I could be humble enough to do that—to be a nice high school teacher. Then you would be trying, and everyone would be throwing spit balls at you!" "I suppose it's somewhat like having children," I remarked. The talk about teaching, and my response to it, brought about a sea-change in our conversation. It emboldened Tom to begin to question me about the cardinal experiences in *my* life—how I have felt about and dealt with them—and what kind of understanding I have reached about the overall sense of the life I have led.

Starzl: Let me ask you this: how hard has it been for you to go through life...to make your way through life?

Fox: Not excessively hard—because I have...somewhat the same sense of tragedy that you have. I have never taken anything that I had in my life for granted. Without being a Pollyanna about it, I feel very grateful...for what my life has turned out to be. I didn't marry. I didn't have children.... That was not by choice.... As to what kinds of psychological factors might have contributed to it...even if I had had years of psychoanalysis, I'm not sure I would have found the answer to that question. These are mysteries.... My life does not seem to have been destined in that particular way. The fact that I had polio when I was young, and that I almost died...gave me a certain relationship to not taking health...and the fact that I survived and flourished, for granted.... I've found enormous happiness in my work and also meaning in it.

Starzl: Is it happiness, or satisfaction? Something so hard can't make you happy, but it can make you satisfied.

Fox: I'm never satisfied. When people ask me, using that current phrase, "Are you comfortable?" I always feel tempted to say, "No, I'm not comfortable, and I don't aspire to be." ...In fact, I think I'd be very disturbed if I were unduly comfortable. The work is not just something that fills up my time; it has a sense of meaning. But it's hard to explain that...because...I don't think I'm going to leave even a toe print in the sands of time.

Starzl: You *have* left a toe print, or a footprint, and not everyone can do that. In fact, very few people can....

Fox: But that's not the point of it really—except perhaps for [what you transmit through] teaching.... Aside from a sharper sense of my own mortality, and the sadness I feel about the illnesses and deaths of contemporaries...the only thing [I find] difficult...at this time in my life is [no longer] to be a full-time teacher.... It's really been sacrificial for me [to give that up].... Even my sense of confidence in my own ideas is somewhat shaken—not because I [previously] had an audience [of students] who sat there as...an applauding claque, but because I had to organize my thoughts to [share and discuss them] with the groups of young people who took my courses.... That contributed to my relationship to my own ideas. And there was a great deal that came back from the students themselves....

Starzl: I'm glad I'm here, because you're teaching me something....

Turning the direction of the questioning back towards Tom, I asked him: "Do *you* have a sense of gratitude?" "I have a great feeling of gratitude," he responded. "I have a great feeling of luck":

> Pure luck dictates what happens in one's life, and I feel like I was lucky. I got to make full cycle. I dreamed of something that was unrealistic and a fantasy, got to do it, found it to be woefully unsatisfactory, and potentially even harmful. That's where you and I sort of lined up, because I agreed with you. I also agreed that people exaggerate[d] [in the affirmations they made about organ transplantation]. I don't believe I did it myself, or at least, I tried not to...because I was writing about how I failed, much more than how I succeeded. So this wasn't a "see what a big boy am I" story.

Starzl professed to be "working hard now...to not aspire to anything.... What I would like to do [he declared] is to be able to just turn my back—I think it's what I want—on all endeavors, and immerse myself in beauty—music perhaps more than anything else—and not care whether I'm treated fairly or unfairly in the minds of those who come behind, or those who are present.... But I don't know very many people who can do that. The reason I am ready to do [it] is that I don't have any other aspirations. I don't have anything to do that I haven't done." Turning his gaze intently on me, he remarked: "I should've thought that maybe you would be very near that plateau."

Philosophical contemplativeness turned to laughter-infused banter as we exchanged notes about how fortunate we felt financially, living as retired university faculty members on our TIAA-CREF incomes. "I never wanted to make a lot of money," he said, and "I've never had anything but a straight salary." But now with our TIAA-CREF pensions, both of us were not only receiving more money per month than we ever had before, but our retirement portfolios made us feel like veritable millionaires. "And I've never owned a car worth more than $10,000!" Tom declared. "I've never even owned a car," I replied. "I've never owned a house. I rent this apartment." "Was your family wealthy?" he inquired. "My father was a self-made man, who was well-to-do," I told him, "but he had Alzheimer's disease in the later part of his life, and the money all disappeared. So, I didn't inherit—one mutual fund, and that's it." "My dad owned a newspaper, but he was tied up in bed," Tom confided. "He was paralyzed [by a succession of strokes]—a quadriplegic for more than ten years. [His money vanished, too.] I wouldn't have wanted anything from him anyway, because I had siblings who I thought would need it more."

Our visit was drawing to a close—but not before Starzl had a chance to share with me what he excitedly termed "the epiphany" that he had experienced since he had ceased to practice surgery. He described it as "the essence of the last ten years of effort in my life": his breakthrough insight into the principle and process by which whole-organ transplants in human beings are "accepted" and "merge" into the bodies of recipients. The best way to understand the epiphany, he said, was to read the three-page epilogue, written for a lay audience, that he had added to the second, 1993 printing of *The Puzzle People*. In this epilogue, he recounted how during the year he had spent working on the book, he had reviewed all the papers about transplantation that he had published over the course of thirty to forty years, with the growing, "nagging" realization that he was describing phenomena without really understanding what they meant.

In spite of all the effort, and all the accomplishments, a very "humbling gap" remained: what had been done had taken place "without the foggiest idea...about how a transplanted organ was able to weather rejection." This remained "an immunological enigma." It occurred to Starzl that what might be done is to ask those "heroic patients" who were "survivors" of the early days of transplantation to return to what he called "the battlefield of their younger days," and to cooperate in being studied. No one refused. "They came to Pittsburgh from all over North America in the spring and early summer of 1992," he wrote, "resembling the tattered remnants of a brigade revisiting a once hostile beachhead"—among them, the longest surviving kidney and liver transplant recipients in the world. "From each of these patients bearing someone else's kidney or liver, and also from more recent recipients of hearts, lungs, and intestines, tiny pieces (biopsies) were removed from the transplanted organs as well as from the patient's own skin, lymph glands, and other organs" (1993:343-344). What Starzl discovered is that in all instances, regardless of which organ had been transplanted, a two-way process of cell migration had taken place: not only had special white cells (leukocytes) moved from the recipient's immune system into the transplant, but the widespread movement of myriads of leukocytes from the donor graft had occurred, and distributed themselves throughout the body of the recipient. "These cells scram, migrate, get out, and go all over the recipient!" he exclaimed.

> Until this discovery was made that you could actually find these donor cells all over, a graft of a kidney or a liver was regarded as a defenseless island in a hostile sea. All of a sudden, you've got a situation where this little defenseless island wasn't defenseless after all. It had its own capability of shooting back, because those cells that you find out there are composite, multi-lineage, [chimeras]....
>
> What you really have when you do an organ transplantation is two warring armies—one of David, and the other of Goliath proportions. The important thing that has got to survive is not the organ; it's those cells—the little David. The cells are the things that induce and maintain tolerance.... You've got a conflict of two immune systems that come to peace with one another.... If the cells disappear...then the organ is gone, and it's going to be promptly rejected....
>
> If the organ survives, that means that the recipient of an organ is physically more intimately connected with that long-forgotten donor of unknown ethnicity [and] unknown sex, of thirty years ago, than any other person in their entire life, with the possible exception of their mother—and probably more intimately connected with the donor than the mother."

But this is precisely what organ recipients experience," I told Starzl. "It coincides exactly with the phenomena that Judith Swazey and I identified very early in our studies of organ transplantation—what we called the 'anthropomorphization' and the 'tyranny' of the gift (Fox and Swazey 1974). Many recipients, we discovered, struggle with the spectral sense that some of the psychic and social, as well as the physical qualities of the donor are transferred with his or her organ into their body, personhood, and life. The impact of these animistic feelings on recipients is increased by the magnitude of the 'gift of life' that they have received, which is of such surpassing significance, that it is inherently unreciprocal. Recipients feel that there is nothing they can do in return that is equivalent to what they have been given. And in the case of cadaver transplants, they often feel guilt over the fact that an unknown donor had to die in order for them to receive his or her organ, and live." "Yes, that's true," was Starzl's reply, confirming our observations:

> It sounds strange, [and] initially I didn't put it that way to any patient groups that I talked to, but somebody picked it up right away. These people of non-technical educational background asked questions like one woman asked: "Does this mean when I put on my lipstick in the morning that I'm touching the cells of this...?" That's exactly what it does mean, because if you biopsied a piece of cheek or lip skin or anything like that, you are going to find donor cells. So that caused many people to really pause at the thought that they would have this kind of a connection. And it was sad for some people.

"What do you think this says about our relationship to one another?" I asked Starzl. "For one thing," he answered, "it breaks down those terrible walls that ethnic groups build up against each other. They don't mean anything when you get down to [this] particular nitty gritty." And he also felt that the "new paradigm," which negated the previously held assumption that a successful transplant was "an alien patch in a homogeneous host"(Starzl, Demetris, Trucco et al. 1993:1127), suggested that that the two sets of white cells—those from the donor and those from the recipient—could become "missionaries" and "peacemakers." As early as 1961-1962, Starzl said, Sir Michael Woodruff "raised the question of whether or not it was possible for two immune systems to co-exist under circumstances in which each would induce tolerance to the other—reciprocal induction of tolerance—leaving both immune systems capable of collaborating in a defense against some outside threat, like infection, for example. I think he's absolutely correct about that."

* * *

Upon his return to Pittsburgh, as he had promised, Tom sent me a copy of the 1993 edition of *The Puzzle People*. On the flyleaf where he had handwritten his thanks for "a very pleasant interlude on December 5" he added: "The epiphany is in the Epilogue." He enclosed a separate xeroxed copy of the epilogue, and marked its last paragraph with a bold, red felt-pen border and arrow. That paragraph read:

> Now, it was time to tremble. We had come upon a cardinal principle whose very simplicity had cloaked its existence and delayed its discovery. Graft acceptance was a sleight of hand, made possible by man's misdirection of the normal defenses of a vigilant but ultimately distractible Nature. To have the fog lift, exposing this clarifying vision, was like being allowed a glimpse of eternity. The moment of tranquility was a fair trade for the thirty-five years of work preceding it. And then it was gone, banished by the next set of questions. (1993:346)[3]

Notes

1. Starzl was recruited by the University of Colorado School of Medicine in December 1961, where he was named chief of surgery at the Denver VA Hospital. Beginning on July 1, 1972 he became chair of the Department of Surgery at the University of Colorado, serving in that position for eight years. On January 1, 1981 he moved to the University of Pittsburgh, to become a professor of surgery and director of the Medical Center's Transplantation Institute.
2. Carla Messikomer, a co-organizer of the colloquium and one of the editors of this book, helped to arrange the interview and attended and tape recorded our conversation. Judith P. Swazey, a co-editor of the book, arranged to have the recording typed and edited the transcript.
3. Starzl also sent me several medical journal papers that describe and analyze his "epiphany" in medical-scientific language (Starzl, Demetris, Murase et al. 1992; Starzl, Demetris, Trucco et al. 1993; Starzl and Zinkernagle 1998).

References

Fox, Renée C. and Judith P. Swazey. 1974. *The Courage to Fail: A Social View of Organ Transplants and Dialysis.* Chicago, IL: University of Chicago Press; 2d ed., revised, 1978; reissued with a new introduction, Transaction Publishers, 2001.

Fox, Renée C. and Judith P. Swazey. 1992. *Spare Parts: Organ Replacement in American Society.* New York: Oxford University Press.

Starzl, Thomas E. 1992. *The Puzzle People: Memoirs of a Transplants Surgeon.* Pittsburgh: University of Pittsburgh Press.

Starzl, Thomas E. 1993. Second ed., with a new Epilogue. *The Puzzle People: Memoirs of a Transplants Surgeon.* Pittsburgh: University of Pittsburgh Press.

Starzl, Thomas E., Anthony J. Demetris, Massimo Trucco, et al. 1993. "Cell Migration and Chimerism After Whole-Organ Transplantation: The Basis of Graft Acceptance" (Special article). *Hepatology* 17:1127-1152.

Starzl, Thomas E., Anthony J. Demetris, Noriko Murase, et al. 1992. "Cell Migration, Chimerism, and Graft Acceptance." (Special article). *The Lancet* 339 (June 27):1579-1582.

Starzl, Thomas E. and Rolf M. Zinkernagel. 1998. "Antigen Localization and Migration in Immunity and Tolerance." (Review article). *New England Journal of Medicine* 339 (Dec.24):1905-1913.

11

What if Food Were a Medicine? The Pediatrician and Childhood Hunger

Deborah A. Frank

As a practicing pediatrician in the inner city, I feel like a bricklayer at an architect's convention—I do not have a sophisticated understanding of the big picture and I cannot articulate the elegance of theory, but I have a lot of grubby practical experience. In this paper I share that perspective and hope that others can address how bricks fit into the grander scheme of the social building. Like a bricklayer, I always work as part of a local work crew: a dedicated multidisciplinary hospital team. I am also a card-carrying member of a national, although not very powerful, union of like-minded physicians and other anti-hunger activists. Locally and nationally we struggle within the constraints of the ancient curse of making bricks without straw—the responsibility of caring for poor children without adequate resources to assure them the quality of life we want for our own children.

My bricklaying expertise was gained as the founder and director of a multi-disciplinary "Grow" clinic at an urban hospital for the past fifteen years, where I have overseen the treatment of approximately 1500 children referred for "failure to thrive." These are children under five years-of-age with clinically significant growth deficits that, in most cases, are attributable either to primary or secondary malnutrition. Some of these children suffer from such Victorian illnesses as tuberculosis, marasmus, and rickets. All have recurring infections, and many manifest disabling developmental impairments. To care for these children, we have been compelled constantly to raise money to support nutritionists and social workers. Since neither the medical nor social welfare system provides these children with sufficiently intensive care or adequate food to restore them to health, we maintain a food pantry. My experiences straddle the highly technical medical world of an urban teaching hospital and the harassed world of the low-tech emergency food provider who is constantly scrounging for peanut butter.

As we do this work, I have found that the religious connotations of feeding the poor are both a blessing and a curse. As Janet Poppendieck (1999) has pointed out in her book, *Sweet Charity*, a sense of religious obligation that crosses denominational boundaries acts as a tremendously powerful force in maintaining anti-hunger efforts and in sustaining many of those who do the work. We in the emergency food network cheerfully and shamelessly work this sense of obligation, preaching guest sermons, talking to Sunday school assemblies, and sending out holiday-specific appeals. My husband's rabbinic colleagues are strongly tempted to develop an urgent previous engagement whenever they see me coming.

Availability of emergency food follows the rhythm of the religious calendar. Donations strain capacity for storage following Yom Kippur and between Thanksgiving and Christmas, are much less at Passover-Easter, and almost non-existent in the summer when the demand is greater because poor children are not receiving school meals, but religious schools are closed for summer and there are no sacred festivals to inspire donations. Religious connotations also allow the broader society to dismiss the social urgency of the problem. Assuring that one's fellow citizens have enough to eat is viewed as a quaint act of particularistic piety like wearing a yarmulke or crossing oneself when passing a church—harmless and even laudable, but of no relevance to those who are not part of that sect, much less to public policy or public health. For reasons I do not understand, this is in striking contrast to the impact of religion on so-called "lifestyle issues" such as reproductive health, sex education, and sexual orientation, where the impact of a much more narrow segment of religious beliefs than those which endorse and motivate anti-hunger efforts act as a political third rail which intimidates many politicians into endorsing legislation at odds with their own world view.

The now discredited journalist Mike Barnicle once referred to me in a broadcast as "Boston's own Mother Teresa," which I took as a reflection on my fashion sense rather than on my moral standing. Nevertheless, it became a label that my colleagues have never let me live down, particularly when I stand in the doctor's conference room swearing in terms that would make a longshoreman blush because yet another act of injustice or incompetence has been perpetrated on one of our patient's families. This linking of anti-hunger work with saintliness, while explicitly complimentary, is implicitly dismissive and yet another mode by which the broader society disowns responsibility. My colleagues and I have repeatedly had the experience of unctuous politicians touring our hospital, shaking us soulfully by the hand and announcing "you are certainly doing the Lord's work here, Doctor," who then vote for policies that suggest that assuring the well being of poor children may be the Lord's work, but it sure isn't theirs! The latent syllogism is that you have to be a saint to care about the well being of poor people. However, most people are cheerfully willing to acknowledge that they are not saints, so it's not their problem.

If one attempts to reframe the problem as one of social justice rather than religious mission, one rapidly loses the aura of sanctity. Our team's Puerto Rican community outreach worker became interested in Afro-Brazilian dancing and started hanging out with the Brazilian community. One day she shyly presented me with a postcard given to her by a Brazilian friend, which now hangs on my office door. The card contains a quote from Dom Helder Camara, a Brazilian bishop: "When I give food to the poor they call me a saint; when I ask why the poor have no food they call me a communist."

Once a very nice woman arrived with generous donations of groceries, and asked me what else she could do for hungry kids. I tactfully suggested that she could contact her state and federal legislators to urge increased funding for WIC (the Supplemental Nutrition Program for Women, Infants, and Children). She replied, "Oh I can't do that, I am a conservative Republican!" I then asked her for a diaper donation, and she eventually became one of the program's most committed volunteers, spending a day each week distributing crackers and crayons to our patients while they waited to be seen. But I never again dared to raise social policy issues with her. Like many other bricklayers, I face the dilemma that if I suggest to people that really caring for children requires a fundamental change in our social/political blueprint, and maybe even a more progressive tax structure, the supply of bricks (in my program's case, money and food) will be promptly cut off and the many families and children who depend on them will be left with even less than before. Even if I believed in theory that permitting increased deprivation of children would ultimately lead to social transformation, which I don't, I could not tolerate emotionally the increased suffering of the patients before me. Moreover, pragmatically, I would worry that many of my patients would not survive to see the dawning of the new day, and many of those who did would be too impaired to participate in it.

However, if I do not try to contribute to changing public policy, I begin to feel like I am only rearranging deck chairs on the Titanic. Advocacy keeps me sane. So how do I address the twin demands of sustaining patient care and trying to push public discourse forward? The distinguished public health physician, Bernard Guyer, once commented to me that "When all you have is a hammer, everything looks like a nail." In my case, one hammer is my clinical experience (which no politician can debate) strengthened by my training in social science. The other hammer is the education I received in the medical/scientific approach to understanding the mechanisms and epidemiology of disease.

I use my clinical experience in a number of ways. First, to give the lie to the assertion that there are really no malnourished children in America, I can always announce blandly that I saw twenty of them in my clinic yesterday. Next, clinical experience often makes painfully obvious problems with public policies that on paper seem entirely sensible. For example, all children, whatever their nutritional status, become ineligible for WIC vouchers for milk and other nutritious foods on their fifth birthday. No doubt it was assumed that by age five children would be in kindergarten and have access to milk and other foods through school meals. However, in Boston, as in most states, there is a rigid school entry policy such that a child who turns five after September is not eligible for public school until the following September. Depending on the month of birth, a poor child may have seamless access to supplemental feeding or may go eleven months with their parents hard-pressed to consistently provide milk and other foods that most families take for granted. Finally, clinical anecdotes give the numbers names and faces. As Dr. Arthur Caplan once cogently remarked to a reporter, "When it is an individual kid, everyone's heart goes out. When it's a proposal to raise your taxes to cover a faceless statistical kid, everyone's wallet slams shut." In this endeavor I have been helped enormously by two things I learned from Renée Fox long ago: that everyone is an expert about their own experiences, and that ordinary people talk poetry if you listen to them carefully and they are talking about something they care about—like their kids. I will always remember the mother who, when asked how she managed to feed her two children at the end of the month, including the malnourished toddler who was my patient, responded, "I prays and I stretches and then I prays and I stretches some more."

Even during the late, lamented period of economic expansion and declining unemployment in 1998, 40 percent of the 12-13 million American children who lived in poverty (with a family income of $16,660 or less for a family of four) experienced recurring episodes of food insufficiency[1] (Nord, Jemison, and Bickel 1999). Until the twentieth century, chronic malnutrition and, indeed, recurrent famine were unavoidable facts of life. Much of the developing world still lacks adequate resources to produce and distribute sufficient food for their own populations, with consequently staggering rates of child malnutrition and child mortality. However, neither lack of food nor lack of infrastructure for distribution can explain nutritional deprivation of poor children in the United States. Childhood hunger in the United States is a consequence of political choices embedded in the complex social meanings of food, charity, and poverty. Of the $55 billion the Personal Responsibility and Work Opportunity Reconciliation Act of 1996—popularly referred to as "welfare reform"—cut, over six years, from income support for poor families, $30 billion came from food stamps and other programs designed to support the nutritional status of the poor. Each year, at both the state and national level, intensive political effort must be expended not to enhance child nutrition programs, but to prevent further cuts in such child-focused programs as WIC, school meals, and childcare feeding.

The problem is further complicated because childhood hunger, like childhood poverty, disproportionately occurs among children of color. Surveys of families with telephones conservatively estimate that 10 percent of African American households with children and 9 percent of Latino households with children under eighteen are not only food insecure, but hungry—i.e. repeatedly experiencing the painful or uneasy sensation caused by lack of food (Hamilton et al. 1997). Since homeless families and the many impoverished families without telephones were not assessed, these figures underestimate the extent of the problem. In spite of much rhetoric to the contrary, it is hard not to perceive that families of color are less valued than others and their suffering is not of compelling interest to politicians, and, more importantly, to the power bases of those politicians.

Fatal starvation is mercifully rare among American children, but nutritional deprivation sufficient to impair health and educational competence is common. Even traditional preliterate cultures recognize that food of insufficient quality or quantity affects the health and survival of all members of the society, but particularly of children and the child in the womb. This ancient popular perception has been buttressed in this century by an extensive body of medical research convincingly documenting that even subtle nutritional deficits influence such important medical outcomes as neural tube defects, birth weight, infant mortality, immune function, and the optimal development of children's cognition and behavior. Some of the associations are extraordinary. Decades after World War II, adults who were infants in utero while their mothers were grossly undernourished during the Dutch hunger winter showed increased incidence of schizophrenia (Susser and Lin 1992). Among children in Florida, iron deficiency anemia in infancy without protein energy malnutrition increases the likelihood that the child will need special education ten years later (Hurtado, Claussen, and Scott 1999).

Strangely, this information about how non-life-threatening deficits of micronutrients in childhood can have profound and lasting effects generates much less sustained public attention than the controversy surrounding whether oat bran lowers cardiovascular risk levels in adults. While the public is perfectly willing to give credence to the impact of nutrition on conditions that they fear may impair their own health as they face the inevitability of old age, they ignore nutritional issues which largely impact young children, particularly if those children are poor.

The problem is complicated further by the paradoxical association of extreme thinness with beauty and wealth among certain groups of adolescent and adult women in our society. As a physical trainer of these women stated in a popular magazine, "Thinness has become a symbol of discipline, power, and control" (Schindehette 1999).

How then do we generate concern for the young, the sick, and the poor whose thinness is the ultimate indicator not of power but of powerlessness?

When I briefly emerge from the fog generated by the interaction of clinical preoccupation and genteel begging and try to synthesize the scientific data, I find myself wondering what the political response would be if we could convince people that researchers had just discovered a miracle drug called foodamycin which decreases premature birth, enhances immune function, and improves school achievement, and that millions of American children are intermittently but repeatedly deprived of this drug both before and after birth. If foodamycin's effects are grounded in science, and they are, letting its availability depend on the haphazard efforts of private citizens of good will is patently inadequate. This becomes a job for experts. We would not dream of suggesting that religious groups and Cub Scouts take Red Cross classes and then provide dialysis to the indigent in renal failure, thus enhancing the "personal responsibility" of the patient and decreasing Medicare costs for the taxpayer.

Moreover, if one buys into the scientific perspective, there is no longer a particular moral stance, other than rational pragmatism, required to underpin efforts at abolishing hunger; it becomes merely a matter of enlightened self-interest like immunization. Feeding people is a lot cheaper than paying for neonatal intensive care for low birth weight babies or than dealing with a generation that is prevented from participating in the information economy for want of adequate nutrition in childhood.

Paradoxically, this scientific perspective is also experienced as empowering by emergency food providers, many of whom have little formal education. I am often asked to address emergency food coalitions in various states to boost morale by explaining to providers that by trying to get families enough to eat they are "really" promoting health, since in our society providing health care is a prestigious activity, while nourishing children is not.

Like all health and social service providers who work with poor families, the physician who cares for malnourished children is confronted with multiple moral and pragmatic dilemmas. What are the implications of medicalizing, however accurately, what is also an issue of social justice? How does one balance one's energy and expertise between meeting the immediate needs of the patients in front of one with the long-term hope of real social change that would greatly reduce the incidence of hunger overall? In advocating for such social change, how far does one dare risk the ire of corporate and individual donors whose support is essential for caring for undernourished children, when the donors, and physicians like me, are themselves the major beneficiaries of the increasing inequality of our society?

Renée Fox taught me, and many others, that there is nothing embarrassingly sentimental or unprofessional about attending to these moral issues and social problems. Our training in these domains energizes us to wrestle with these issues rather than withdraw in despair. Her students may never change the world, but they are not going to stop trying.

Note

1. Food insufficiency is technically defined by a family's inability to obtain a consistent supply of food of adequate quality and quantity for normal health and activity through socially acceptable methods.

References

Hamilton, Willam L., John T. Cook, William W. Thompson, Lawrence F. Burgon, Edward A. Frongillo, Christine M. Olson, and Cheryl A. Wehler. 1997. *Household Food Security in the United States in 1995: Summary Report of the Food Security Measurement Project.* Washington, DC: United States Department of Agriculture, Food and Consumer Service, Office of Analysis and Evaluation.

Hurtado, Elyse K., Angelika H. Claussen, and Keith G. Scott. 1999. Early Childhood Anemia and Mild or Moderate Mental Retardation. *Am. J. Clin. Nutr.* 69:115-119.

Nord, Mark, Kyle Jemison, and Gary Bickel. 1999. *Measuring Food Insecurity in the United States, Food Assistance and Nutrition Research Report No. 2.* Washington, DC: United States Department of Agriculture, Food and Rural Economics Division, Economics Research Service.

Poppendieck, Janet. 1999. *Sweet Charity.* New York: Penguin Books.

Schindehette, Susan. 1999. Going to Extremes. *People* 52:110-120.

Susser, Ezra S. and Shang P. Lin. 1992. Schizophrenia After Prenatal Exposure to the Dutch Hunger Winter of 1944-1945. *Archives of General Psychiatry* 49:983-988.

12

Uncertainty and Changing Trust Relationships in Medicine

David Mechanic

Trust, the expectation that others will act as expected consistent with status and role and meet their responsibilities to us, is fundamental to the idea of society. Although most sociological theorists have not explicitly treated trust as a central frame for their work, it is implicit in most major theories of social relations. Trust-related concepts were used by such classical theorists as Toennies, Durkheim, Simmel, and Weber in explaining how social order was established and maintained (Misztal 1996). Luhmann (1979), Parsons (1949), and Barber (1983), among others, elaborated more directly on the integrative and facilitative functions of trust, while rational choice theorists such as Coleman (1990) and Elster (1989) treat trust as a basis of action and cooperation. Whatever the conceptualization, it seems plain that trust is the glue that holds collectivities together.

To the best of my knowledge, Renée Fox never used trust as her primary organizing frame. But it asserts itself in almost every one of her studies, from patients and physicians on an experimental metabolic unit (Fox 1959) and organ transplantation (Fox and Swazey 1974) to her work on informed consent, bioethics, uncertainty, health professional socialization, and the two cultures of Belgium (Fox 1988).

My own forays into the area of trust are modest and are motivated by the rapid transformation of health care, the growth and increased penetration of managed care, and many future medical uncertainties (Mechanic and Schlesinger 1996; Mechanic 1998a, 1997, 1996). While trust is central to all social relationships, it has had particular salience in medical care, where large inequalities in expertise exist between doctor and patient, where persons with serious illness and life-threatening disorders are highly dependent on their care providers, and where macro health care changes are undermining long-established assumptions about roles and responsibilities.

The work I report on here has been largely exploratory, using different methods to examine varying aspects of trust relationships in medical care. Among these have been relatively informal inquiries of health care leaders about the importance of trust and what their institutions were doing about its apparent erosion. I have visited some interesting programs as well to learn more about them. Our project has also interviewed ninety patients with serious life-threatening or debilitating illnesses about their trust in their doctors and the factors that sustain or weaken such trust. Among these patients are women with breast cancer, patients with chronic Lyme disease, and persons with serious and persistent mental illnesses. Although coping with each of these uncertain conditions has unique aspects, there is remarkable concordance in the factors that promote or undermine trust in treatment situations. Since much of the public unhappiness with medical care focuses on the changes brought by the growth of HMOs and managed care, we have also surveyed a national sample of medical directors of such organizations about trust issues and programs. We build on other work of colleagues who are engaged in similar efforts to understand how to develop a more effective and humane health care system.

The Health Care Transformation

Health care in the United States is undergoing large and rapid changes in response to cost pressures and ideological influences. In the past decade we have seen rapid privatization and consolidation of health care companies, a focus on competition and the medical marketplace, and the widespread implementation of a range of management structures, approaches, and strategies. In this process much power has shifted from physicians and their professional organizations to health care entrepreneurs and managers. Third parties are increasingly involved in overseeing and altering treatment plans between doctors and their patients. Through physician capitation and a variety of incentives, medical roles have been shifting from the traditional ideal of patient advocacy to one of allocation. Both physicians and patients report frustration and distrust with these new arrangements. In a recent survey, 51-61 percent of respondents in light and heavy managed care arrangements reported that they were very or somewhat worried that the health plan would be more concerned about saving money than about the best treatment for them when they are sick, as compared with only 34 percent in traditional plans. More than half of the respondents in managed care did not trust the health plan to "just about always" do the right thing for their care (Blendon, Brodie, Benson et al. 1998). These responses are consistent with other surveys indicating significant erosion of trust in medicine and the society more generally (Blendon, Hyams, and Benson 1993; Lipset and Schneider 1987; Nye, Zelikow, and King 1997). There is widespread public skepticism about the truthfulness and reliability of health plans, the media, and government, as well as a precipitous decline over time in the belief that most people can be trusted (Lipset 1995).

There is substantial evidence that erosion of trust is not simply a reflection of medical care alterations, but is symptomatic of broader changes in modern society and the growth and penetration of the mass media (Lipset and Schneider 1987; Nye et al. 1997; Lipset 1995). No social institution has gone untarnished, and growing distrust has been documented around the world under political, economic, and medical systems very different from our own (Nye et al. 1997). As social trust diminishes, people turn back to their primary relations with whom they have extended kinship ties and relationships and who they believe are less likely to mislead or betray them (Putnam 1993; Fukuyama 1995). Medicine is an interesting case because it falls between primary and more formal relationships and because the relationship between doctor and patient has traditionally been seen as an important instrument for achieving many of the important goals of medical care. Patients, particularly those who face serious illness, invest much more emotionally than they do in most other secondary relationships. The doctor-patient relationship is seen as a vehicle to address highly personal psychosocial issues and as a basis to achieve important behavioral changes.

For our purposes, it is important to distinguish between social and relationship trust. Most of the work on trust in medicine deals with relationship trust and how trust is built between doctor and patient over time. In contrast, social trust refers to both symbolic and real ties between individuals and organizations. Social trust may be built on experience with community institutions or may be primarily reputational. In the first instance, persons make judgments about institutions based on their experience with them. Experience with large and complex institutions like hospitals, health plans, and large medical groups are segmented and partial, but people seem willing to generalize from small samples of such experience to judgments about the organization as a whole.

Judgments of social institutions with which persons have no personal experience are shaped by a variety of influences. Persons first depend on their primary relations for information. Thus, the experience of relatives, friends, coworkers, and one's physician have high credibility. In choosing a doctor, hospital, or health care plan, such informants are found to be far more influential than health plans, report cards, or government (Lubalin and Harris-Kojetin 1999; Robinson and Brodie 1997). Images of institutions are also shaped by the media, and some institutions have particularly high reputational standing, such as the Mayo Clinic, Johns Hopkins, or the Harvard Medical School. Most health plans and many hospitals and medical groups advertise to build their public reputations. It is difficult to assess the influence of these efforts since the public has little trust in health care advertising (Isaacs 1996).

Trust can also be seen as an attitude or disposition, a product of temperament, social development, and personal histories. People differ substantially in their willingness to openly trust in new relationships. As a patient in one of our studies described her behavior: "I'm a pretty trusting person when it comes to people in general. I think I just have a wait-and-see attitude. I trust somebody until they do something I realize was untrustworthy" (Mechanic and Meyer 2000). Members of the public express very different attitudes in surveys about whether they trust most people. The fact that reported trust in others changes over time (Lipset 1995) suggests that this measure is more than simply a measure of disposition.

Trust is multi-dimensional and also usually qualified. We understand that we can trust others in some ways but not in all ways. The essence of trust is uncertainty and risk, since trust is always a prediction about a future that might not be realized. As the stakes rise people enter trust relationships more carefully. Trusting strangers with a small sum is different than trusting them with one's fortune; disclosing ordinary information about oneself is different from disclosing one's innermost secrets; and choosing a doctor for a routine complaint is vastly different than such a selection when critically ill. Risk assessment studies suggest that people tend to be risk averse. Thus, negative feedback about risk may have disproportionate effects.

There are a number of important dimensions of interpersonal trust in physicians, but most patients primarily focus on three: technical competence, interpersonal competence, and advocacy. Patients have a well-developed conception of interpersonal competence and even use interpersonal cues as a source of information about technical competence. Patients also greatly value the idea that the doctor is their agent, committed to pursuing their interests (Mechanic and Meyer 2000). We have also questioned patients about confidentiality, control, and disclosure issues. Confidentiality is widely assumed in medical practice and appears problematic primarily for persons with highly stigmatized problems. Physician disclosure and control have not been issues for most patients because of their limited understanding of new health care arrangements. However, when financial arrangements between health plans and physicians are explained to them, they tend to strongly disapprove.

The Effect of Organizational Changes on Trust

There are a variety of challenges to social trust and interpersonal trust both in general and in specific relation to changes in the financing and organization of our medical care system. Many social scientists have written about what they believe to be an increasing erosion of social capital (Putnam 1995). The concept of social capital is now commonly used in explaining patterns of illness and death, health care mobilization, and as a basis of the social solidarity needed to bring medical coverage and care to the disadvantaged. With strong emphasis on the market and individualism, the sense of community and concern about others appears to have weakened. Despite a decade of economic growth and vitality, the uninsured population has continued to grow without a public outcry.

In the United States and elsewhere there is evidence of disillusionment with government, cultural cynicism, and lack of confidence in the reliability of leaders, experts, and others in positions of authority (Blendon et al. 1993; Lipset and Schneider 1987; Nye et al. 1997; Lipset 1995). In the U.S., the cultural battles of the 1960s, and the Vietnam War, did much to undermine the credibility of authority figures. Perhaps more important is the growth of mass media and its instant accessibility, providing negative, disconfirming, and conflicting images of much that goes on in our social institutions. The media markets negativity and scandal, and psychological research demonstrates that negative images have a more powerful impact on public conceptions than favorable portrayals (Kasperson, Golding, and Tuler 1992). Nor has there been a lack of widely publicized violations of public trust that feed public perceptions. With the privatization and commercialization of medicine, and the publicity given to selfishness and fraud, it is not difficult to understand the precipitous drop in confidence in medical leaders and health plans.

Managed care, involving a variety of structures, strategies, and approaches to more appropriately distribute care, is a case in point. With the privatization and centralization of managed care organizations, a large diversity of practices are now encompassed under a single rubric. With the hundreds of millions of transactions taking place, there inevitably will be errors of judgment, negligence, and even fraud as there have always been. But now the media can more readily frame anecdotes of abuse using a single symbol, and misdeeds are often generalized to an entire industry (Mechanic 1997). Thus, what were once the errors or greed of individual doctors, hospitals, or laboratories are now broader indictments. These tendencies are encouraged by television and other media that build interest around anecdotes and human interest stories.

Individual clinicians, unlike health care plans, have been more insulated from these broader forces, but changing medical arrangements also challenge interpersonal trust. Interpersonal trust develops in voluntary associations over time as participants get to better know one another and feel more confident of their predictions of how others will behave. Studies of trust in physicians find, as expected, that choice and continuity of care are important influences contributing to trust (Thom et al. 1999; Kao et al. 1998), but both have been restricted in recent years. Most employers select their employees' health plan and offer no health plan choice; less than half the population have such choices. To most patients, however, physician choice is more important than plan choice, but as employers change plans and physician networks are modified, patients may be more restricted in their physician choices and their ability to remain with preferred physicians. Moreover, managed care approaches such as the use of gatekeepers and restrictions of access to specialists have also frustrated patient choice. Thus, the changes that have taken place have diminished the conditions for interpersonal trust, although much trust in personal physicians remains.

Other factors also may reduce the conditions of trust. Clinicians report pressures to work more rapidly. Yet trust develops through communication that allows time for careful listening and feedback. Both patients and doctors commonly complain about insufficient time which may impede effective communication central to good doctor-patient relationships.

Time that doctors spend with patients, however, has not decreased as many believe. In a study of time doctors spent in visits with patients between 1989 and 1998, we found that time increased over the ten-year period for primary and specialty care, for HMO and non-HMO patients, for new and continuing patients and for those with more and less serious conditions (Mechanic, McAlpine, and Rosenthal 2001). A further analysis of 1999 data found the pattern of increasing time continuing.

The gap between perceptions and reality requires explanation. Several factors probably contribute. As health plans compete for patients and patient loyalty they understand that satisfaction is important. They monitor patient satisfaction and convey expectations to doctors concerning their performance. Doctors understand the importance of time for patients. With increased information in the media, the Internet, and direct advertising, patients come with more information and questions. Physicians need to spend more time explaining options, answering questions, and correcting inaccurate information. Doctors also are increasingly expected to deal with prevention and many other life issues. While they appreciate that expectations are often unrealistic, they understand their importance and try to do what they can. But this takes time. Also, with employers changing health plans, and changing networks of care, more patients may have to change doctors, disrupting doctor-patient continuity. New patients, who doctors do not know, invariably require more time than patients with whom doctors have continuing relationships.

As patients encounter utilization review and denial of physicians' treatment recommendations, they may come to understand that their physicians do not fully control their treatment and may wonder how aggressively their clinicians advocate for them. Doctors may need more time to explain managed care procedures and to reassure patients that they are acting as their agents to the greatest extent possible. Third party involvement in treatment plans may also raise questions about privacy and confidentiality. Moreover, as patients increasingly learn about the economic incentives given to clinicians to stay within utilization targets, they may have more reason to question their physicians' motivation or their advocacy.

Some believe that trust is not all that important, and perhaps even counterproductive. They point to the many types of failures of medical care and suggest that patients who trust too easily will be duped. They argue for patient activism, independent information seeking, and second-guessing the doctor. They understand that lack of trust results in suspicion, but believe that some suspicion is a good thing. Of course, trusting too much or too easily can be foolish. Appropriate regulation if properly structured can provide a foundation for trust and help sustain it.

There is much regulation of medicine, and careful selection, training, and licensing of physicians. One can assume that because of such entry restrictions, the random patient seeing a random doctor can expect a reasonable level of competence. Trust reduces transaction costs and the need for elaborate and costly regulations. More importantly, trust facilitates effective communication, patient disclosure and cooperation in treatment, and makes it more possible to achieve useful health-related behavior changes. Medical care is in part an important psychosocial influence process that is impossible without reasonable levels of trust. Nevertheless, it is important and appropriate to inquire as to the appropriate balance between trust and regulatory mechanisms necessary to allow trust to develop without too much risk.

Concepts of Trust among Patients with Serious Illness

The routine decision to trust one's doctor involves small risk. Such risk increases substantially when individuals face serious and life-threatening conditions where the quality of care can have large impact on function, quality of life, and life itself. Our interviews with patients indicate that while they may enter trusting relationships with doctors on the basis of reputation and advice of relatives and friends, their trust is cautious and qualified (Mechanic and Meyer 2000). As in other interpersonal situations, trust builds over time as patients have opportunities to gauge the competence and responsiveness of the clinician. Sick patients feel highly dependent on their doctors, and unequal in their knowledge and understanding, but they impose their own common sense tests in appraising the doctor. Patients explicitly describe testing their doctors—as one patient put it, "Well, first of all I hit them with something. I see how they come back at me. If they evade the issue or they ignore it or something else, then they're not to be trusted" (Mechanic and Meyer 2000).

Patients know best the doctor's interpersonal competence and such competence is the basis on which they begin to make other trust judgments as well. In characterizing such competence the words patients choose most commonly are "listening," "caring," "concern," and "compassion." It is clear from their descriptions that these are not simply empathic responses but measurable forms of demeanor and behavior. Patients commonly describe demeanor by terms such as "condescending," "arrogant," "friendly," "patronizing," "respectful," and "attentive." They discuss behaviors such as "abruptness," "eye contact," "reassuring," "sensitive," and "nonjudgmental." What is most interesting about these characterizations is that they commonly involve teachable skills and need not be simply seen as aspects of personality or the "art of medicine" (Scott et al. 1995).

Patients, of course, care a great deal about technical competence, but they are much less able to judge it. Thus, they indirectly assess competence through the clinician's capacities and the expected progress of their illness. When they speak of capacity, the words most commonly chosen are education, credentials, intellect, and expertise. But they also impose empirical criteria on physician behavior such as double-checking, keeping current, thinking ahead, and having access to newer information. Patients also make judgments about the progression of their illnesses and whether matters are proceeding as they should. They identify lack of technical competence by the fact that they are not getting better, or that they feel worse. They also make judgments about misdiagnoses, being given the wrong medicine, and the failure of the clinician to pick up on relevant information.

The other dimension of particular salience to patients is the doctor's agency and fiduciary responsibility. Patients trust doctors who they believe are on their side, advocate for them, fight for their best interests, do everything in their power, and put themselves on the line. As noted earlier, many patients are not fully conversant with the changes accompanying managed care. But many of those who are sick have already come to understand that doctors are losing control. They know that increasingly doctors are pressured, restricted, interfered with, dictated to, limited, and hassled. They all know that some treatment claims are denied. Under these conditions, patients don't lose trust but rather evaluate the physician by how hard they believe he/she will advocate in their interest.

HMO Responses to Trust Issues

Health plans understand the importance of trust and are alarmed at the strong backlash against managed care practices. It is frequently suggested that the industry shares the low point in public esteem with the tobacco industry and that in both cases the public is receptive to having the government impose regulations and sanctions. A recent Kaiser Family Foundation/Harvard School of Public Health National Survey found that more than half the public had an unfavorable opinion of tobacco companies, oil companies, HMOs, and health insurance companies as compared with only 25 percent who had unfavorable views of hospitals and 17 percent who had unfavorable views of doctors (The NewsHour with Jim Lehrer et al. 2000). Eighty-five percent of the public favored legislation that would regulate HMOs (Kaiser Family Foundation/Harvard School of Public Health, Post-Election Survey 2001).

We surveyed the medical directors of HMOs in the United States to assess what they were doing about this problem (Mechanic and Rosenthal 1999). After much effort, we were able to gain the cooperation of 42 percent of potential respondents. This is a disappointing response rate but the sample is reasonably representative of HMOs nationally and of varying types of HMOs. The survey queried medical directors about some twenty-six types of programs that had been identified in my earlier surveys of medical leaders (Mechanic 1996) and that were believed to have some value in building and maintaining trust. We first asked the directors whether their HMO had a program of each type, and if it did, how useful they believed the program to be. Almost all the HMOs made specific efforts to improve patient satisfaction and most used focus groups. Other common programs, reported as present in at least two-thirds of HMOs, were mediation for dispute resolution, the use of patient clinical pathways, confidentiality awareness programs, formal support programs for patients and families, patient representative/ombudsmen programs, and sponsorship of community development. Types of programs believed to be most useful in encouraging trust were specific efforts to improve patient satisfaction, patient representatives/ombudsmen programs, and formal support programs (Mechanic and Rosenthal 1999).

Sponsorship of such programs varied by group/staff HMOs (like the traditional Kaiser-Permanente model) versus other types, between nonprofit and profit HMOs, and between HMOs independent of chains versus those that were part of chains. Group/staff HMOs were more likely to have a variety of these programs as compared with other types of HMOs, and they were more common in nonprofit than in for-profit organizations, and in organizations that were not part of chains. This pattern persisted even when controlling for other factors such as enrollment size and market characteristics. The most distinctive differences, however, were between the group/staff model and other types of HMOs.

Group/staff model HMOs have both a significant advantage and a significant liability. Because care is given in large group settings under a relatively unified management, it is more possible to develop organizational strategies at the level of the provider group to deal with patient issues and improve care. Some of the most interesting examples of innovative care practices, professional teamwork, effective use of practice guidelines, chronic disease management, and patient and family education are found in such organizations. These organizations also give more attention to provider interpersonal competence, ethics consultation, and related issues (Mechanic and Rosenthal 1999). The significant liability of such organizations is the restriction of patient choice to a limited number of physicians. In part, these organizations may need to give greater attention to interpersonal competence and patient relations because such areas are more problematic in closed panels.Group/staff models, however, are increasingly a smaller proportion of the managed care sector and most recent growth has been in network/IPA models and preferred provider organizations. These are typically virtual networks with small groups of doctors working out of their own premises and maintaining membership in a number of different HMOs. Such conditions make it much more difficult to put in place a range of organizational innovations that improve the management of care and build trust. The trust issue is abated to some degree in these large virtual networks because patients often have a fairly extensive choice of primary care physicians and can shift easily if they are dissatisfied. Such choice provides a safety mechanism for dealing with patient dissatisfaction but not necessarily for putting in place effective care management systems. The belief is that real time medical information networks will ultimately serve the same purpose, but this remains to be demonstrated.

As I have proceeded in this study I have encountered some extraordinary people and some truly innovative and exciting ideas (Mechanic 1998b). There is an extraordinary amount of talent and innovation in our health care system, but typically these are expressed in local programs developed by people on the scene who are not only not visible nationally, but who are generally not even known in their own institutions. In our highly pluralistic system we have no established ways to identify innovative programs and disseminate them widely, and this issue deserves much attention. We also have to do better in systematically evaluating innovative programs and assessing their strengths and weaknesses. It is significant that few of the programs identified had been evaluated, and the common belief that they contributed usefully to trust was more a matter of faith than evidence.

References

Barber, Bernard. 1983. *The Logic and Limits of Trust.* New Brunswick, NJ: Rutgers University Press.

Blendon, Robert J., Mollyann Brodie, John M. Benson, Drew E. Altman, Larry Levitt, Tina Hoff, and Larry Hugick. 1998. "Understanding the Managed Care Backlash." *Health Affairs* 17(4):80-94.

Blendon, Robert J., Tracey S. Hyams, and John M. Benson. 1993. "Bridging the Gap between Expert and Public Views on Health Care Reform." *Journal of the American Medical Association* 269(19):2573-2578.

Coleman, James S. 1990. *Foundations of Social Theory.* Cambridge: Harvard University Press.

Elster, Jon. 1989. *The Cement of Society: A Study of Social Order.* New York: Cambridge University Press.

Fox, Renée. 1959. *Experiment Perilous: Physicians and Patients Facing the Unknown.* New York: Free Press.

Fox, Renée. 1988. *Essays in Medical Sociology: Journeys into the Field.* New Brunswick, NJ: Transaction Publishers.

Fox, Renée and Judith P. Swazey. 1974. *The Courage to Fail: A Social View of Organ Transplants and Dialysis*. Chicago: University of Chicago Press.

Fukuyama, Francis. 1995. *Trust: The Social Virtues and the Creation of Prosperity*. New York: Free Press.

Isaacs, Stephen L. 1996. "Consumers' Information Needs: Results of a National Survey." *Health Affairs* 15(4):31-41.

Kaiser Family Foundation/Harvard School of Public Health. 2001. *Post-Election Survey: The Public and the Health Care Agenda for the New Administration and Congress*. MenloPark, CA: Kaiser Family Foundation. January.

Kao, Audiey C., Diane C. Green, Nancy Davis, Jeffrey P. Koplan, and Paul D. Cleary. 1998. "Patients' Trust in Their Physicians: Effects of Choice, Continuity, and Payment Method." *Journal of General Internal Medicine* 13(10):681-686.

Kasperson, Roger E., Dominic Golding, and Seth Tuler. 1992. "Social Distrust as a Factor in Siting Hazardous Facilities and Communicating Risk." *Journal of Social Issues* 48(4):161-187.

Lipset, Seymour M. 1995. "Malaise and Resiliency in America." *Journal of Democracy* 6(3):4-18.

Lipset, Seymour M. and William Schneider. 1987. *The Confidence Gap: Business, Labor and Government in the Public Mind*. Baltimore: Johns Hopkins University Press.

Lubalin, James S. and Lauren D. Harris-Kojetin. 1999. "What do Consumers Want and Need to Know in Making Health Care Choices?" *Medical Care Research and Review* 56:67-102, Supplement 1.

Luhmann, Niklas. 1979. *Trust and Power*. New York: John Wiley.

Mechanic, David. 1996. "Changing Medical Organization and the Erosion of Trust." *Milbank Quarterly* 74(2):171-189.

Mechanic, David. 1997. "Managed Care as a Target of Distrust." *Journal of the American Medical Association* 277(22):1810-1811.

Mechanic, David. 1998a. "The Functions and Limitations of Trust in the Provision of Medical Care." *Journal of Health Politics, Policy and Law* 23(4):661-686.

Mechanic, David. 1998b. "Public Trust and Initiatives for New Health Care Partnerships." *Milbank Quarterly* 76(2):281-302.

Mechanic, David and Mark Schlesinger. 1996. "The Impact of Managed Care on Patients' Trust in Medical Care and Their Physicians." *Journal of the American Medical Association* 275(21):1693-1697.

Mechanic, David and Marsha Rosenthal. 1999. "Responses of HMO Medical Directors to Trust Building in Managed Care." *Milbank Quarterly* 77(3):283-303.

Mechanic, David and Sharon Meyer. 2000. "Concepts of Trust Among Patients with Serious Illness." *Social Science and Medicine* 51(5):657-668.

Mechanic, David, Donna D. McAlpine, and Marsha Rosenthal. 2001. "Are Patients' Office Visits with Physicians Getting Shorter?" *The New England Journal of Medicine* 344(3):198-204.

Misztal, Barbara A. 1996. *Trust in Modern Societies: The Search for the Bases of Social Order*. Cambridge: Polity Press.

Nye, Joseph S., Jr., Philip D. Zelikow, and David C. King, eds. 1997. *Why People Don't Trust Government*. Cambridge: Harvard University Press.

Parsons, Talcott. 1949. *The Structure of Social Action*. New York: Free Press.

Putnam, Robert D. 1993. *Making Democracy Work: Civic Traditions in Modern Italy*. Princeton: Princeton University Press.

Putnam, Robert D. 1995. "Bowling Alone: America's Declining Social Capital." *Journal of Democracy* 6(1):65-78.

Robinson, Sandra and Mollyann Brodie. 1997. "Understanding the Quality Challenge for Health Consumers: The Kaiser/AHCPR Survey." *Joint Commission Journal on Quality Improvement* 23(5):239-244.

Scott, Robert A., Linda H. Aiken, David Mechanic, and Julius Moravcsik. 1995. "Organizational Aspects of Caring." *Milbank Quarterly* 73(1):77-95.

The NewsHour with Jim Lehrer/Kaiser Family Foundation/Harvard School of Public Health. 2000. *National Survey*. September.

Thom, David H., Kurt M. Ribisl, Anita L. Stewart, Douglas A. Luke, The Stanford Trust Study Physicians. 1999. "Further Validation and Reliability Testing of the Trust in Physician Scale." *Medical Care* 37(5):510-517.

13

The Social and Moral Commitments of a Physician-Writer

Robert Klitzman

While I was a medical student, Robert Coles compiled a volume of William Carlos Williams' doctor stories, and wrote in an introduction that Williams "bring[s] to us ironies, paradoxes, inconsistencies, [and] contradictions" about medical work (Williams 1984)—all of which, I think, can enable a writer or a physician-writer to comment on social and moral issues he or she faces. Coles included in the volume an excerpt from Williams' autobiography that in some ways moved me more than the stories themselves. Recently, I went back and looked at these words again, and they seem as fresh and true to me today as they did then—fifteen years ago. Williams wrote:

> "...as a writer I have never felt that medicine interfered with me but rather...it was my very food and drink, the very thing which made it possible for me to write. Was I not interested in man? There the thing was, right in front of me. I could touch it, smell it...oh, I knew it wasn't for the most part giving me anything very profound, but it was giving me terms, basic terms with which I could spell out matters as profound as I cared to think of..."

In short, a physician-writer can comment on universal aspects of human life, beyond the world of medicine alone.

Williams continued, in a passage that I typed out during my internship and taped to the wall over my desk: "When at times we see through the welter of evasive or interested patter, when by chance we penetrate to some moving detail of a life, there is always time to bang out a few pages. The thing isn't to find the time for it—we waste hours everyday doing absolutely nothing at all—the difficulty is to catch the evasive life of the thing, to phrase the words in such a way that stereotype will yield a moment of insight. That is where the difficulty lies." Those insights, I think, are fundamentally social and moral—not just aesthetic.

In medical school and through internship and residency, I began writing short pieces of literary non-fiction about my experiences with patients, to make sense of the experiences—seeing patients get sick and die—and to help me keep my eyes beyond the scut work each day to the larger human themes with which I was ultimately involved.

I write partly to remember patients. As a medical student, many of them remained with me after they died. I recall the first time I tried to help resuscitate a patient. It was in the emergency room, and despite our efforts, the intern eventually "called the code" and the nurse "pronounced the patient." The physicians hurried away, leaving a few nurses and me with the body to clean up the bloodstained gauze pads, pull out the catheters and tracheal tube, and to tie a tag with the patient's name and chart number to his big toe. It was all too matter of fact for me. I couldn't just walk away. I wrote a story about what had happened—it ended up being one of the pieces in my first book, *A Year-long Night: Tales of A Medical Internship* (Klitzman 1989).

As an intern, my first patient was "Miss Steiner," a proud, feisty elderly woman who refused her medication, or to have blood drawn. She fought with me, yet afterwards, the other interns and I still referred to " Miss Steiner's Old Room," in remembrance of her. Another woman with a terminal disease battled with me daily over cold medicine and other mundane matters, fighting with me rather than yielding to the onslaught of her disease. Theirs were poignant stories, often of pain and courage, and I wrote them to remember them, to memorialize them—not to have them die.

Other patients struck me with the strength of their hope and faith—more than I often had at times. One woman came into the emergency room, having been picked up by the police after wandering the streets at 4 am in a nightgown, lost. She knew neither her name nor address nor had any identification on her. She had a severe expressive aphasia, probably from a stroke. She was still on our ward but we had no other treatment to provide her, and we didn't know what to do with her. There was nowhere to send her. She helped staff with simple mechanical chores such as tying rubber bands around laboratory order slips, and sat with patients who needed company.

She regained a few fragmented words. "Home...home..." she would say, grasping my arm. I cared for her, and then had to move on, too. As I said goodbye to her for the last time she looked up at me, and kissed me on the cheek—the first time a patient ever had. Her head shook. "Last..." she said. 'Last..."

"Last what?" I asked.

She didn't answer.

I wanted to remember her, too—not to let the story of her life pass with her—to be a witness. Eventually I learned her name, through some detective work, and she went to a nursing home. She has tried to escape several times, but remains there.

Similarly, during my residency in psychiatry, I found myself repeatedly astonished and sometimes appalled by what I saw. I found myself mediating conflicts between patients and their families, and between patients and myself, discharging or hospitalizing patients against their will, deciding to "make patients DNR"—ordering do not resuscitate in the event of cardiac or respiratory arrest. I wondered who I was in my twenties to be doing these things.

Each day, we debated at length with nurses over whether the door to the ward should be open or locked. The doctors, who had legal responsibility, preferred it to be locked. The nurses, who spent their whole day on the ward interacting with patients, preferred to have it open. I felt we were arguing over other things besides the door—over notions of freedom in patients' lives, and power over patients and between nurses and physicians. Yet we never spoke of these things directly.

My social conscience sometimes conflicted with my capacities as a physician—treating homelessness, confronting cutbacks, telling patients they could no longer be seen because their insurance coverage had run out. Over several hospitalizations, for example, I treated a man who had bone cancer and had become addicted to his pain medications. His family in Florida had kicked him out, and he was now homeless, sleeping on park benches or in shelters. Strangers regularly stole his money or his cane. When his coverage ran out, I had to kick him out into the street again, too. My supervisor told me to give him only the address of a shelter—which my patient already knew. He continued to come to the hospital occasionally as an outpatient. Then one day, he died—a possible overdose. A social worker called to invite me to a small funeral service being held at a neighborhood temple. From the agencies, shelters, soup kitchens, and hospitals my patient hobbled to, he had pieced together a support system for himself. Ironically, only now might he be given a resting place he never had when he was alive. Writing can make us and others—readers in and outside of medicine, including policymakers—more aware of the larger social issues he and others face.

The limitations in our knowledge often amazed me as well. I was disturbed about performing electroconvulsive therapy (ECT)—sedating a patient to unconsciousness, then pressing a little red button on "the black box," as it was called, and zapping electricity through his or her skull. No one knew how the treatment worked, but it somehow did. I was once again stunned by the power we had over patients' lives. Some patients agreed to ECT on the ward, but once in the ECT suite, seeing the machines, resisted. We had to persuade and cajole them. I was left confused by the power. Yet patients—paranoid and depressed to begin with—often ended up changed and grateful in the end. Still, the coercion carried a price. These rites of passage—of wielding subtle and not so subtle violence—charted our development as professionals, and increased awareness of them can help physicians and those in training avoid becoming aloof or distant. The "detached concern" about which Renée Fox (1988:51-77) and others have written—the right balance between detachment and concern—is hard to achieve and maintain day in and day out as stresses mount.

It can be difficult to separate personal from professional feelings and responses, and not let the two interfere with one another. A patient of mine with a borderline personality disorder, for example, kept cutting her wrist while on the ward, despite my efforts to help her. Then she called me up at night at home. She frustrated and angered me—raising "counter transference" issues. Other trainees complained of "borderlines" all the time. It is easy to become hardened. I wrote about these experiences to try to understand them, leading to my book *In a House of Dreams and Glass—Becoming a Psychiatrist* (1995). I sensed that if I was surprised by what I saw, others outside the profession would probably be as well. The techniques of novels and short stories enable a writer to capture the poignant and often subtle but telling details, revealed, for instance, in odd passing comments. Once late at night, a resident said to me, "something just came into the emergency room"—that is, a "thing."

Psychiatric supervisors accidentally referred to trainees as patients—all of which revealed underlying attitudes.

I have received numerous letters, phone calls, and emails from students who have read these two books, wondering if they should become doctors or psychiatrists. Others told me the books helped them navigate through difficult experiences with supervisors. Patients and family members have written to me that these books have helped them better understand doctors or therapists. Writing can also correct stereotypes in the media and elsewhere about patients and physicians. Too often, movies and novels portray psychiatrists, for example, as either charlatans or as wise sages or saints who can practically read minds and, in a few words, alter entire lives. The reality lies somewhere in between. Writing can enhance both public and professional education about medicine, both of which are vital.

The year I began medical school, 1981, also marked the beginning of the HIV epidemic. Through the course of my training I observed the complicated social and psychological as well as medical devastation caused by this disease. At least prior to 1996, and the widespread use of protease inhibitors, patients faced widespread death in their own lives, and in those around them. I began to interview them about their experiences, which became the basis of a book, *Being Positive: The Lives of Men and Women with HIV* (Klitzman 1997).

People with HIV still had hope, though researchers couldn't understand how or why. Interviewing patients and hearing their stories, I sensed answers. Patients spoke of lost dreams, lost life, losses of self, a sense of disintegration. Yet they also entered a larger social movement, "HIV land," as one patient called the HIV community, that gave them a vocabulary, words, and thus a framework, a sense of meaning and supports, more than doctors could offer. As one woman told me, "in my AIDS residence, I hang out only with the positive people. The negative people there bring me down." The negative people were angry and depressed. To be positive was to be upbeat, and was considered good. In HIV land, the valences of positive and negative become reversed.

Patients wondered "why me," and whether HIV was somehow their fate. They faced feelings of guilt over their lives, over sexual behavior or drug use, and searched for meaning. Again and again, what they talked about was the importance of spirituality in their lives, something doctors generally don't discuss.

One man, for example, told me how he prayed to St. Jude, the Saint of Hopeless Causes. He believed God would help him, despite what the Catholic Church said about his being gay; and he believed his former lover was in heaven, and spoke to him. "God isn't ready for me," he told me. "There will survivors in this epidemic, just as in war and the Holocaust. Other people bear their crosses, HIV is mine." The metaphors were not those of medicine. As physicians, we don't speak to patients about spirituality, but it was the central concern of patients themselves.

Writing can also reveal and reflect to us how we construct disease, and the assumptions we make.

Before attending medical school, I conducted fieldwork among the Stone Age Fore group in the Eastern Highlands of Papua New Guinea, studying the kuru epidemic. As I described in my book, *The Trembling Mountain: A Personal Account of Kuru, Cannibals and Mad Cow Disease* (1998), the Fore believed the disease was caused and could be cured by sorcery, while Western medicine believed the disease resulted from an infectious protein or prion transmitted through cannibalistic feasts. One day, my guides introduced me to a man who told me he could cure the disease. I wondered what I could possibly learn from him. He explained that he dispensed herbs, which I knew had been tested at the NIH and found to be ineffective. He uttered an incantation, and prescribed that for one week the patient was not to drink water, eat any salt, or touch a member of the opposite sex.

As the disease had wiped out most of the population in some areas, anyone with headaches, backaches, or minor pains now automatically feared they had kuru. These cases, which I labeled as misdiagnoses or hypochondriasis, presumably constituted his cures. Yet none of the patients whom I had diagnosed with the disease had responded to his treatment. Why then didn't he and the other Fore see a problem? I asked him. "Very simple," he responded. "They didn't follow my advice. They drank water or ate salt or touched a member of the opposite sex." In short, they were noncompliant. He blamed failures not on the treatment but on the patients. No one ever called the treatment itself into question.

The Fore believed kuru was caused by kuru stones. A sorcerer allegedly wrapped a possession belonging to his victim—a nail clipping or even a potato peeling—around a stone, and cast a spell on it. Such stones had been dug up and said to have caused disease. When

I explained that kuru resulted from a very small living thing, smaller than an insect, they asked to see it. I couldn't show it to them. They asked what it looked like. I said we weren't sure. "Had I seen it?"

"No."

They all laughed at me. "Kuru is caused by kuru stones," they said. "Besides, if you white men think you know what causes Kuru, why haven't you cured it? We've cured the disease. You haven't!"

When I returned to the U.S. and attended medical school, I began to hear similar arguments—treatment failures blamed on patients' poor compliance or low motivation. I saw treatments of dubious efficacy prescribed. Writing can provoke us to see ourselves and what we do more clearly.

I have tried to bring together techniques of literary non-fiction with sociological methods of participant observation. Good writers are good sociologists. A narrative approach to social and moral issues also follows from recent work in the social sciences, as in anthropology and the work of Clifford Geertz and others, using narrative and "thick description" to convey aspects of a culture otherwise missed. Narrative can enable us to enter the worlds of others, to see and become more sensitive to other points of view. Writing can give voice to patients who cannot speak.

Writing can serve, too, as an antidote to medicine's belief in its own empiricism—the need to find a right answer. Literature is about the absence of right answers—the ways people grapple with conflict, the ironies and suffering, and the prices paid for success. It addresses feelings, confusion, and pain absent from textbooks and peer reviewed journal articles, and can present not only the visible, but the invisible and unspoken.

The tradition of physician-writers is long: Rabelais, Chekhov, Arthur Schnitzler, William Carlos Williams, and the German poet Gottfried Benn, not to mention those who attended medical school at least briefly, such as James Joyce, Gertrude Stein, Somerset Maugham, and Walker Percy.

Yet tensions exist, too, between being a writer and being a physician. Problems arise—ethical and logistic—such as having time to do both. And maintaining at times dual perspectives, seeing events from contrasting viewpoints—wearing constant bifocals.

An important antidote is having mentors. I am very fortunate to have been a Robert Wood Johnson Foundation Clinical Scholar at the University of Pennsylvania, and to have worked closely with Renée Fox, who was that and much more. She has an extraordinary appreciation of, and sensitivity to, the shared language of patients, physicians, and poets, and her encouragement to explore these terrains has been vital to countless students and myself.

References

Fox, Renée C. 1998. *Essays In Medical Sociology.* New Brunswick, NJ: Transaction Publishers.

Klitzman, Robert. 1989. *A Year-long Night: Tales of a Medical Internship.* New York: Viking Press.

Klitzman, Robert. 1997. *Being Positive: The Lives of Men and Women With HIV.* Chicago: Ivan R. Dee, Inc.

Klitzman, Robert. 1995. *In a House of Dreams and Glass: Becoming a Psychiatrist.* New York: Simon and Schuster.

Klitzman, Robert. 1998. *The Trembling Mountain: A Personal Account of Kuru, Cannibals, and Mad Cow Disease.* New York: Plenum Trade.

Williams, William C. 1984. *The Doctor Stories.* NY: New Directions.

III

Bioethics, Sociology, and Medicine

14

Renée Fox, Human Experimentation, and Therapeutic Innovation: A Career of Values and Observations

Victor Lidz

One of Renée Fox's remarkable characteristics is the originality and insight of her empirical observation. She is constantly the ethnographic observer, whether in conducting formal research or in living everyday events. When she is not engaged in formal participant observation, she becomes what I have called an observing participant (Lidz 1991), examining the situations she accesses through her personal social roles. Her constant observation and interpretation of the surroundings is connected to the insightfulness of her formal research. As observing participant she rehearses for the role of participant observer. More deeply, however, she adds to the fund of personal experience that provides "working capital" for her discernment and sensitivity.[1]

My first encounter with Renée came some seven years before I met her in person. As a college junior in 1960, I took a first true course in sociology, titled simply "The General Theory of Action," with Talcott Parsons. For the reading period assignment, Parsons allowed each student to read one of several then-recent empirical studies carried out with the theory of action, and then report on it critically in response to a question on the final exam. I chose *Experiment Perilous*, Fox's first book (1959), and spent a memorable two days immersed in the world of research physicians and patients as they confronted the trials of extreme treatment regimens accepted as hoped-for alternatives to death. It was likely the first participant-observation study that I had read. The memory of being captivated by the human dilemmas it portrayed is still vivid.

Experiment Perilous established a mode of analysis that Fox has used in practically all of her writings and teaching. Her study was one of social change, namely, how clinical research develops new knowledge and creates grounds for changing medical practice. She focused mainly on the dynamic, ever-changing institutional complex of clinical research, then much smaller and simpler than today, yet the same in basic structure. Her analysis concentrated on *conflicts* between social values. A primary conflict was between the clinician-investigator's investment in developing new knowledge and the duty of all medical practitioners to care for patients as effectively as possible. The clinical investigators and the medical practitioners were, in the Ward F-Second of Fox's research, the same individuals, viewed as filling roles that were different but overlapped.

Tensions between the values of advancing knowledge and of caring for patients created stresses that each physician had to manage within himself or herself (Fox 1974, Introduction to Paperback Edition). All members of the staff reported experiencing dilemmas about the extent to which patients could be asked to participate in burdensome experimental protocols that might advance knowledge of their diseases, but were unlikely to help them as sick individuals. At times, when physician-investigators resolved these dilemmas in different ways, the tensions between the two underlying value-complexes created interpersonal as well as intrapersonal conflicts. Some members of the staff identified more strongly with the values of advancing knowledge, while others clung more strongly to those of patient care. Yet, all of the physician-investigators recognized the legitimacy of, and identified personally and professionally with, both sets of values. Tension and conflict were generated only about disagreements over the balances or relative priorities between the two value-complexes under the circumstances of particular study plans.

Clinical research, in Fox's treatment, drew legitimation for the privilege of employing risky procedures from both the investigational and the patient care value complexes. The physician-investigators, clinical staff, and, indeed, patients on Ward F-Second shared beliefs that research should improve clinical care and that investigational treatment should often benefit patients who received their medical care on the unit. The physician-investigators were acutely aware that the availability of patients with select metabolic disorders and the will to take part in research protocols created special opportunities for their research and, hence, careers. They were motivated to provide the best care and treatment possible, and the patients thus had reason to obtain treatment at this research center despite the discomforts and burdens of participating in its studies. Many patients held hopes—or shreds of hope—that Ward F-Second might achieve breakthroughs in the treatment of their conditions in time to save their lives. Others realized that there was virtually no chance that their lives would be saved by a quick breakthrough, but found personal meaning in facilitating research to save the lives of future patients.

In Fox's analysis, Ward F-Second was enlivened not only by brilliant minds and a distinguished record of innovation, but more deeply by the significant stress placed on the legitimating value-complexes of research and patient care. When study protocols failed, patients were subjected to burdensome or even painful procedures, or deaths occurred among favorite patients, and stress often pervaded the ward (Fox 1959, especially Chapters II to IV). In this environment it was routine for patients to die, but the deaths of some patients created greater stress. Patients who had earlier gained favorable results from investigational procedures or who had been outstanding in bearing up to the pains and discomforts of difficult protocols were particularly hard to lose. Their deaths were often especially burdensome for other patients as well as the nurses and physicians. Moreover, there were differences in the responses of the physicians. The fellows, other young physicians, and those who identified more strongly with the values of patient care felt losses more deeply. The senior physician-investigators tended to sustain a medical stoicism in the face of losses, even ones that were deeply felt. However, Ward F-Second maintained solidarity—among the medical staff, among patients, and between staff and patients—by reemphasizing commitments to the values of investigation and patient care in the face of losses and stress.

In Fox's discussion the clinician-investigator is an existentialist actor caught in moral dilemmas and trying to reach workable resolutions under trying circumstances. Doubt and uncertainty of outcomes condition every effort to resolve the dilemmas. The clinician-investigator strives to create knowledge that will help entire categories of patients in the long run, but must decide on research protocols for particular patients in the immediate setting. With uncertainty about the outcomes of a new protocol, how can the physician determine what burden of suffering can be imposed on patients to evaluate a new approach to treatment? What might be justified if the treatment provides a cure or at least months or years of melioration of an illness will not seem justifiable if the patient derives no benefit or is harmed. What about the burdens of new testing procedures? They may produce findings helpful in devising treatments for future patients, yet the knowledge may prove useless in care of the very patients who suffered the pains entailed in development of the new tests. Belief in the values of clinical investigation helps the physician to live through such dilemmas, while the values of patient care serve in these cases to limit what the physician may feel justified in undertaking.

The patient is also an existential actor trying to resolve moral dilemmas under conditions of doubt and uncertainty (Fox 1959, Chapter IV). The patients on Ward F-Second typically knew that they were facing courses of declining health, growing disability, and death in the short to moderate term future. In the face of dimming hopes for continued health and life, they, too, were supported by the values of investigational medicine. They took comfort in believing that "everything possible" was being done to care for them. Often they agreed to undergo arduous tests and treatments because the new procedures carried the meaning of "everything possible." Often they participated in investigational treatments out of vicarious identification with future patients who would be successfully treated for the same conditions. Thus, the patients, too, resolved their existential dilemmas and in some cases gained a sense of control over their declining conditions through profound identification with the values and culture of clinical investigation. They expected, believed in, and derived meaning for their remaining lives from medical progress. In some cases, patients adapted to their clouded futures by identifying deeply with their physicians, learning a great deal about their metabolic disorders, the chief strategies being pursued to develop new treatments, and the contributions of the Ward F-Second investigators.

Fox noted that the work of Ward F-Second also had broad cultural resonance (see especially Fox 1959, Chapter VIII). Some of the innovations developed on the ward were noted by the public as well as by the medical profession and patients with metabolic disorders. The press widely reported the first bilateral adrenalectomy followed by the administration of "miracle" drugs to sustain the patient. The transformation of a dangerous procedure into a life-preserving treatment received public celebration. In turn, the attention and celebration gave the investigators confirmation of the value of their work and thus reinforced their professional commitments. The special meaning of life-saving innovations within American popular culture and the impact of that meaning on the growing institutions of clinical research are themes that Fox has traced through the last fifty years of medical history.

Under the glare of intense publicity and widespread public acclaim, the late 1960s and early 1970s saw the emergence of "heroic" and "extraordinary" treatments now often seen as the prototypal procedures of modern, high-technology medicine (Fox and Swazey 1974). Kidney, liver, heart, and lung transplants, chronic dialysis, bone marrow transplants, the newer and more intensive forms of chemotherapy for various cancers, coronary artery bypass grafts, angioplasty and stenting for blocked coronary arteries, the procedures of microsurgery for repair of organs and the reattachment of severed limbs, and genetically engineered and reproduced medications have all been developed as successful treatments by, approximately, the last generation of clinical investigators. These highly technical procedures, requiring truly specialized practitioners to conduct them, have in key respects restructured medicine. The specialists who largely replaced the general practitioners in the first two-thirds of the twentieth century are in many areas of medicine now being replaced, or at least supplemented, by the subspecialists. General cardiology is giving way in part to specialties for reading echocardiagrams, conducting stress tests, performing angioplasties, etc. Specialists in ALS or MS have emerged in neurology, in HIV/AIDS, in infectious diseases, in bone marrow transplantation, in hematology-oncology, in Hepatitis B or C, in gastroenterology, and so forth.

Renée Fox and her colleague, Judith Swazey, have together devoted over thirty years to chronicling and analyzing some of the most dramatic developments in this transformation of medicine. Their books, *The Courage to Fail: A Social View of Organ Transplants and Dialysis* (1974, 1978) and *Spare Parts: Organ Replacement in American Society* (1992), carry forward the mode of analysis that

Renée developed in *Experiment Perilous*. We find in the newer works the same emphasis on the values of clinical investigation and patient care and a similar highlighting of the existential dilemmas involved in investigational patient care. From the era of *Experiment Perilous*, through the periods of *The Courage to Fail* and *Spare Parts*, to the present, investigational medicine, though it has grown immensely more sophisticated and specialized, adheres to the same institutional and evaluative foundations and presents the same existential problems for the clinical innovator. As the title *The Courage to Fail* underscores, existential courage is needed to risk failure when patient lives are at stake. Such courage is needed by patients and their families as fully as by the physician, as demonstrated in the case studies of *The Courage to Fail*. Yet, some clinician investigators can have an excess of this virtue. As shown by the first attempts to implant artificial hearts, courage that overrides the need for thorough preparation and realistic assessment of barriers to success can result in premature ventures, tragic error, and painful failure (Fox and Swazey 1974, Chapter 7; Fox and Swazey 1992, Chapter 5).

The Courage to Fail differs from *Experiment Perilous* in underscoring vulnerabilities of the institutions of investigational medicine. The early phases of transplant surgery, particularly of heart transplantation, emerged under a glare of publicity that was unprecedented in the history of medicine. The judgment that some surgeons exercised in planning early transplants was affected by the public and professional acclaim, instant fame, and adulation they received and by the prospects, in a competitive environment, for attracting the funds to develop large and prominent institutes. A race to be first with new procedures emerged, and then to be among the largest and most famous centers conducting them. A star system followed, supported by medical schools and hospitals that sought to secure their own prominence as well as vast new resources by capitalizing on the fame of leading transplant surgeons. Several surgeons emerged as charismatic figures who ventured, at times with Faustian boldness, upon transplant procedures that were unlikely to achieve frequent success until better means of controlling the rejection process were developed. Fox and Swazey (1974, 1992) show that in several cases the innovators' personal decision-making and the collective decision-making of their medical teams went beyond courage to injudicious optimism. The case of the Jarvik 7 artificial heart and the patient Barney Clark was perhaps the most egregious instance of a highly publicized, intensely dramatic, but inadequately prepared surgical venture (Fox and Swazey 1992, Chapter 5).

In several fields, including kidney, cardiac, and liver transplantation and chronic hemodialysis, initial boldness was followed by a moratorium. High rates of failure suggested that caution needed to replace courage until such technical problems as rejection of transplanted organs could be resolved. Fox has been particularly interested in the phenomenon of a moratorium because it represents the collective and institutional decision that a justifiable balance of innovation and quality of patient care cannot in the immediate future be achieved (Swazey and Fox, "The Clinical Moratorium" in Fox 1979). It imposes a halt on a type of procedure because of a shared understanding that harm to patients is sufficiently certain that the possibility of gaining new knowledge cannot justify use of the procedure. A moratorium also shifts the burden of proof to the investigator who proposes the restart of a procedure to demonstrate that a new development has improved the chances for favorable outcomes. In transplant surgery, the advent of cyclosporine proved to be the development that changed the outlook on patient outcomes and ended the moratoria. As Fox and Swazey show in the first chapter of their 1992 book, cyclosporine, a medical rather than surgical innovation, transformed the era of *The Courage to Fail* into the era of *Spare Parts*.

The moratoria of the 1970s also dampened much of the publicity and cultural fervor that attended "heroic" procedures. Although extraordinary publicity and widespread glorification had attended the early transplant procedures, there had also been an undercurrent of confusion about, distrust of, and opposition to such radical procedures. Some of the negative reactions derived from religious concerns over tampering with life-giving organs, particularly the heart, which in cultural terms was viewed, beyond being a physiologically active organ, as an essence of individual life (Fox 1979: 115-121). The emergence in the late 1960s of the criteria of "brain death" that permitted the harvesting of organs for transplantation from patients who were breathing and had pumping hearts, still circulating blood, but who were deemed to be medically dead, occasioned much negative public reaction. Fears were voiced that some patients might be declared dead for the convenience of transplant surgeons or to benefit richer patients who could afford transplant operations. Other reactions to early attempts at transplants addressed the high rate of failure, the apparent suffering of the patients, and the enormous resources devoted to the care of small numbers of profoundly ill persons, even as the country's system of medical care devoted too few resources to basic and inexpensive public health measures (Parsons, Fox, and Lidz, 1974; Lidz 1984). The moratoria showed the public that thoughtful medical judgment was being exercised. The public was reassured that the well being of patients would not be sacrificed to procedures with little chance of success, that innovation would go forward only when qualified specialists collectively judged that the opportunities for success were reasonable, and that the star system and the charisma of a small number of star physicians would not be permitted to undermine the regulatory aspects of medical institutions.

Reassuring as the moratoria were for both the medical profession and the public, the later 1970s saw the emergence of a new mechanism of regulation and social control for clinical research (Fox 1979, Parts VI and VII). The vast growth of the system of clinical research, the public unease regarding care for patients under investigational protocols, and the increasing proportions of clinical research supported by the National Institutes for Health and other federal agencies together resulted in a system of Institutional Review Boards (IRBs) and, for many studies, Data Safety Monitoring Boards, to conduct formal, collective, and documented review of federally funded clinical research and, indeed, nearly all organized research with living human subjects. Over the past thirty years, the system of formal review to protect the interests and well being of human subjects has grown into a vast complex of institutions. It now encompasses a core set of ethical guidelines, such as the Belmont Report (National Commission for the Protection of Human Subjects of Biomedical and Behavioral Research 1979); thick and growing volumes of research regulations in the Code of Federal Regulations; first hundreds and now thousands of local IRBs at universities, hospitals, agencies of state and local government, research institutes, and social service agencies; thousands of institutional administrative offices keeping track of review documentation; and, hardly least, vast effort on the part of tens of thousands of investigators and study coordinators who prepare the protocol documents, including consent materials, that they are required to submit for IRB review.

To the surprise of some, the IRBs have not had a peaceful history. They were originally established with the idea that they would operate within the cultures of their local institutions and communities, applying locally defined and codified standards for protection of patients and other human subjects. Soon, however, the federal regulations set forth to define essential terms and elements of the review system, such as clinical research, human subjects, the duties of IRBs, the proper and necessary processes of review, and classes of subjects requiring special protection (e.g., children, pregnant women, prisoners, the mentally disabled), began to grow. The assurance documents through which local institutions obtain federal approval from the Department of Health and Human Services (DHHS) for their IRB policies and procedures became ever more standardized. The authority of IRBs, their procedures, their formal guidelines for the conduct of research with human subjects, and the standards of review that they impose on research generally became restatements or paraphrases of applicable sections of the Code of Federal Regulations. Most of the assurances began to specify that IRB review and standards of protection for human subjects would extend not only to federally funded research, but to all human subjects research conducted by institutions that accept federal research funds.

Over the past several years, the office in DHHS that supervises IRB operations has greatly increased both the number and the stringency of its site visits to research institutions. Several leading research universities and medical schools have had harsh sanctions imposed on them for failure to fulfill the terms of their assurances to DHHS for protection of human subjects. In some highly publicized cases involving leading centers of biomedical research, including Duke University and Johns Hopkins University, the sanctions have included a formal halt to all ongoing studies until shortcomings have been fixed. In most of the cases in which major institution-wide sanctions have been imposed, notably at Duke University, the shortcomings identified by federal officials have not involved the quality of judgment exercised by the IRBs themselves, but the failure of institutional officials to provide the administrative support needed to operate thorough review processes. Yet, IRBs across the country are at present acutely aware that their policies, procedures, and reviews are under federal scrutiny by officials who are skeptical of the quality of their work and empowered to stop research at their institutions if site visits were to uncover evidence of inadequately supervised studies.

IRBs have also faced controversy within their institutions. Academic IRBs in particular have drawn nearly constant criticism for seeming to restrict the investigational freedoms of faculty members. Many faculty members, particularly in the humanities and social sciences, regard freedom of investigation as closely akin to freedom of speech and conscience, and hence resent any limitations imposed on it. Faculties in clinical fields, by contrast, are more likely to perceive review of investigational protocols as akin to the supervision they receive for all clinical work. Their complaints about IRBs focus less on the principle of review than on the detailed requirements regarding elements of the protocols and consent documents that they must submit for review and on the levels of review to which their studies are subjected. To clinical faculties, the packages of documentation they must submit for review appear to grow exponentially in volume, the number of required forms, the standard elements that should be described in each protocol, the exacting verbal formulae that must appear in consent forms, and, hardly the least problematic, the time consumed between submitting materials and receiving permission to initiate studies. Members of IRBs feel an unrelenting heat of implicit if not explicit criticism from their colleagues, a heat that is especially bothersome when it comes from esteemed investigators. Not infrequently, IRB members feel pressure from heads of clinical services, department chairs, and even chief administrators to expedite the review of scientifically or budgetarily important research. IRB members learn that their efforts to maintain focus on the central purpose of protecting human subjects from inappropriate risk of harm are often complicated by other issues entailed in the review of certain types of protocols. Such issues include protecting their institutions and individual investigators from risk of legal suit; making sure that their institutions do not accept statements of liability for harm to high risk subjects (e.g., terminal cancer patients receiving experimental medications known to be toxic as last resort therapies); smoothing the way for doctoral students to conduct dissertation studies; creating records to document that reviews of high risk protocols have been thorough; and facilitating the progress of scientifically promising investigations and studies. Depending on how they are managed, issues of these kinds may distract the review process from a proper focus on protection of human subjects or may give it valuable depth and nuance.

In my experience, IRB members try to maintain a balance between diffidence about the risk of infringing on the investigational freedoms of colleagues and a conviction that thorough protection of human subjects requires firm exercise of IRB authority. One need not serve on a medical school IRB for very long before one encounters protocols that raise concerns: surgical studies that propose to implement high risk procedures with little preparation for handling inevitable adverse outcomes; medical studies that would withdraw patients from standard medications and assign some of them to placebos in order to evaluate an experimental drug given to the others; psychiatric studies that include no methodical procedure for assessing the ability of schizophrenic patients to provide genuinely informed consent; criminal justice studies that do not take into account the coercive settings of probation or parole offices in which they solicit the participation of subjects; or social scientific studies that do not plan to inform subjects in advance that interviews will include personal and sensitive questions about their sex lives, criminal acts, or dependence on illicit drugs. The energy with which IRB members impose rigorous standards of review is typically rooted in the experience of having protected patients or other subjects from initial research plans that include serious risks to health and well being or the principle that participation in research should be fully voluntary.

The vast majority of studies are approved once a number of fixes have been made to planned procedures and consent documents. The high proportion of successful fixes indicates that, despite tensions, there is generally an effective working relationship between investigators and IRB members, who, in many cases, are the same individuals in different social roles. However, nearly every experienced member of an active IRB has a number of "war stories" to tell about the dangerous or insensitive protocols that unthinking colleagues had planned to implement. Reciprocally, investigators too have "war stories." Their stories concern studies delayed for months over minutiae of indemnification agreements with sponsors, protocols lost in the complex administrative shuffling of paperwork, or disputes over the words a consent form uses to describe risks of a study, provisions in case subjects are injured, or alternative treatments available to patients who decline to participate in research (most of whom will never be shown the consent form).

Fox's writings, from *Experiment Perilous* to *Spare Parts*, enable us to understand why medical IRBs, their procedures, and members are subjected to so much stress and conflict. IRBs in clinical institutions have jurisdiction over the points of conflict between the values of therapeutic innovation and the values of clinical care for patients. The difficult, stressful, and chronic issues of ethical judgment that she identified in *Experiment Perilous* are in the contemporary medical institution often aired in the forum of the IRB meeting. Of course, IRBs do not and cannot monopolize thought or ethical expertise regarding the limits of medical innovation and research. All investigators and many non-investigators with important roles in clinical services have their thoughts and expectations about these issues, often ones created without the burdens of decision-making that weigh on IRBs. The fact that ideas and expectations about freedom of investigation and the ethical responsibilities of clinical researchers are strongly held by nearly every participant in the modern medical institution—from senior faculty to house staff, from hospital administration to ICU nurses, from patients to their anxious family members—adds unavoidable stress to the IRB's relationships with its many constituencies.

It is common for IRB members and administrators today to refer condescendingly and sometimes disbelievingly to clinical research conducted before the era of IRBs as completely unregulated. They often speak of "wild and woolly" times before there were any protections for human subjects. Fox's research documents that this is a false characterization. There was regulation—not infallible, though generally effective—but it relied far more heavily on informal institutionalization of ethical standards. Investigators as individuals or in small groups had to balance the values of scientific innovation against the values of patient care in their own consciences and act accordingly. In difficult situations, they might consult chiefs of services, senior colleagues, associate deans for research, or their own counterparts at other medical centers, but they generally did so without any formal obligation.

In my own judgment, and from my personal experience as a research subject in the informal era[2] and a researcher and IRB member today, it is not apparent that the former system was less effective than the current system. To be sure, there were monumental lapses—most infamously, the Tuskegee syphilis study, due in large degree to the racism of the era. Other famous lapses, such as the CIA's experimentation with LSD on uninformed subjects, and the Defense Department's experimentation on the effects of radiation from atomic weapons using enlisted men under orders to participate, would likely have escaped formal human subjects review even if the present system had existed then. In general, the informal system appears to have been quite effective, given the smaller volume of research conducted forty or fifty years ago. However, it does not follow that the mechanisms of IRB review are not essential today. With the far greater volume and more rapid pace of research, it seems all but certain that informal procedures for the protection of human subjects would fail to prevent myriads of significant ethical lapses.

Although, among sociologists, Renée Fox has been the leading researcher of investigational medicine and high technology medical care, she has not been its apologist. It is true that her profiles of several outstanding innovators, for example, Norman Shumway, Denton Cooley, or Thomas Starzl, have highlighted their charismatic qualities and been interpreted by others as predominantly favorable (Fox and Swazey 1974).[3] However, she has consistently emphasized the need to maintain social control over the enormously complicated processes of medical innovation. Moreover, she has in particular attended to the special difficulties of making social control effective when it must limit the activities of prominent, self-confident, charismatic innovators who are extremely influential within their own medical centers. The penultimate chapter of *Spare Parts* bears the classic title "Who Shall Guard the Guardians?" but attention to that issue runs throughout Fox's writings. Moreover, she has consistently raised the issue of whether heroic procedures that consume large quantities of resources in treating the desperately ill are wise or ethical investments for a society that, despite its wealth, fails to provide basic primary care for substantial portions of its population (Fox 1979, Parts VI and VII; Fox and Swazey 1992). Why has American society and its system of medical care and research tolerated a growth over the past twenty years in what Fox and Swazey call "medical indigence" (Fox and Swazey 1992, Chapter 8)? In what ways are the heroic successes of medical innovation linked to the failure to improve health care for the medically indigent?

Fox has shown more richly than any other social scientist that it is not possible to understand the direction, focus, or concerns of research medicine without examining the broad cultural contexts in which the value-conflicts between investigation and patient care are played out. Part of her demonstration has rested on comparative analyses of medical science in the United States and in Belgium, where she conducted studies over some thirty years (Fox 1979, Part IV; Fox 1994). Belgium is a modern society and provides up-to-date medical care for its citizens, but has not been an innovator in the heroic procedures that have been so prominent in American medical research and has been far slower to adopt heroic measures in the years since they have become proven treatments. Belgium is not only smaller than the U.S., but it also invests smaller portions of its national economic resources in medical care. Yet, such measures as life expectancy show that in overall medical care of its citizenry Belgium achieves similar results to the U.S. Moreover, it has progressed further in overcoming medical indigence and has done so with comparatively modest investment of resources.

The different balances between medical innovation and equalizing access to medical care in Belgium and the U.S. are consequences of their respective value systems. American social values are highly individualistic and entrepreneurial, whereas Belgian values give priority to a variety of particularistic solidarities (Fox 1979, Part IV). In Belgium, there is comfort—for political leaders, for medical practitioners, and for the citizenry—if quality care is available to the members of the particular group (ethnic, religious, linguistic, class-based, or local) with which an individual identifies. Through a complex political balancing act among particularistic groups, care has been made reasonably accessible to all. In the U.S., by contrast, cultural resonance gives special meaning to the heroic procedures. American culture is fascinated by the charismatic and entrepreneurial innovators who developed them. It has also been fascinated by the drama of the gravely ill or injured person's struggle with death. Death is often viewed as defeat, and hence special evaluative significance is attributed to the use of all possible resources to master or stave off death (Parsons and Lidz 1967). Use of heroic measures to overcome death has become more and more thoroughly routinized. Investment in the capacity to provide what were once extraordinary measures, such as heart, liver, and kidney transplants, has grown rapidly. By contrast, investment in low technology measures to protect health, such as smoking cessation programs, primary care for the entire population, or balanced nutritional education, languishes. Aside from specialized and politically isolated discussions of public health, measures of the latter type rarely figure in the public's or the medical profession's conception of "best" medical care. Our leading medical centers are uniformly the ones that provide a wide array of high technology procedures, but only inconsistently the ones that invest heavily in comprehensive care for their local communities. Even with public debate over patients' rights and ineffective health insurance mechanisms, the medically indigent do not figure prominently in planning for improved medical institutions. Any plan of insurance to secure access to medical care for the citizenry at large continues to be viewed as tainted by anti-individualistic socialism. Health maintenance organizations and other health insurers come under attack whenever they try to limit subscribers' access to any form of care, even unproven experimental treatments or extraordinary procedures that have shown little benefit.

I offer two brief conclusions to this discussion of Renée Fox's writings and teachings. One pertains to the implications of her work for general sociology, the other more specifically to the social scientific understanding of medical institutions.

First, the conventional wisdom in sociology has held for a generation that any focus on values will bias research and understanding against the all-important phenomena of conflict, change, and dynamic forces. A focus on values is claimed to lead inexorably to an emphasis on stability and consensus. Fox's writings and teachings demonstrate that just the opposite is true. Study of commitment to values requires attention to limits on their implementation. It requires attention to the boundary or borderline situations in which other value commitments predominate. It thus entails consideration of tradeoffs and conflicts between or among distinct value-complexes, as in the case of the limited but sometimes fateful conflicts between the values of medical investigation and the values of medical care. The study of conflict among values also leads directly into the domain of existential moral or ethical judgment and, with it, the domains of feeling, affect, and emotion. Fox's writings show that this dynamic approach addresses institutional change in a truly insightful way. The reader who compares the institutionally simple world of clinical research on Ward F-Second, the era of heroic innovations analyzed in *The Courage to Fail*, and the medical institutions described in *Spare Parts* will see an exceptionally powerful and insightful portrayal of social change.

Second, two and three decades ago, one often heard the criticism that Fox's writings were concerned only with rarified settings of high technology biomedical research. They described doctors who were an elite of innovative practitioners at leading medical centers and their patients. It was argued that they had little application to the settings in which ordinary patients receive care and treatment from everyday physicians. True as this may have seemed in past decades, changes in medical institutions have made Fox's research more broadly applicable to the routines of care and treatment. Many of the procedures about which she wrote thirty, twenty, and ten years ago, for example, heart valve replacements, coronary artery bypass grafts, chronic renal dialysis, bone marrow, kidney, liver, and heart transplants, and complex strategies of chemotherapy for cancers, are now routinely provided services.

The physicians who conduct these procedures remain elites in the profession of medicine, but are no longer rare charismatic figures breaking with accepted standards of practice. There are now many of them and they are thoroughly trained subspecialists, organized in national associations, working within well-defined medical roles, and adhering to refined standards of practice. They continue further to refine standards of practice, often invoking an ideal of evidence-based medicine, and a large expansion in the volume of high technology research has resulted. The quantity and scale of studies, complexity of protocols, and numbers of collaborating medical centers have all grown vastly. A consequence has been a need to enroll many more patients and therefore integrate research more closely with the routines of medical care and treatment.

The ethical dilemmas of clinical investigation have, as a result, become matters large proportions of medical professionals, hospitals, clinics, medical schools, and patients face frequently and even routinely. The emergence of IRBs and other regulatory institutions has been closely bound up with these developments. Ethical issues that seemed rarified on Ward F-Second are today experienced on a very large scale. Renée Fox's analyses of the enduring ethical dilemmas and conflicts of clinical investigation are thus an increasingly salient resource for understanding contemporary medical reasoning and practice.

Notes

1. I recall the occasion some thirty years ago when I was first struck by one of the ways Renée's observations related to her personal experience. In the summer of 1971, our former teacher and colleague Talcott Parsons arranged a get-together for the three of us to plan the essay that became "The Gift of Life and Its Reciprocation" (Parsons, Fox, and Lidz 1972). My wife and I were coming east from Chicago in late July to show off our baby daughter to family and friends. Talcott and his wife, Helen, were on vacation at their farm in New Hampshire, and Renée met Talcott in Cambridge during one of his visits to his office and drove up to the farm with him for a few days' stay. My wife, Katharine, our five-week-old daughter, Liberty, and I arrived at the Parsons' farm around 10:00 a.m. Talcott, Renée, and I worked in Talcott's small study for a few hours on a sunny and very warm morning, reviewing ideas for the paper, planning the sequence in which they should be presented, and deciding who would draft what parts. As we finished our discussion, Helen announced lunch in the garden. Soon we were sitting at a redwood picnic table in the partial shade of an umbrella of trees. My wife had put the baby on her small sheepskin blanket on the grass near the table. As we ate and talked, Liberty was lying on her stomach and trying to lift her head to watch us. We were deeply engaged in conversation, but Renée suddenly said, "Look how hard Liberty is working to keep her head up! I know how hard it is for her. You have all forgotten, but I can remember how difficult it is to learn to hold one's head up."

   Renée was referring to her own rehabilitation from the bulbar poliomyelitis she had contracted when a college student. She had relearned basic motor skills and bodily controls as a young adult, and therefore had specific memories of the difficulties involved. The others of us had learned such basic skills two years or so before, consolidating the mental schemas necessary for organized memory. What struck me then was that Renée was able to use her experience following polio as a basis for empathetically understanding what Liberty was doing in a manner that simply did not occur to the rest of us.

   So I have found Renée Fox's insight over the years acutely observed and empathetic to her subjects, often in dimensions that do not occur to others. Whether in her writings, in discussions among colleagues, in the classroom, or simply in telephone conversation, her observations often express a distinctive understanding of others, even as compared with the views of other distinguished social scientists or medical researchers. Her understanding has been especially important in elucidating the respective burdens of patients and investigators in the situation of research medicine as it has evolved over the past fifty years. Like her observations of my daughter, this understanding has often been rooted in her own long and arduous experiences as a patient. However, other dimensions of her personal experience are also involved. Often she speaks in the voice of one who has conducted fieldwork in the midst of the post-colonial Congolese civil wars of the 1960s, or one who studied sociology in Harvard's interdisciplinary Department of Social Relations at the peak of its creativity, or one who followed the early development of transplant surgery in close connection with its several charismatic founders (Fox 1979, Introduction). She converts personal experience of all kinds into a ground of interpersonal understanding.

2. When an undergraduate, I was a subject of psychological research conducted in 1959-62 at Harvard University by Henry A. Murray and protégés that is often mentioned as a study involving deception and stress that IRBs would likely not approve in the current system of review. It is briefly described in Robinson (1992: 337-338) and was recently criticized in the popular press by Chase (2000). In no discussion I have read or heard has the care with which study participants were debriefed and supported for a few hours after the stressful events been acknowledged—nor has the individual attention that each subject received from Murray himself and his co-investigators over the three-year period of the study. Although current IRB standards provide new protections, I have not seen a contemporary experimental design that includes development of close and supportive relationships between subjects and investigators comparable to Murray's practice.
3. Judith Swazey has reminded me that she and Renée Fox removed the chapter "A Sociological Portrait of the Transplant Surgeon" from the second edition of *The Courage to Fail* (Fox and Swazey 1978) because of the misinterpretation it received from many readers.

References

Chase, Alston. 2000. "Harvard and the Making of the Unabomber." *Atlantic Monthly*, June.

Fox, Renée C. 1979. *Essays in Medical Sociology: Journeys into the Field*. New York: Wiley- Interscience.

Fox, Renée C. 1959. *Experiment Perilous: Physicians and Patients Facing the Unknown.* Glencoe, IL: Free Press.

Fox, Renée C. 1974 (paperback edition). *Experiment Perilous: Physicians and Patients Facing the Unknown.* Philadelphia: University of Pennsylvania Press.

Fox, Renée C. 1994. *In the Belgian Chateau: The Spirit and Culture of a European Society in an Age of Change.* Chicago: Ivan R. Dee.

Fox, Renée C. and Judith P. Swazey. 1974. *The Courage to Fail: A Social View of Organ Transplants and Dialysis.* Chicago: University of Chicago Press; 2nd edition, revised, 1978.

Fox, Renée C. and Judith P. Swazey. 1992. *Spare Parts: Organ Replacement in American Society.* New York: Oxford University Press.

Lidz, Victor. 1984. "Community and Medical Institutions in America." *Listening: Journal of Religion and Culture*, 19 (2): 128-142.

Lidz, Victor. 1991. "The Sense of Identity in Jewish-Christian Families." *Qualitative Sociology*, 14 (1): 77-102.

National Commission for the Protection of Human Subjects of Biomedical and Behavioral Research. April 18, 1979. "The Belmont Report; Ethical Principles and Guidelines for the Protection of Human Subjects of Research." *Federal Register.*

Parsons, Talcott, Renée C. Fox, and Victor Lidz. 1972. "The Gift of Life and its Reciprocation." *Social Research*, 39: 367-415.

Parsons, Talcott and Victor Lidz. 1967. "Death in American Society," pp. 133-170 in *Essays in Self-Destruction*, edited by E. Schneidman. New York: Science House.

Robinson, Forrest G. 1992. *Love's Story Told: A Life of Henry A. Murray*. Cambridge, MA: Harvard University Press.

15

Religious Sources for Debates in Bioethics

Jonathan B. Imber

What remains of trust in doctors owes its contemporary force to two remarkable inheritances: from Protestant deliberations on character, office, and profession; and from Catholic reflections on medically and morally complex cases.[1] Both Protestant and Catholic inheritances have been recycled in ways that make their more specific historical identities now difficult to recognize. An historically Protestant insistence that manner always reveals motive has only cynical appeal in an era in which the big stakes are on the manner of delivery of services and related economic motives. Physicians are more uncertain today about the meaning of their vocation, despite immense scientific and technological progress, because their authority is no longer what it once was, either personally or culturally.

The idea of vocation, in its post-Protestant expression, has been gradually effaced, leaving only traces of embattled conscience, psychologized as stress. A strong determination to give the medical career a solid professional and business foundation, in what came to be called by the middle of the twentieth century medical economics, paralleled professional efforts to publicize the physician as caring and competent. At the American Medical Association meetings in San Francisco in 1950, Louis de Rochemont's documentary film, "M.D.—The U.S. Doctor," debuted, the first of a new series known as "The Reader's Digest on the Screen." Described in the pages of *The Journal of the American Medical Association*, the 39-minute film "depicts the state of the nation's health by reviewing medical progress, tracing the education required for a physician, highlighting the work and interests of the American Medical Association, revealing how research surges onward and describing the life of a rural practitioner" (*JAMA* 1950:746). Publicity was rapidly to become the major strategy for maintaining the "public image" of the profession.

Along with efforts to maintain better public relations, administrative leaders in medicine recognized how the problem in communicating medical progress was related to the explosion in information that made such progress possible. When *Current Medical Digest* published its first issue in October 1933, its editor, Samuel M. Wagaman, described an image of doctoring that seventy years later requires little qualification: "Busy practitioners, with insistent demands upon their time, have little opportunity to select or the facility in translation of such literature as is essential to familiarity with the trend of contemporary medical thought" (Wagaman 1933:9). The idea that doctors were overwhelmed by the growth of knowledge influenced the profession's approach to communicating its goals to the public. The power of the AMA was not simply economic but also decisively cultural, aiding the profession in gaining the public trust for a considerable period of time.

Beneath these multiple layers of scientific and professional growth, new calls to the physician's conscience were raised among a generation of physicians—largely white, male, and Protestant—who took for granted that they were trusted by virtue of their professionalism as much as by their demonstration of skill. The medical profession's moral authority, that is, its capacity to be morally persuasive either individually or collectively, was undermined by various cultural and legal challenges that marked the 1960s and that led to a general decline in expectation about the physician's duty with respect to ever more intimate matters. A revival of the form of Catholic casuistry of the past—pastoral medicine—appeared coincident with a spiritual exhaustion in the meaning of the physician's career.[2] But in the afterlife of the admonitory traditions of Christian morality, the casuistical content was literally reinvented.

The Protestant Decline in Moral Authority

By the middle of the twentieth century, the physician's vocation found its post-Protestant vernacular in the professional focus on the "medical career," leaving little of the Protestant and admonitory inheritance about individual character as part of the meaning of that career. The long-standing assumption that the 1950s were a peaceful prelude to the disruptive 1960s cannot be maintained with respect to the types of challenges that were already forming in the larger society soon after the Second World War over such matters as sexual mores. Oliver Wendell Holmes's *Elsie Venner* (1869), which a century earlier had exposed the tensions between religious and medical authorities in New England, was superseded by a new and more vivid contrast between individual and community authority over matters of privacy and rights. Grace Metalious's best-selling novel, *Peyton Place* (1956), another New England "exposé," titillated while it subverted the authority of community over and against the rights of individuals.

To be effective, Metalious's lowbrow mocking of moral hypocrisy required a central figure in authority, who, not coincidentally, was the town doctor, Dr. Matthew Swain. Faced first with the decision of whether to perform an abortion for his patient, who is accused of killing her stepfather who raped her, Dr. Swain must then breach confidentiality in order to avert a harsh verdict against her. In the 1957 film by the same name, the physician is placed at the center of the drama's conclusion. Dr. Swain's righteous indignation over the community's unwillingness to face up to its gossip-ridden, rumor-mongering ways, is the only celebrated form of condemnation in the entire film. The legacy of Puritan hypocrisy was at last exposed and exhausted, and the physician was appointed the guardian of the community's conscience. The busy-bodies of Peyton Place were no longer, even ostensibly, the guardians of moral rectitude, but were instead depicted as the suppressers of and whisperers about uglier treacheries, including abuse, rape, and abortion. In the impending era of sexual liberation, the resort to abortion, the exposing of abuse and rape, and the fights against sexual discrimination and harassment would all supplant an earlier reticence, later condemned as a form of denial, about such matters.

The seeming inevitability of those changes can be illustrated in the deeper binds in which the guardians of moral rectitude found themselves when challenged by the dual powers of the marketplace and of a citizenry made restless by the alleged hypocrisies of social and sexual conventions. After its release in paperback, *Peyton Place* was banned in the state of Rhode Island. In 1963, The United States Supreme Court ruled against the Rhode Island Legislature's empowering of a Commission "to educate the public concerning any book...or other thing containing obscene, indecent or impure language, or manifestly tending to the corruption of the youth as defined [in other sections] and to investigate and recommend the prosecution of all violations of said sections" (*Bantam Books v. Sullivan* 1963). The Rhode Island Commission had been given no specific authority to prosecute, but the Court's majority, reversing the opinion of the Rhode Island State Supreme Court, left the clear impression that the Commission's power to intimidate was unacceptable.

Concurring in the result brought by the majority, Associate Justice Tom C. Clark observed that the legal challenge had been the result of "certain inept phrases in the notices sent out by the Commission" about obscene materials. He criticized the Court for dropping a "demolition bomb on 'the Commission's practice' without clearly indicating what might be salvaged from the wreckage" (*Bantam Books, Inc. v. Sullivan* 1963). Clark's observation was poignant in its implications about the Commission's authority to denounce a book as distinct from any power to curtail and prosecute the distribution of materials deemed harmful to the young. The Rhode Island Commission's feeble and ill-guided attempts to address profound changes in American mores were decisively resisted, setting the stage for further judicial rulings, for example, on prayer and abortion, that would challenge the authority and effectiveness of public institutions and professions. In effect, the high post-Protestant authority of the Supreme Court paralleled the popular art of Grace Metalious: both were condemning the efforts to condemn in the old way. The admonitory function of cultural and legal elites was inverted, assigning blame to the accusers rather than to those accused. This inversion had implications for the role that physician judgment would play in what were deemed to be more matters of public morals than medical expertise.

The collective efforts at stemming the tide of alleged indecency were symptoms of, rather than solutions to, the emerging problems of authority in a host of moral matters that no longer seemed as clear as they once had under the Protestant dispensations of character and culture. The idealizations of personal character and public culture could not withstand the powerful assaults from above and below out of which arose a nonjudgmental, if not purely relative, standard about individual moral conduct. The declining significance of Protestant authority, exemplified in the caricaturing of an older Protestant judgmental authority, created a vacuum of sorts within specific institutions and professions. Medical economics, which represented by the mid-twentieth century the exhaustion of the inheritance of Protestant insistence about the links between character and conduct, was easily caricatured as blatant self-interest (thus impugning character), opening the way for a new medical ethics as an apologetics for medical conduct in distrustful times.

From Pastoral Medicine to Bioethics

Sociologists and historians study the nature and changing character of normative or cultural consensus. Historians, and particularly social historians, in recent decades have been interested in how consensus is challenged and transformed. Sociologists also have regularly studied the dynamics of such changes, sometimes melding their commitments for change with their understandings of it. Over this same time, sociologists have come to view consensus as intellectually uninteresting, unless it is a kind of pathological consensus of the sort that raises anxieties, for example, in connection with cults, whether they are religious or political. Historians and sociologists have developed an animus toward *understanding* non-pathological consensus and long-standing traditions as well as the stability and endurance of social institutions and social forms over time.

Despite this contemporary animus, the canonical history of sociology is fully indebted to an early and sustained focus on the stabilizing forces of religion. The religious sources for debates in sociology can be briefly summarized: Auguste Comte, who coined the word "sociology," hoped to make "sociocracy" the final, stable form of human civilization. Sociologist-priests would gather positive knowledge about the best forms of social organization, and they would establish themselves, on the basis of such knowledge, as infallible keepers of social order. T.H. Huxley, the great Victorian polemicist for science, was among the first to notice that Comte's Religion of Humanity was "Catholicism without Christianity." The Swiss philosopher Hans Barth, in his neglected work, *The Idea of Order*, remarked without attribution to Huxley that "The philosophical and political system of positivism is a Catholicism without Christian content" (1960:128). Finally, the most arresting observation about Comte's legacy comes in F.A. Hayek's *The Counter-Revolution of Science* (1952), in which the Comtean ambition is regarded as a precursor to twentieth-century totalitarianism. Even though the debates about the political implications of totalitarianism have receded, the meaning of "Catholicism without Christianity" has resonance for how we understand the management of individual conduct based upon the role of institutions.

Viewing the historical development of religious influences on medical matters during the past century, "Catholicism without Christianity" is what bioethics is. Like sociology, bioethics has sought, quite appropriately in the minds of most bioethicists, to distance itself from the claims of institutional and collective forms of religious authority. When Daniel Callahan wrote *Abortion: Law, Choice, and Morality* (1970) he did not seek the *nihil obstat* or the *imprimatur* of the Catholic Church. For that matter, John T. Noonan, now a federal judge in California, remembered in the abortion debate for his work on drafting a human life amendment in the late 1970s, did not publish such work under the Church's imprimatur (Noonan 1978). This is not to say that either Callahan, or certainly Noonan, are Catholics without Christianity. But it is a sociological observation about their relative distance from conducting their work under the official auspices of the Church. They have pursued different kinds of commitments to defining normative order apart from, but by no means excluding, religious authority. Church doctrine does exist on many important bioethical subjects but is, by virtue of its origins, at odds with one specific secular mission of bioethics, which is to serve as mediator and expert in complicated medical-scientific, legal, and public controversies.

The Catholic sources for debates in bioethics have been influential, sociologically speaking, in *how* deliberations are conducted rather than in *what* answers are reached. Both Callahan's and Noonan's efforts are at once related to and distinct from the tradition of pastoral medicine out of which they arose. The definitive work on this tradition and the earlier forms of Catholic reasoning on medical morality is David F. Kelly's *The Emergence of Roman Catholic Medical Ethics in North America* (1979). His work describes the influential nature of Catholic teaching as recently as forty years ago and the continuing efforts since then by Catholic moralists, including Callahan and Noonan, to be influential beyond the Church's doctrinal teachings.

The Catholic source begins and ends in efforts to create a pedagogy for answering morally complex medical questions for both

Catholic and non-Catholic institutions. Father Charles J. McFadden's *Medical Ethics* (1946), issued by the medical publisher F.A. Davis, was intended initially for the moral instruction of nurses. By its third edition in 1955, the entire text had "been adapted to suit the needs of pre-medical students, medical students, doctors, and nurses" (p. xiii). By then, Father McFadden realized that his work was part of a larger effort to interpret natural law and divine positive law (that is, revelation) for the entire moral domain of medicine. The book contained the following declaration on the reverse side of the title page: "The '*nihil obstat*' and '*imprimatur*' are official declarations that a book or pamphlet is free from doctrinal or moral error. No implication is contained therein that those who have granted the '*nihil obstat*' and '*imprimatur*' agree with the contents, opinions, or statements expressed." This declaration with its perplexing disclaimer placed Father McFadden's efforts both within and beyond the Church. The clear implication was that both natural law and divine positive law stood above and guided specifically Catholic doctrine and were thus intended to be instructive to and binding upon all regardless of religious belief.

The tradition of natural law does not serve Catholic thinking alone. The Protestant theologian Paul Tillich in 1955 characterized the differences in doctrines of natural law between Catholicism and Protestantism: "Catholicism believes that the natural law has definite contents, which are unchangeable and are authoritatively stated by the Church (cf. The fight of the Roman Church against birth control). Protestantism, on the other hand, determines, at least today and in this country, the contents of the natural law largely by ethical traditions and conventions; but this is done without a supporting theory, and therefore Protestantism has the possibility of a dynamic concept of natural law. It can protest against each moral content which claims unconditional character" (Tillich 1955:131).[3] The specific inheritance of bioethics, as an emerging tradition in its own right, began with Catholic questions that pertained to "definite contents" but challenged the "unconditional character" of prevailing Catholic answers.

One line of criticism of bioethical thinking has been made about its rather relentless focus on autonomy and rights, among other distinctly American preoccupations. A different tack might take into account the intellectual framework in which bioethical deliberations generally have been conducted. As a largely normative as distinct from empirical enterprise, bioethics has long gained notice by its appeal to a kind of enlightenment casuistry in which Immanuel Kant and David Hume substitute for and supersede Saints Augustine and Thomas Aquinas. But this transition from the teachings of the Church Fathers to the teachings of the Enlightenment Fathers conceals something of the methodological implications of appealing to any authority, whether religious or secular. When Stephen Toulmin (1982) observed how philosophical ethics was saved by the practical conundrums of medicine, he appreciated better than most what was at stake institutionally in the longer run. It would be the modern hospital and modern university (and its applied humanists) rather than the contemporary Church that would serve as central sources of a new contemplative ideal out of which some semblance of authority over medicine in particular would develop. There are now three forms of managed care in America: governmental, corporate, and bioethical. The last of these is by far the most trusted, as compared to the other two. Many in bioethics attribute this trust to their alleged disinterest, itself a form of guidance.

During the second half of the nineteenth century, physicians equated medical morality with the material and organizational interests of their professional practice. At the same time, more narrowly Catholic deliberations on medical morality, in the form of what was then called pastoral medicine, went virtually unnoticed by the mainstream medical profession. The decisive matters for Catholic physicians and moralists of the late-nineteenth century (such as abortion, sexual sterilization, and specific operations such as craniotomy and Caesarean section) would become far more decisive and divisive issues for American medicine and politics during the last quarter of the twentieth century. Specific kinds of medical practices that were peripheral to professional interests would be catapulted to the center of normative conflict beyond professional interests, pulling the profession along the way and often into the fray.

Intrigued by the role of pastoral medicine in the history of medical ethics, the well-known bioethicist Robert Veatch (1995) proposed several important arguments about how to understand the relative influence of religious traditions on medical morality. He pointed out that the first Code of Ethics of the American Medical Association, adopted in 1847, must be seen as distinct from the Catholic tradition of pastoral medicine with its deliberations on specific medical-moral matters. Those physicians who formulated the 1847 Code took no interest in the Catholic moralizers, and vice versa. In Veatch's rendition, they were two ships passing in the night.

Veatch's argument depends on the assumption that "Protestant thought in the mid-nineteenth century showed no concern about the ethics activities of the AMA" (Veatch 1995:123). Protestantism, Veatch argued, was central in the phenomenon of religious revival and the work of temperance, abolition, and charitable work, especially during and after the Civil War. This is an entirely straightforward and accurate depiction of the social movements within Protestantism, which led to the range of public debates that define much of nineteenth-century American history. But Veatch ignored the key social characteristic of American professional medicine in the same period. The American Medical Association was the embodiment of American Protestant concerns. It was demographically a Protestant professional association. The Code it promulgated addressed matters we now call medical etiquette, while Catholic thinkers, by virtue of a different intellectual inheritance more central to very longstanding Church preoccupations, were already addressing matters we now call ethical.

By the middle of the twentieth century, the Protestant character of medical etiquette was parodied by the Episcopal priest Joseph Fletcher in *Morals and Medicine*: "The extant literature on it [medical ethics] consists for the most part in homilies on the bedside manner and such calculated questions of propriety and prudence as shined shoes, pressed trousers, tobacco odors, whether to drink Madeira, and the avoidance of split infinitives! It is composed, in a phrase, of manuals or exhortations on competitive success" (1954:6). Fletcher was correct, in his time, to observe that the decorum of physicians was, in their opinion, crucial to the preservation of professional authority. This was a consummately Protestant professionalism that appeared to bring little publicly to bear in the way of reflection and analysis on those matters addressed in the Catholic traditions of pastoral medicine. In its endorsement and elaboration of such ideas as vocation and professionalism, Protestantism made individual conscience, rather than the Church, the locus of decision-making about complex cases. Abortion is the central example. It does not figure in the AMA Code but was nevertheless of great concern to Catholic moralists in Europe and to Protestant physicians who taught in the elite American medical schools of the time.

Veatch's analysis did not address the fact that the same Protestant profession that remained silent in its Code about abortion also led the crusade, as James Mohr described it, to outlaw abortion in the United States in the latter half of the nineteenth century (Mohr 1978). Mohr, too, had a difficult time reconciling the fact that elite Protestant doctors were leaders *against* abortion, while Protestant clergymen appeared all but silent on the matter. About abortion, then, there was a silent Code, an indifferent Protestant clergy, an outspoken Catholic casuistry, and an activist Protestant medical profession, which formed the seemingly contradictory aspects of a rising public consensus.

Abortion was not a matter of public debate in 1850 (any more than it was in 1950), but the historiography, with few exceptions, of nineteenth-century abortion anachronistically seeks to find twentieth-century post-*Roe v. Wade* validations for liberalized abortion practice. A seemingly indifferent Protestant clergy served as a good illustration of Protestant indifference generally. Yet abortion was, at that time, practiced in ways that came to be viewed as threatening not simply to the authority of physicians but to the safe and effective practice of medicine. Rather than citing clerical indifference as the key to Protestant acceptance of abortion, the question Mohr and others should have asked is why the Protestant clergy did not *resist* the criminalization of abortion led by Protestant doctors. The reason is because the societal or normative consensus was already clear—abortion was understood in Christian terms as a sin. In contrast to a Protestant, civil society approach to defining public morality about abortion, the Catholic tradition allowed for a framework of debate about abortion in particular circumstances. By the middle of the twentieth century, for Protestant physicians, whether abortion was legal or illegal mattered more than any disputations from natural law about specific cases. The Catholic framework inspired Daniel Callahan's earliest efforts in bioethics, regardless of where he came out specifically on the matter of abortion.

Insiders, Outsiders, and Bioethics

Like the term "sociology," bioethics is a neologism: a new word coined for the purpose of crystallizing a new way of thinking, often about old problems. Comte's vision of positivism, a philosophy and science that would provide guidance to the administration of society, finds parallels in the normative approaches in bioethics. That no comparable efflorescence of intellectual oversight has developed for professions and occupations other than medicine suggests a deeper connection between sociology and bioethics than is revealed at first sight by the broadness and abstractness of the former and the relatively narrow and concrete focus of the latter. I will devote the remainder of this essay to some comparisons between these fields.

The institutional success of bioethics cannot be underestimated. Already several attempts at canonical-like histories of the field have been written, including David J. Rothman's *Strangers at the Bedside* (1991), Albert R. Jonsen's *The Birth of Bioethics* (1998), and most recently, M.L. Tina Stevens' *Bioethics in America: Origins and Cultural Politics* (2000). Rothman defined bioethics as "outside" medicine. In the Epilogue, he concluded that "Outsiders to medicine, more conspicuously and successfully than physicians, now define the social and ethical questions facing the profession and set forth the norms that should govern it" (Rothman 1991:247). He assumes, as most contemporary observers of medicine do, that physicians were once principally responsible for defining the social and ethical questions facing the profession and that an evermore wary and disenchanted public took the control of medical decision-making from them. This might be called the "civil rights" view of recent medical history, and in that sense is true insofar as physicians have become answerable to a host of outsiders, including courts and legislatures, clinical epidemiologists, feminists, and bioethicists.

In another sense, outsiders in previous times were not so much excluded from the processes of medical deliberation as they were insistent that physicians embody their cultural expectations about trust and duty. The doctor who in 1950 was anxious about tobacco odors or the shine on his shoes was not exemplifying behavior absent in the population—on the contrary, what I have described as Protestant preoccupations were decisive because they fused motive with action in the public mind. Rothman's portrayal of the recent history of the profession confirms that there was once a much greater correspondence between the motives of outsiders and insiders. Representative outsiders, far from being hostile to medicine, were intent upon finding ways to ride the wave of enthusiasm that was created by medical-scientific discoveries and treatments.

What is different today is how the critique of medical professionalism is understood. The problems that sociologists uncovered, for example in the work of Eliot Freidson and others, rarely proceed to litigation in the courts. Sociologists reported empirical findings about the organization of medical practice, about the nature of the physician-patient relationship, and about the socialization of doctors into their profession, often with the hope of achieving normative transformations in these areas. These empirical approaches had little to do with the interests of individual patients or physicians, and this is important to remember when examining how bioethics succeeded in gaining public notice far more effectively than sociology in the past few decades. On the other hand, sociologists did have a strong sense of advocacy about the seeming indifference of medical professionals to patient needs, about inequities in health care delivery, and about the corporate power of professionals generally. The remarkable force of contemporary feminism is impossible to understand apart from the fusion of such advocacy with empirical "horror" stories in medicine.

Bioethicists, as they emerged with a distinct identity, may have shared much of the "civil rights" enthusiasm with their sociologists-in-arms, at least initially. But to achieve institutional effectiveness, they had to take up old subjects in new ways. The empirical study of abortion in 1969 started from the reality of its criminal character,[4] but the normative study of it in 1970 by Daniel Callahan began on a much different premise. Rather than assume, as many sociologists did, that the pursuit of women's rights around abortion was primarily a matter of advocating for and furthering the interests of a social movement, those philosophers, humanists, and theologians who examined the question sought a change in how to *think* about the problem. Callahan's singular achievement was to lead the way in changing the normative contexts in which life and death issues were raised. Such contexts were much easier to change than social ones, and in any case, redefining the normative contexts would invariably lead to changes in the empirical realities defined by such contexts. Sociologists, by seeking first to describe empirical realities, were expected to define the norms in relation to those realities as well. Changing the norms was itself a kind of advocacy.

What developed is now a legacy of institutional transformation so profound and so systemic that all debates about life and death matters in American society are indebted to the formulations of normative contexts by the most well known bioethicists. These are contexts that enable *other* professions, most conspicuously law and medicine (but also journalism), to reorganize strategies of transformation and normalization according to each emerging dilemma. In the law, the odd confluence of Protestant medical opposition to abortion along with Catholic moral reasoning against it ended decisively when the Supreme Court no longer regarded the professional interests as paramount. The Court did not completely disestablish those professional interests, and it left the question of access to be a perennially empirical rather than normative matter. At the same time, each changed normative context has opened the way for the possible study of new empirical contexts, though it appears that such developments as stem-cell research and human cloning will be more normatively than empirically important in public debates for sometime to come. That is to say, the unintended empirical consequences of permitting or forbidding this or that innovation will be observed as opportunities to propose new normative contexts in which to consider them, there being no empirical authority, such as the Church, to define limits, as it has historically.

Bioethicists are the consummate insiders to this process of normative, then empirical, transformation. But they possess no special institutional authority. Indeed they eschew it as a matter of professional pride, thus conveying a broad, indeed, catholic sense of what Max Weber demanded of sociology: value neutrality. Sociologists would be the first to point out that such disinterest, in practice, has its interests nonetheless. But this kind of disinterest, insofar as ascertaining what is happening in the empirical world, means that advocacy can be separated from observation. On the other hand, a disinterestedness about values themselves is something unique to democratic societies in which so many questions once deemed by consensus to be moral matters have been transformed by consensus to be matters of rights. In the process, the simplification of principles that are said to be in conflict has made for the rapid and effective communication of otherwise complex and often confusing issues. As Paul Tillich foresaw in the case of Protestant natural law, and as Joseph Fletcher recognized in filling the old bottles of Catholic casuistry with the new wine of liberal Protestant indeterminacy, which used to be known as antinomianism (Andrew 2001), the professional success of bioethics has come in a sleight of hand that gives guidance about the questions that should be asked without claiming authority over, much less responsibility for, the answers that should be given.

I have not raised or addressed here the distinctive place of Jewish voices and concerns in the advising of the medical profession or the rise of bioethics, as the institutionalization of contemporary bioethics clearly has been accelerated by concerns central to the Catholic tradition. But the extraordinarily rich tradition of Responsa in the various traditions of Judaism, from biblical times on, defines a historically important way in which matters of conscience and action in medicine have been adjudicated for Jews in particular. Such Jewish contributors as Immanuel Jakobovitz (1975), Fred Rosner (Rosner and Bleich 1975), Willard Gaylin, cofounder of the Hastings Center, and Leon Kass, head of the Bush Administration's Council on Bioethics, represent an important part of the overall story of the relationship between religion and professional authority (see also Elon 1971:131-142).

This phenomenon of moving from the normative to the empirical (e.g., the method of bioethics), as distinct from the empirical to the normative (e.g., the method of sociology), illustrates the limits of both philosophical ethics and social-scientific research. Neither can provide definitive answers to the problems of human existence, and each has, in its own way, been associated with many types of false promises along that line. Bioethics is at the beachhead of modern mass communication about the dilemmas of scientific and medical innovation, with only residues of resistance remaining in the older fronts in this cultural struggle to define the purposes and limits of human life. Social science has a different mission than philosophical ethics, yet each has some reason to look back in time for sources that may help provide such purposes and limits. That these sources were historically defined as religious should not be viewed in hindsight as merely sectarian debates that have been superseded by the advocacy of social movements, in the case of sociology, or the refinement of Enlightenment thinking, in the case of philosophical ethics. On the contrary, resistance to innovation, whatever its source, is an able guide to a research agenda in empirical sociology, just as the appearance of doctrine from Church sources and the arguments from anti-secular bioethicists should be a good guide to mainstream bioethics.

A Personal Postscript:

I have written this essay mindful of the work and contributions of Renée C. Fox, my mentor, teacher, advisor, and friend for close to thirty years. She understood earlier and more profoundly than any other sociologist that the moral mandate of ethnography is to report the truth of circumstances in human life. The impetus to do so in the context of medicine was once to achieve some collaborative consensus between those who served in medicine and those who were served. Collaboration gave way to social movement forces in the transformation of medical norms, on the side of sociology, and to litigation in the courts and new laws by legislatures, on the side of bioethics. One cannot lament this realistically, except to observe that the incursions into medicine over the past quarter-century, whether by government, business, or experts (now ethical experts) have largely displaced the authority of the individual practitioner. Such displacement is bound to have its own empirical and normative unintended consequences over time, and it will be the task of younger observers to report the truth of these new circumstances as they unfold.

Notes

1. The argument condensed here is developed extensively in Jonathan B. Imber, *Trusting Doctors: The Decline of Moral Authority in American Medicine*, forthcoming.
2. Social science research on the physician's career during the 1950s and 1960s focused on physician socialization and on the quality of physician training. In the latter case, researchers examined empirically the factors that contributed to or interfered with the length of training of doctors. I refer here to a spiritual exhaustion in the meaning of the physician's career, not to indict that research in any way, but rather to place it in the context of the rising tide of normative research that would follow under the eventual rubric of bioethics. For empirical research on socialization at that time, see Robert K. Merton, George Reader, and Patricia L. Kendall, eds., *The Student-Physician: Introductory Studies in the Sociology of Medical Education* (Cambridge, MA: Harvard University Press, 1957); Howard Becker et al., *Boys in White: Student Culture in Medical School* [1961] (Rutgers, NJ: Transaction Publishers, 1997); and Renée C. Fox, "Is There a 'New' Medical Student? A Comparative View of Medical Socialization in the 1950s and the 1970s," in *Essays in Medical Sociology: Journeys into the Field* (New York: John Wiley, 1979), pp. 78-101. For empirical research on the quality of medical practice as determined by career-path choices, see Fremont J. Lyden, H. Jack Geiger, and Osler L. Peterson, *The Training of Good Physicians: Critical Factors in Career Choices* (Cambridge, MA: Harvard University Press, 1968).
3. For an extensive discussion of Protestant and Roman Catholic approaches to ethics, see Gustafson (1978).
4. See Nancy Howell Lee, *The Search for an Abortionist* (Chicago: University of Chicago Press, 1969). Howell, a sociologist, studied social networks and the differential access to abortion.

References

Andrew, Edward G. 2001. *Conscience and Its Critics: Protestant Conscience, Enlightenment Reason, and Modern Subjectivity*. Toronto: University of Toronto Press.

Bantam Books, Inc. v. Sullivan, 372 U.S. 58 (1963).

Barth, Hans. 1960. *The Idea of Order: Contributions to a Philosophy of Politics*. Translated by Ernest W. Hankamer and William M. Newell. Dordrecht: Reidel.

Callahan, Daniel. 1970. *Abortion: Law, Choice and Morality*. New York: Macmillan.

Elon, Menachem. 1971. "Jewish Law and Modern Medicine," in *Jewish Law in Ancient and Modern Israel, Selected Essays with an Introduction by Haim H. Cohn*. Hoboken, NJ: KTAV Publishing.

Fletcher, Joseph. 1954. *Morals and Medicine: The Moral Problems of: The Patient's Right to Know the Truth, Contraception, Artificial Insemination, Sterilization, Euthanasia*. Princeton: Princeton University Press.

Gustafson, James M. 1978. *Protestant and Roman Catholic Ethics: Prospects for Rapprochement*. Chicago: University of Chicago Press.

Hayek, F.A. 1952. *The Counter-Revolution of Science: Studies on the Abuse of Reason*. Glencoe, Ill.: Free Press.

Holmes, Oliver Wendell. 1869 [1861]. *Elsie Venner*. Boston: Field's, Osgood.

JAMA [Journal of the American Medical Association]. 1950. Vol. 143 (8, June 24):746.

Jakobovitz, Immanuel. 1975 [1959]. *Medical Ethics: A Comparative and Historical Study of the Jewish Religious Attitude to Medicine and its Practice*. New York: Bloch Publishing.

Jonsen, Albert R. 1998. *The Birth of Bioethics*. New York: Oxford University Press.

Kelly, David F. 1979. *The Emergence of Roman Catholic Medical Ethics in North America: An Historical – Methodological – Bibliographical Study*. New York: Edwin Mellen Press.

Metalious, Grace. 1956. *Peyton Place*. New York: Julian Messner, Inc.

Mohr, James C. 1978. *Abortion in America: The Origins and Evolution of National Policy*. New York: Oxford University Press.

Noonan, John T. 1978. *A Private Choice: Abortion in America in the Seventies*. New York: Free Press.

Rosner, Fred and J. David Bleich, eds. 1979. *Jewish Bioethics*. New York: Sanhedrin Press.

Rothman, David J. 1991. *Strangers at the Bedside: A History of How Law and Bioethics Transformed Medical Decision Making*. New York: Basic Books.

Stevens, M. L. Tina. 2000. *Bioethics in America: Origins and Cultural Politics*. Baltimore: Johns Hopkins University Press.

Tillich, Paul. 1955. "Moralisms and Morality from the Point of View of the Ethicist," in *Ministry and Medicine in Human Relations*, edited by Iago Galdston. New York: International Universities Press.

Toulmin, Stephen. 1982. "How Medicine Saved the Life of Ethics." *Perspectives in Biology and Medicine*, 25(4):736-750.

Veatch, Robert M. 1995. "Diverging Traditions: Professional and Religious Medical Ethics of the Nineteenth Century," in *The Codification of Medical Morality: Historical and Philosophical Studies of the Formalization of Western Medical Morality in the Eighteenth and Nineteenth Centuries, Volume Two; Anglo-American Medical Ethics and Medical Jurisprudence in the Nineteenth Century*, edited by Robert Baker. Dordrecht: Kluwer.

Wagaman, Samuel M. 1933. *Current Medical Digest* 1 (1, October):9.

16

Sociology and the De-moralization of Bioethics

Howard L. Kaye

Outwardly, the enterprise of bioethics appears to be thriving. It has become an accepted and growing academic field, an established part of medical education, a recognized and even mandated part of clinical practice. Bioethics programs, institutes, journals, professional associations, conferences, committees, and commissions continue to proliferate, and the range of issues addressed by bioethicists continues to expand. Beyond the field itself, public, governmental, and corporate interest in and support of bioethics remains strong, as does coverage in the national media.

Inwardly, however, there are signs of confusion and even discontent with the development and present state of bioethics. At the great gathering in 1995 of the four leading bioethics associations—The American Society of Law, Medicine and Ethics; Society for Health and Human Values; Society for Bioethics Consultation; and the American Association of Bioethics—the field's most prominent spokesman, Arthur Caplan, acknowledged in his address that bioethics is "a field that has no idea what it is" and "no sense of self-definition" (quoted in Marker 1995:36). More pointedly, a number of those who have been actively involved with the enterprise of bioethics from its beginnings in the late 1960s, and who have played prominent roles in its development and spread—people like Daniel Callahan, Leon Kass, and Renée Fox—have expressed a certain dissatisfaction, even dismay, over what the field has become, despite its outward success. According to these founding figures, with the growth and professionalization of the field have come important changes in how bioethical issues are approached, and in the role that bioethical debate has come to play. What is disheartening to them, and to others in the field, is the extent to which issues identified for ethical analysis are being examined in an ever-more narrow, specialized, and technically-oriented way, focusing on procedural solutions to particular problems, while the broader issues and implications—whether we call these existential, metaphysical, spiritual, or social—are separated out and marginalized (Callahan 1999:280-285; Capron 1999:297, 313; Churchill 1999:255-257; Crigger 1998:208-209; Fox 1994:53; Kass 1990:6-7; Rosenberg 1999). As Renée Fox, for example, points out, we may debate procedures and regulations designed to facilitate the procurement and utilization of transplantable organs, but the moral and cultural implications of such proposals (e.g., the desacralization and commodification of the human body) and the unambiguous "goodness" of the practice itself are not adequately discussed (Fox 1994:41; Callahan 1999). If such "proceduralism," as Alexander Capron terms it (1999:297), continues to dominate the field, it will not be long before today's broad debates on the morality of physician-assisted suicide and cloning will also become essentially questions of *how* they are to be done, not whether or not they *should* be.

For those with long memories, who have observed the life cycle of various contentious bioethical debates, a certain weariness, even fatalism, is difficult to avoid. Writing in 1992, Leon Kass, for example, recalled the "progress" achieved over the previous twenty-five years of biomedical development and bioethical debate:

> In the...years since I began thinking about these matters, our society has overcome longstanding taboos and repugnancies to accept test-tube fertilization, commercial sperm-banking, surrogate motherhood, abortion on demand, exploitation of fetal tissue, patenting of living human tissue, gender-change surgery...the widespread shuttling of human parts, assisted-suicide practiced by doctors, and the deliberate generation of human beings to serve as transplant donors... Perhaps more worrisome than the changes themselves is the coarsening of sensibilities and attitudes, and the irreversible effects on our imaginations and the way we come to conceive ourselves. (Kass 1992: 85).

From such a perspective, it is hard to avoid the judgment that bioethics has become de-moralized, and reduced to little more than our ritual act of hand-wringing with which we wash away our lingering moral concerns, thereby freeing ourselves to do whatever some among us want to do (Callahan 1996:3).

For both Callahan and Fox, this de-moralization of bioethics reflects, in part, what they see as the "secularization" of the field. What they are referring to is not simply the dramatic decline in the prominent role initially played by theologians and other religiously trained and "musical" intellectuals in the early years of bioethics. Nor do they wish to suggest that religious doctrines and religious authorities were explicitly appealed to by the founding generation of bioethicists in staking out their particular positions on the issues of the day. Instead, they argue that bioethics became "secularized" in the sense that the sort of issues and concerns traditionally expressed by religiously-influenced intellectuals—concerns about human hubris and the proper limits to human freedom; reverence for the natural order of things and the special dignity of man; and the values of charity, compassion, and brotherliness—have been pushed aside as more secularly-minded philosophers and lawyers have entered the fray, with their foci on individual rights, principlism, and procedural justice (Callahan 1990:2; Fox 1994:52-54; Kass 1990:6-7; Walters 1985).

Oddly enough, Callahan's own intellectual trajectory seems, at first glance, to embody the very secularization he has come to decry (Walters 1985:13). Disturbed by Pope Paul VI's stand on birth control, and increasingly alienated from his former Catholic faith, Callahan's involvement in biomedical issues and in the establishment of the Hastings Center (the Institute of Society, Ethics, and the Life Sciences) in 1969 seemed to be purely secular in orientation, a turning away from his former faith in favor of his academic training in analytic philosophy (Walters 1985:13). As Callahan later noted:

> Was it not obvious...that moral philosophy, with its historical dedication to finding a rational foundation for ethics was well suited to biomedical ethics, especially in a pluralistic society? Just as I had found I did not need religion for my personal life, why should biomedicine need it for its collective moral life? (1990: 2)

However critical of the Church's positions, and however committed to the great modern quest for such a rational, secular morality, Callahan soon became "alarmed by the apparently unthinking ways in which biomedical knowledge and technologies were being taken up and disseminated" (1996:19). To express that alarm, Callahan found himself drawing on the insights and perspectives of the religion whose beliefs he had explicitly rejected. Like the literary intellectuals and social theorists of the Victorian age, who had experienced a similar loss of faith, Callahan has attempted to cling to the moral kernel of his former faith while dispensing with its dead spiritual husk in the hope of finding some rational, secular means of sustaining that moral vision. But Callahan's efforts have proven no more successful than those of a George Eliot or a Herbert Spencer. The problem is due not simply to the necessity of addressing a broad public in a pluralistic society in a purely secular manner, but to the stubborn fact that moral kernels do not seem to thrive without the faith which nourishes them (Callahan 1990: 2).

In addition, as Renée Fox and Leon Kass note, many of the theologians and religious individuals drawn to bioethics have appealed, not to their religious traditions, but to purely secular notions of individual freedom and autonomy as their highest values, which made them indistinguishable from their areligious colleagues (Fox 1994:52-53; Kass 1990:6-7). For every theologian or religiously influenced participant who worried about human attempts to "play God" through various biomedical interventions, there was another equally religious figure proclaiming man to be "God's co-creator" and free to do as he thought good. For every Paul Ramsey, there was a Joseph Fletcher. Even a three-year project on "Genetics, Religion, and Ethics" organized by the Institute of Religion and the Baylor College of Medicine, which brought together 260 religiously sensitive physicians, researchers, ethicists, and theologians to explore the ethical and religious significance of the Human Genome Project (HGP) could arrive at no consensus on precisely what religion could contribute to the discussion of the HGP's ethical, legal, and social implications. In a bland and meaningless "Summary Reflection Statement" produced after three years of work, all that could be said was that "religious traditions are a rich source of knowledge and practical wisdom concerning human life" and that "religious voices should be heard and respected in discussion of delicate and difficult moral issues associated with genetic research and counseling" (Nelson 1994:29). What prevented the formulation of any more substantive position was not simply the tensions between scientists and theologians or the diversity of religious denominations represented, but the diversity of moral stances within the same religious denominations.

With the issues and themes traditionally associated with religion muted by the demands of pluralist discourse, drowned out by secular philosophers and lawyers, and canceled out by equally religious voices, bioethics has come to focus on the more immediate practical issues at hand. Shifting from an interdisciplinary quest for moral guidance, including both secular and religious perspectives, to a search for consensus based on a rational, secular morality, and then settling for the least common denominator among a plurality of irreconcilable positions and for a narrowing of focus to procedural matters, bioethics finally approaches the abandonment of ethical judgment altogether. What we are left with then often seems to be little more than resignation papered over with regulation, as bioethics becomes a kind of mediation service for conflicting interests (Jonsen 1993:S4), each of which is to be listened to with "detached neutrality" (Callahan 1990:4).

The report of the National Bioethics Advisory Commission on *Cloning Human Beings* (1997) exemplifies this endpoint in the evolution of the bioethical enterprise: the demoralization of bioethics. After the usual parade of experts of all varieties and perspectives and a "broad...cross-section of the community," the only point around which consensus could be achieved (the least common denominator) was the current unacceptability of cloning given the direct physical risk to any fetus produced in this manner. Acting as seemingly neutral mediators, the commission weighed the arguments for and against the practice of cloning and considered them to be equal, thereby canceling each other out (p. ii). The nearly unanimous public concern, even "revulsion" (p. 3) over the prospect of human cloning was essentially discounted as ill-informed and irrational, rooted in the public's "gross misunderstanding of human biology and psychology" (pp. 32, 68-69, 83). In addition, the NBAC argued that because the objections raised to human cloning, however universal, are justified through appeals to a variety of ethical and religious viewpoints, no one of which is "universally, shared by all Americans" (p. 93)—a state of affairs which is hardly surprising since the NBAC deliberately solicited a diversity of viewpoints—they could not reach a "common evaluation" of the issue (p. 93). But by choosing the impossible standard of total intellectual and ethical unanimity for making such judgments—in effect giving each American veto power over any attempt to condemn the practice—the NBAC insured that no such judgment could possibly be made. Finding itself unable to reach such a "common evaluation" (p. 93), the NBAC offered what they explicitly term a "political judgment" (p. 93), not a moral one: a temporary ban on human cloning (three to five years) during which time the physical risks to fetuses could be reduced through scientific advances, and the "irrational" fears of a scientifically ignorant public could be diminished through public education efforts and the natural process of evanescence which we have observed so many times before in connection with other, once alarming practices (e.g., in vitro fertilization and surrogacy).

While James Childress, a member of the NBAC, insists that the decision to recommend a temporary ban on human cloning also rested on moral grounds—the belief that it is unethical at this time to attempt to produce a child in this way, because of uncertainty about the safety of the procedure—the text clearly demonstrates that a mixture of motives was at work. To the extent that Childress is correct (the report does speak of ethical considerations at points; see p. 82), the position taken by the commission reflects the lowest common moral denominator among its members and hardly represents a position of moral rigor. Instead, it is a safe position, taken in order to avoid addressing the morally more fundamental and socially more important question: whether or not producing children in this fashion is morally acceptable and ought to be permitted. In addition, prudential political considerations (a fear of public outrage) clearly weighed heavily on the commission (p. 93).

While the NBAC did call for continued "discussion and evaluation" of the concerns raised about possible psychological, moral, and cultural harm associated with cloning, their hope and expectation seemed to be that the controversy would simply go away in time without the need to make any fundamental moral judgment. Indeed, by now we all know what the end result of such discussions will likely be: a stalemate amounting to tacit acceptance as long as the proper IRB is consulted and the proper consent form signed. For reasons such as these, a number of bioethical commentators have come to view the enterprise as performing a kind of "ideological" function (Jennings 1998:258) by providing "academically [and legally] respectable rationales for questionable behavior" (Bosk 1999:64; Callahan 1990:4; 1996; Churchill 1999:256-257, 269; DeVries 1995:127; Kass 1990:8; Rosenberg 1999:38-39, 42).

To help counteract such tendencies, sociology can, I believe, play an important role of the sort once played by religion, in keeping alive "enduring questions of meaning" and the necessity of moral choice (Callahan 1999:280; Fox 1994:93). In light of sociology's reputation as the most amoral of sciences and its limited involvement with bioethics to date, such a claim seems odd. In fact, many sociologists engaged in the study of issues touching on bioethical questions, such as Renée Anspach (1993), in her account of treatment decisions in neonatal intensive care units, and Charles Bosk (1992), in his ethnography of genetic counseling, argue that sociologists must limit themselves, however reluctantly, to describing *what* goes on and *how* decisions are made, leaving moral judgments to the professional ethicists (DeVries 1995; Devries and Conrad 1998:250). To do otherwise seems to compromise sociology's already fragile claims to scientific status. In addition, recent interest in developing a "sociology of bioethics" has focused on the social and cultural factors influencing the development and functioning of the field as a whole and its mode of dealing with particular issues, while deliberately leaving questions of "ought" aside. Such a sociology of bioethics, as one practitioner has noted, is characterized by "disinterested analyses motivated by sociological curiosity, the questions asked [being] basic questions about social organization" (DeVries 1995:120; DeVries and Subedi 1998).

Certainly such efforts can make a valuable contribution to the bioethical enterprise, as well as to the discipline of sociology, but they reflect a limited understanding of both what sociology can be and what it can contribute to the difficult task of making moral judgments. To most investigators, the "sociology of bioethics" refers to the "social causes" of bioethics, i.e., the social forces at work in the origin and development of the field, in the sorts of issues selected and not selected for bioethical analysis, in the decisions arrived at, and in the principles articulated. The recent analysis of John H. Evans (2000), for example, helps us to understand some of the sociological reasons for the triumph of principlism in American bioethics, beyond the demands of secular pluralism. Drawing on Max Weber's concept of formal rationality, Evans argues that principlism was victorious, not because it was the best approach ethically, but because it was the best approach rationally. Principlism "takes the complexity of actually lived moral life" and grinds it down into a coarse meal to be weighed on the four approved ethical scales—autonomy, beneficence, nonmalfeasance, and justice—simplifying bioethical decision-making by rendering it calculable, predictable, impersonal, and politically useful (Evans 2000:32-33).

Easily taught and applied, principlism also proved useful in training the large number of "ethicists" necessary to operate the proliferating IRBs and hospital ethics committees in a rational, bureaucratic fashion. Once established, principlism has become the dogma in which cadres of bioethicists have been schooled, so that other approaches have become virtually unthinkable (Evans 2000).

Evans's analysis reminds us not only of the reductionism that principlism entails, but also of the facts that other approaches remain theoretically possible, and that other questions remain worth asking. But what approach ought we to favor? What stance ought we to take on the bioethical issues of the day? Here Evans's analysis, like that of most sociologists, is silent.

In a similar fashion, other social scientists engaged with bioethics have brought to light cultural biases in the dominant, principlist approach, grounded in the celebration of personal autonomy (Fox and Swazey 1984; Kleinman 1999; Wertz 1998; Wolpe 1998); political and economic biases in the selection and construction of bioethical issues (Guillemin 1998; Light and McGee 1998); and the social and organizational biases that interfere with what bioethicists have set forth as proper ethical conduct (Anspach 1993; Barber et al. 1973; Bosk 1992; Christakis 1999; Gray 1975; Guillemin 1998). Such analyses can help bioethicists become more aware of their "blind spots" and of the manifold influences that color their judgments. Sociology can also help bioethicists become more sensitive to the contexts in which patients and biomedical personnel act and react, and to the complexities and ambiguities involved in real life ethical dilemmas. By doing so, sociology can help bioethicists achieve the kind of "effective, reasoned and independent" stance, to which they aspire (Bosk 1999; DeVries and Conrad 1998).

A second meaning and focus of the "sociology of bioethics" has been on the "social consequences" of bioethics. What has been emphasized in such accounts has been the "ideological" function of bioethics in rationalizing the interests of biomedical investigators and institutions, and the clientele that they serve. While granting that bioethics has had a significant impact on medical practice, curtailing physician autonomy and achieving some acknowledgement of patient rights, sociologists often argue that bioethics has lost its critical edge and has been "co-opted." Rather than challenging the dominance of medical perspectives, institutions, and interests, bioethics too often serves to reconcile patients and the broader public to them (Bosk 1999:64; Churchill 1999:256-257; 269; DeVries 1995:127; DeVries and Conrad 1998:236-237, 246; Jennings 1998:258; Rosenberg 1999:38-39, 42). Here, too, the contribution of sociology is designed to help bioethicists function more effectively and independently by providing information about the unintended, and possibly undesirable, consequences of their efforts and judgments. In doing so, sociology remains essentially silent about moral judgments—about what ought to be done—besides offering a critique of professional dominance, institutional power, and corporate interests of the sort which, given the political orientations of most sociologists, is not unexpected (DeVries and Conrad 1998:234; Light and McGee 1998:6).

Whether focusing on social causes or social consequences, sociology remains essentially an adjunct to bioethics, a source of information and criticism, which is largely ignored by bioethicists and by the courts (Capron 1999), but not a source of moral guidance: a task that is still left to bioethicists, despite their increasing reluctance to perform it. More recently, there have been a few tentative efforts by social scientists to question this disciplinary division of labor, but not very persuasively (see Zussman 2000; Nelson 2000).

There is, however, another way in which sociology can contribute to the enterprise of bioethics. As the work of Renée Fox in particular demonstrates, "sociology of" can also refer to "the social meaning of," and it is by exploring the social meaning of bioethics that sociology can perform a moral task, of the sort more religiously grounded intellectuals once performed in bioethics.

Fox freely acknowledges that her efforts in the realm of bioethics have "never been academically detached" (Fox and Swazey 1992: 199). On the contrary, in both her ethnographic accounts of various therapeutic innovations and in her broader discussions of bioethics and its dominant issues, she has always pushed beyond the immediate issues at hand in order to bring to light the more fundamental moral and cultural questions they raise, and the implications of the answers offered, both those explicitly given and those tacitly made. By doing so, she has treated bioethics not only as an interdisciplinary effort to grapple with the difficult moral issues associated with modern biomedicine, but as a marker of where we are culturally and where we appear to be headed; i.e., as both a sign of, and contributor to our present moral confusion and impoverishment (Fox and Swazey 1984; Fox 1994).

Her work shows us that in addition to the issues of organ procurement and the proper distribution of scarce resources, the overzealous practice of transplantation and its celebration expresses a "relentless, hubris-ridden refusal to accept limits" and a "technocratizing" of the body, both of which are pervasive in contemporary biomedicine and are potentially dehumanizing in their effects (Fox and Swazey 1992:199-210). Her work reminds us that in addition to the issues of reproductive rights and the freedom of scientific inquiry, the development of new reproductive technologies both expresses, and adds to, our fundamental confusion over questions of identity, family, and parenthood, and over just how human we wish to remain. In sum, her research demonstrates that the seemingly isolated, specialized, and autonomous decisions made within the walls of hospitals and clinics are not only subject to a broad range of social, economic, and cultural influences, but resonate with meanings which are felt throughout social life in ways we must consider carefully. Do we really think, for example, that the effects of legalizing physician-assisted suicide will be contained within the walls of hospitals and will remain a matter of personal choice, and that the routine and guiltless taking of human life will leave our sense of life's sacredness undiminished?

Efforts such as these can serve moral forces in the only way which, as Max Weber tells us, is available to a science like sociology: by helping us to gain clarity about the possible consequences and ultimate meanings of our actions, so that we might choose and act more responsibly. In doing so, sociology can serve as a kind of conscience for bioethics at a time when it is most in need of one.

To illustrate, it is useful to return to the NBAC's response to the concerns raised by the prospect of human cloning. Noting that anxiety about the possible psychological harm to children produced through somatic cell nuclear transfer has often been cited as grounds to ban the practice, the NBAC sets out to evaluate these concerns. They do so by asking if there is "a moral or human right to a unique identity, and if so would it be violated by this manner of human cloning?" (p. 67). Given the existence of homozygous twins and the ability of such twins to develop as separate and distinct individuals—however difficult this might be—the answer appears to be no.

Other philosophers, however, have argued that the situation of naturally occurring homozygous twins and cloned generic "twins" separated in time would be profoundly different because the cloned "twin" "knows, or at least believes he or she knows" what he or she is supposed to do and be (pp. 67-68). To this the Commission responds by asserting that no "right to ignorance" or "right to an open future," if it exists, would be violated, because: (1) arguments about how a cloned child might feel are speculative, and because such feelings would be "directly related to certain specific cultural values," they would likely be highly variable; (2) if, indeed, a cloned child felt oppressed by his genetic identity and phenotypic expectations, he would be in error, and guilty of "the crudest genetic determinism"; (3) "What such a twin is likely to believe will depend on the facts that emerge and what scientists and ethicists claim" (pp. 67-68). Therefore, such anxieties and arguments are not sufficiently persuasive to count.

In rejecting the concerns so frequently expressed, the NBAC makes a number of assertions—concerning the implications of genetic sameness, the interpretations offered by scientists, and the reactions of the broader public—with which a sociologist might well take issue. To a sociologist (rather than to a philosopher) the fundamental issue is not whether some putative right, invented by a philosopher, is violated, but what effect might cloning have on the life of copies (their identity, their treatment by others, their happiness or misery) and on the society around them. Given that no such cloning has yet occurred, its impact on copies and on their society is necessarily speculative, but this hardly invalidates the effort to foresee and avoid possible dangers. Speculations may be more or less plausible, and the consequences foreseen may be more or less grave. If, after due deliberation, an anticipated danger seems reasonably possible and potentially devastating in its effects, then wisdom and prudence rightfully suggest that it is better not to wait for empirical evidence in the form of disaster.

As the NBAC notes, the psychological and social impact of cloning may well be "directly related to certain specific cultural values." But this is certainly a topic about which social scientists might have something valuable to say, which would help us to anticipate the impact of cloning in the American cultural context. Indeed, in light of the oft-analyzed premium that American culture places on expressive individualism, personal autonomy, authenticity, and the self's liberation from all "external" constraints (see for example Bellah et al. 1985), the potentially harmful emotional impact of cloning should be apparent. Whether scientifically correct or not, it is likely that both the child produced by cloning and the surrounding community will view the cloned child as at least *intended* as a copy and will act on that basis. As I have argued elsewhere, individuals who select particular genotypes to be cloned for some phenotypic ends will very likely attempt to manipulate environmental influences for the same purpose. If they succeed, they will have added to the oppressive burden of expectations endured by the duplicates, but if the experiment fails and the duplicates diverge from the longed-for phenotype, the bitter disappointment of parents and the suffering of what have now become "defective copies" will have been enhanced (Kaye 1998:487-488). Either way, the actions of the parent(s) cruelly threaten the child with a loss of freedom, individuality, and love: precisely those values appealed to in order to justify the practice.

The NBAC also asserts, entirely without evidence, that what copies and others will likely believe "will depend on the facts that emerge and what scientists and ethicists claim." From a sociological point of view, however, this claim is doubly naïve. To think that what the public believes is so easily determined by the claims of experts, however rigorously grounded those claims may be, is hardly born out by either historical evidence or empirical fact—as evolutionary biologists have learned. In addition, such a claim reflects a social determinism as crude as the genetic determinism that they decry.

Finally, to think that what scientists will present to the public will simply be the "facts" about genetics and human development is empirically false. If the public adheres to the "crudest genetic determinism," the fault lies not simply with the scientific ignorance of laymen, but to a great extent with the efforts of our over-zealous scientists and irresponsible science journalists, who, for over forty years, have been trumpeting such biological reductionism. Driven by deeply-held philosophical commitments to biological determinism, fantasies of total mastery over all life, longings for immortality, and more sober pecuniary interest, scientists such as Francis Crick, James Watson, Joshua Lederberg, Jacques Monod, E. O. Wilson, Richard Dawkins, and Steven Pinker have been hammering home the message that our genes make us who we are—a message reinforced by every headline celebrating the alleged discovery of the latest human gene (Kass 1999; Kaye [1986] 1997; Midgley 2000; Nelkin and Lindee 1995). So pervasive is this genetic determinism that it now appears to be self-evident truth. Even the NBAC's report can criticize the "erroneous belief" in "genetic determinism" in one sentence and then immediately assert in the next that "genes play an *essential* role in the formation of…behavioral characteristics," without noticing any contradiction (p. 32; emphasis added).

From a sociological point of view then, the risks discounted by the NBAC seem graver and more likely to occur; the correctives proposed by the commission, less trustworthy and effective than they believed; and the aspirations of those advocating the development and practice of human cloning, less rational and admirable than they allowed. In light of such analyses, the scales of judgment might well appear to be less balanced than the NBAC claimed, thereby permitting a reasoned moral judgment to be made.

As religion once did, sociology can remind us that bioethical issues may involve far more than individual rights. Developments in biomedicine may have social, psychological, and cultural consequences that are difficult to foresee; they may involve fundamental issues of our humanity, our obligations to one another, our sense of a life worth living, and the meaning of our lives. Sociology can help us to address such issues and to grasp the elements of belief, fantasy, hubris, irrationality, ideology, and idolatry even in the seemingly scientific and rational stances of physicians and researchers. Sociology can help broaden our moral vision, enabling us to see what is at stake, not only in single, discrete bioethical issues, but also in their cumulative effects, and in their connections with social and cultural developments outside the sphere of biomedicine. By doing so, sociology can, at its best, actually help us to choose and act more wisely (Campbell 1990; Fox 1994; Fox and Swazey 1984; Kass 1990, 1999; Midgley 2000; Wind 1990).

References

Anspach, Renée R. 1993. *Deciding Who Lives: Fateful Choices in the Intensive-Care Nursery*. Berkeley: University of California Press.

Barber, Bernard, John J. Lally, Julia L. Makarushka, and Daniel Sullivan. 1973. *Research on Human Subjects: Problems of Social Control in Medical Experimentation*. New York: Russell Sage Foundation.

Bellah, Robert N., Richard Madsen, William M. Sullivan, Ann Swidler, and Steven M. Tipton. 1985. *Habits of the Heart*. Berkeley: University of California Press.

Bosk, Charles L. 1992. *All God's Mistakes: Genetic Counseling in a Pediatric Hospital.* Chicago: University of Chicago Press.

_____. 1999. "Professional Ethicist Available: Logical, Secular, Friendly." *Daedalus* 128 (4):47-68.

Callahan, Daniel. 1990. "Religion and the Secularization of Bioethics." *Hastings Center Report* 20, (4; July/August):2-4.

_____. 1996. "Calling Scientific Ideology to Account." *Society* 33 (May/June):14-19.

_____. 1999. "The Social Sciences and the Task of Bioethics." *Daedalus* 128(4): 275-94.

Campbell, Courtney S. 1990. "Religion and Moral Meaning in Bioethics." *Hastings Center Report.* 20(4): S4-S10.

Capron, Alexander Morgan. 1999. "What Contributions Have Social Science and the Law Made to the Development of Policy on Bioethics?" *Daedalus* 128(4): 295-325.

Christakis, Nicholas A. 1999. "Prognostication and Bioethics." *Daedalus* 128(4):197-214.

Churchill, Larry R. 1999. "Are We Professionals? A Critical Look at the Social Role of Bioethicists." *Daedalus* 128(4): 253-74.

Crigger, Bette-Jane. 1998. "As Time Goes By: An Intellectual Ethnography of Bioethics," pp. 192-215 in *Bioethics and Society: Constructing the Ethical Enterprise*, edited by Raymond DeVries and Janardan Subedi. Upper Saddle River, NJ: Prentice Hall.

DeVries, Raymond. 1995. "Toward a Sociology of Bioethics." *Qualitative Sociology* 18 (1): 119-28.

DeVries, Raymond and Peter Conrad. 1998. "Why Bioethics Needs Sociology,"pp. 233-237 in *Bioethics and Society: Constructing the Ethical Enterprise*, edited by Raymond DeVries and Janardan Subedi. Upper Saddle River, NJ: Prentice Hall.

DeVries, Raymond and Janardan Subedi, eds. 1998. *Bioethics and Society: Constructing the Ethical Enterprise*. Upper Saddle River, NJ: Prentice Hall.

Evans, John H. 2000. "A Sociological Account of the Growth of Principlism." *Hastings Center Report* 30(5): 31-38.

Fox, Renée C. 1994. "The Entry of U.S. Bioethics into the 1990s: A Sociological Analysis," pp. 21-71 in *A Matter of Principles? Ferment in U.S. Bioethics*, edited by Edwin R. Dubose, Ronald P. Hamel, and Laurence J. O'Connell. Valley Forge, PA: Trinity Press International.

Fox, Renée C. and Judith P. Swazey. 1984. "Medical Morality is Not Bioethics—Medical Ethics in China and the United States." *Perspectives in Biology and Medicine* 27(3; Spring):336-60.

_____. 1992. *Spare Parts: Organ Replacement in American Society*. New York: Oxford University Press.

Gray, Bradford H. 1975. *Human Subjects in Medical Experimentation*. New York: Wiley Interscience.

Guillemin, Jeanne. 1998. "Bioethics and the Coming of the Corporation to Medicine," pp. 60-77 in *Bioethics and Society: Constructing the Ethical Enterprise*, edited by Raymond DeVries and Janardan Subedi. Upper Saddle River, NJ: Prentice Hall.

Jennings, Bruce. 1998. "Autonomy and Difference: The Travails of Liberalism in Bioethics," pp. 258-69 in *Bioethics and Society: Constructing the Ethical Enterprise*, edited by Raymond DeVries and Janardan Subedi. Upper Saddle River, NJ: Prentice Hall.

Jonsen, Albert R. 1993. "The Birth of Bioethics." *Hastings Center Report* 23(6; November/December):S1-S4.

Kass, Leon R. 1990. "Practicing Ethics: Where's the Action?" *Hastings Center Report* 20 (1; January/February):5-12.

_____. 1992. "Organs for Sale? Propriety, Property, and the Price of Progress." *The Public Interest* 107 (Spring):65-68.

_____. 1999. "The Moral Meaning of Genetic Technology." *Commentary* 108(2): 32-38.

Kaye, Howard L. [1986] 1997. *The Social Meaning of Modern Biology: From Social Darwinism to Sociology*, 2nd edition, New Brunswick, NJ: Transaction.

_____. 1998. "Anxiety and Genetic Manipulation: A Sociological View." *Perspectives in Biology and Medicine* 41(4):483-90.

Kleinman, Arthur. 1999. "Moral Experience and Ethical Reflection: Can Ethnography Reconcile Them? A Quandary for 'The New Bioethics.'" *Daedalus* 128(4): 69-97.

Light, Donald W. and Glenn McGee. 1998. "On the Social Embeddedness of Bioethics," pp. 1- 15 in *Bioethics and Society: Constructing the Ethical Enterprise*, edited by Raymond DeVries and Janardan Subedi. Upper Saddle River, NJ: Prentice Hall.

Marker, Rita. 1995. "The Woodstock of Bioethics." *The Human Life Review* 21(1): 35-52.

Midgley, Mary. 2000. "Biotechnology and Monstrosity: Why We Should Pay Attention to the 'Yuk Factor.'" *Hastings Center Report* 30(5): 7-15.

National Bioethics Advisory Commission. 1997. *Cloning Human Beings: Report and Recommendations of the National Bioethics Advisory Commission*. Rockville, MD.

Nelkin, Dorothy and M. Susan Lindee. 1995. *The DNA Mystique: The Gene as a Cultural Icon.* New York: W. H. Freeman and Company.

Nelson, J. Robert. 1994. *On the Frontiers of Genetics and Religion*. Grand Rapids: Wm. B. Eerdmans.

Nelson, James Lindeman. 2000. "Moral Teachings from Unexpected Quarters: Lessons for Bioethics from the Social Sciences and Managed Care." *Hastings Center Report* 30 (1): 12-17.

Rosenberg, Charles E. 1999. "Meanings, Policies, and Medicine: On the Bioethical Enterprise and History." *Daedalus* 128(4):27-46.

Walters, Leroy. 1985. "Religion and the Renaissance of Medical Ethics in the United States: 1965-1975," pp. 3-16 in *Theology and Bioethics*, edited by E.E. Shelp. Boston: D. Reidel.

Wertz, Dorothy C. 1998. "International Research in Bioethics: The Challenges of Cross-Cultural Interpretation," pp. 145-65 in *Bioethics and Society: Constructing the Ethical Enterprise*, edited by Robert DeVries and Janardan Subedi. Upper Saddle River, NJ: Prentice Hall.

Wind, James P. 1990. "What Religion Can Offer Bioethics." *Hastings Center Report* 20 (4):S18-S20.

Wolpe, Paul Root. 1998. "The Triumph of Autonomy in American Bioethics: A Sociological View," pp. 38-59 in *Bioethics and Society: Constructing the Ethical Enterprise*, edited by Robert DeVries and Janardan Subedi. Upper Saddle River, NJ: Prentice Hall.

Zussman, Robert. 2000. "The Contributions of Sociology to Medical Ethics." *Hastings Center Report* 30(1): 7-11.

17

The Moral and the Medical: The Stakes of Social Experience

Arthur Kleinman

The point of this paper can be put into a seemingly simple but, as I hope to demonstrate, thickly textured aphorism: *the moral, the political, and the medical are inseparably bound together through the stakes of collective and subjective experience.* Understand this tripartite nexus and you appreciate the stakes of experience, or, put contrariwise, get at what is at stake in experience and you thereby understand how the moral, the medical, and the political interfuse. On the one side lies an issue for the social sciences of health and medicine; turn it around and the medical social sciences illumine a central condition for moral theory about ordinary social life. A paper on this topic seems appropriate for a volume honoring Renée Fox because, throughout her major books, there is the strong sense of a deep moral and religious core to social life, a core that serious illness concentrates and medical practices realize. Here is Renée Fox, in the introduction to the 1974 edition of her classic 1959 book, *Experiment Perilous*, a work of profound poignancy as much as a social analytic *tour de force* about uncertainty in the face of "inexorable illness, human experimentation...suffering, and death":

> Ward F-Second plunged me into a world of extreme stress... In this shared predicament, along with physicians and patients, I had to find ways of coming to terms with the existential implications of that 'perilous experiment,' the anguished emotions it aroused and the ethical dilemmas it posed... The major intellectual challenge with which Ward F-Second confronted me was that, to my knowledge, no first-hand sociological study of illness, medical experimentation with human subjects, or the psychosocial dynamics of therapeutic innovation had ever been made. Not only was there no precedent for such an inquiry, but its legitimacy was questionable. Neither the moral justification for this type of study nor its social scientific meaningfulness was established (p. 9).

Twenty-three years later, after having reflected on the "undaunted striving of modern medicine to control death" (Fox and Swazey 1978:377) and engaging the poignant conflicts entailed in its ability to do so, she wrote, disenchanted, "What I regard as profanation is observable, for example, in the movement away from the conception of human organ transplantation as a gift of life, the movement toward the commodification of organs that is taking place, and the reduction of the body to 'only a thing-in-the-world' that this commodification implies" (1996:262).

These words authorize a return to the subject of this essay: the moral (here understood to extend from the secular to the sacred), the political, and the medical and what is at stake in social life. Social theorist Bryan Turner has claimed that much of contemporary social science, in his view, turns its back on the downright precariousness of social experience and the attention-focusing ontological frailty of persons, substituting in its place what he condemns as merely "ornamental sociology" (Personal communication May 1998). When the French social theorist Pierre Bourdieu (1990) refers to the practical sense of the field, he has something akin in mind: namely, that the dangers of collective and personal existence make men and women everywhere acutely oriented to their local worlds, with a sense of threat. This same orienting idea can be found in the writings of John Dewey, William James, and other pragmatist writers as well as among continental phenomenologists from Maurice Merleau-Ponty and Max Scheler to Arnold Gehlen and Helmut Plessner. The German social historian Thomas Nipperdey (1974, 1979) has put it this way: the task of the historian and the social scholar, he observed during the battle of the historians in Germany a decade ago, is to return to the past the anxiety and uncertainty and danger it held as it was actually lived.[1]

I take this to be what hundreds of ethnographies and social histories describe, that local worlds of experience are dangerous, that the infrapolitics of ordinary life turn on things that are so deeply at stake for people that they often feel, with considerable justification when one looks at the historical and cross-cultural record, that their ways of life and very existence are at stake. Michael Oakeshott, the political philosopher, in his resonant volume *Experience and Its Modes* (1978), sums up by arguing that the practical activity of experience puts things that matter most to us under challenge or threat such that "the practical comprises all that we mean by a moral life." In this view even the transcendent needs to be understood as part of the overwhelming practicality of social life. As I read these words, I take them to reflect a social science perspective that the moral aspect of social life is not in and of itself about "the good" in the sense of transcendent value, but rather that what is at stake in collective and personal experience—say, for example, status, resources, relationships, survival—describes the particular moral processes of a local community or institution, though the moral processes in turn may be quite remote from and even inimical to "the good" in a transcendental sense. That is to say, local values as interpreted in the ordinary encounters of social life may be dangerous, threatening, even unethical. For what they are about is not some ideal or universal, but rather the practical particularities of our relationship to power and its consequential effects. The moral and the political, in this sense, are conceptually inseparable. What is at stake is the politics of the everyday. The moral, in this ethnographic sense, is about expedience, compromise, scapegoating, and inequality, as much as it is about endurance, solidarity, and empathy. Betrayal, resentment, and revenge are as much a part of such local moral processes as are remorse, regret, and the sensibility to be of use to others. Seen this way, moral experience challenges the philosophers' aphorism that one cannot derive an "ought" from an "is." The normative and descriptive are held to be entirely separate, on that influential philosophical truism. But for the historian and the ethnographer this is simply wrong. Local worlds are always messy conglomerates of "is" and "ought," which are inseparable in moral experience.

This is a side of experience that is quite different from what we mean when we talk about ethics. Unlike the moral processes of social experience, which are everywhere locally positioned and partisan—a view from somewhere—ethics is said to be about the aspiration for and struggle to realize translocal or universal values—the view from nowhere. We require the perspective of ethics because, while many of us would question whether there ever has been or can be a view from nowhere (an ethics ungrounded in particular contexts), nonetheless ethical deliberation is what shows that locally lived values may be inhuman and unethical; we only know moral processes as such if we have the sensibility of translocal values. Ethics itself of course has, like all things made by men and women, feet of local clay. But reaching for something outside the local is crucial and, as illustrated by the comparative enterprise itself, is a feasible if thorny and controverted undertaking. We need the perspective of local moral processes as well, however, because much of the time ethical deliberation is utopian, uncontextual, and comes close to being irrelevant to local experience. And here is where the moral and the political relate most centrally to the medical.

As the moral is to the ethical so is illness experience to disease processes. Illness experience, as I have written in *The Illness Narratives* (1988) and other places, is about the choke and sting of symptoms, their material impact on persons and relationships, their metaphorical extension outward into work and family and inward into the imaginative interstices of the self. Symptoms and functional limitation, and the rest of illness experience, are caught up in local categories and institutions. They are perceived, lived, expressed, and responded to in the subjective and interpersonal space of a local world of interconnecting networks, social and economic inequality, cultural hierarchy, and political power. Hence the illness experience of diabetes, ischemic heart disease, breast cancer, or depression is an intrinsic part of moral experience, of which it may be one of the things that clarifies what is most at stake. So understood, illness experience is always a moral experience. And using the same analysis advanced above, as a moral experience it gets taken up in the infrapolitics of local worlds, the social dynamics of power. Class, race, ethnicity and other social categories affect and are affected by illness. They create a social course in interaction with the disease process. For example, an illness experience can have serious effects on work, career, spousal and parenting roles; it often brings significant financial burden; it threatens social relationships; and it frequently engenders a search for meanings. It may threaten norms and transform emotions and sense of self. This then is one of the ways that the moral, the political, and the medical come together.

But this would be an incomplete understanding of this triadic relationship, as Renée Fox and others have demonstrated through the study of medical institutions. It is not that illness experience is the only aspect of health and medicine that gets taken up in the nexus of the moral and the political. That health is organized by moral-political processes is manifest by the moral and political economy of disease causation and health maintenance, which places that one-fifth of the globe's population who live in extreme poverty and who experience the greatest social inequality at much greater risk of morbidity and mortality. It also is visible in the gradient of health status that is worse for those living in societies with the steepest differential between rich and poor. The political and moral economy of tuberculosis as seen inside Russian prisons is but one example; these are the world's most powerful breeding grounds for MDRTB (multidrug resistant tuberculosis). But the politics and moral economy of American prisons also offer a powerful illustration *vis-a-vis* HIV/AIDS, which can be said to be, in the world's richest and most technologically advanced nation, endemic in this setting (see, for example, Chen, Kleinman, and Ware 1994; Desjarlais, Eisenberg, Good, and Kleinman 1995; Farmer 1991).

Disease processes, and the physicians, nurses, and researchers who deal with them, are also part of this nexus. The framing of disease via biomedical categories bears historical and cultural specificity, but those categories carry moral values and are appropriated in the political process in communities. The institutional arrangements of care-giving are shaped so powerfully by economic and political processes that ours is an era of financial and managerial revolution in services that has altered fundamentally medical work, the training of medical students and residents, and the institutional demands on researchers. These managerial and economic changes reflect and express what is at stake in each of these domains of practice, teaching, and research. What matters most today is not the same as what mattered most in the same domains when I was a medical student and active practitioner in the 1960s and 1970s.

But there is one detail worth pursuing because it has been of abiding interest to our honoree, even during times when it was a politically and professionally incorrect interest for her to hold. Both moral processes and ethical deliberation have their religious sides. It is not just that religionists have contributed in the most basic ways to ethics, but that the aspiration for translocal ethical values is deeply rooted in theological traditions and the religious institutions that sponsor them. Religious ritual and devotional practices in general are particular examples of local moral processes. And these are processes that forge the contingent subjectivity of our era in which the "healthy" self has replaced the suffering self of an earlier era in the Judeo-Christian tradition as a salvific subject, with all of the changes in institutions and ideology that that implies. With the possible exception of "no pain, no gain" in sports, suffering today in American society does not carry the moral weight and religious meanings it has had in earlier eras, and that has both experiential and theological significance, as Joan Kleinman and I explained in a *Daedalus* issue on *Social Suffering* (1996). Hence, the argument advanced about the moral, the political, and the medical extends to religion. Indeed, it is rarely certain when this continuum of social experience from the moral to the religious stops on one side or the other: the processes are open-ended and imply that both may be involved, even when formal institutional trajectories seem separate.

In a time when global flows of images, finance, commodities, and people are extensive and bring intensive pressure to bear on local worlds, when migrations have created widespread diasporas, and technology and law are increasingly transnational, there is added reason for the utility of a social science perspective on values that brings moral processes and ethical claims into dialogue. Human rights discourse is an example of such transnational ethical claims. But to be availing, such discourse must engage the contextual reality of local moral processes, where the often hyper-autonomy of global concerns for the "rights" of the individual is confronted by culturally legitimated communal obligations and transpersonal responsibilities. Uncertain as the outcomes of such interactions between contrasting claims must always be, surely it is only through such a dialogue that the ethical and moral aspects of values can be worked out. It is precisely this dialectical scenario that speaks to the on-the-ground reality that local worlds are permeable to global forces to a substantial and perhaps unprecedented degree and are often intensified by global flows, while transnational processes take on their influence in disparate local settings. Thus, the approach I am advancing would seem to be especially apt to engage health and health care in this period.

What are we to do with this understanding, whose lineaments have been clear for many decades? I would suggest that there are two large issues that should be addressed. The first is the failure of ethnographers and social historians to make this knowledge accessible to laypersons and health professionals in forms that they can understand and use. Our knowledge is loculated. We write largely for each other. We exude confidence in overly sophisticated understandings that elude laypersons and that are off-putting to professionals—not so much for what we have to say as for the way we say it. We need to refigure how our knowledge is transferred and popularized, especially that knowledge that cuts against the grain not only of the globalized political economy and the culture it so powerfully shapes, but of the profession of medicine and much of the health care industry. This is a fundamental challenge to our pedagogy that I see no evidence of being adequately addressed.

Second, the knowledge base I have described has substantial potential for social theory, moral theory, and bioethics. Here again there are problems in the receptivity and responsiveness of these domains to the findings we have to offer. When I first proposed a course on moral theory from an anthropological perspective to the Core Curriculum Committee at Harvard College I was informed, somewhat diffidently, by the then chair of philosophy, that moral theory could not be taught from the standpoints of anthropology. Another illustration comes from the field of stigma studies of mental illness. Much work in this field takes its origin from Goffman's greatly influential, yet to my mind still inadequate, social psychology of stigma as resulting from the discrediting of persons who then feel discreditable for the stigmatizing mark (material or symbolic) they bear—a somewhat circular argument. Edgerton's *Cloak of Competence* makes much the same point about the spoiling of identity among those with mental retardation, who, when confronted with the pseudo-mutuality of mainstreaming, are forced to disguise limitations they realize cannot be hidden (1967). Closely in tune with this approach is the understanding of stigma that comes from symbolic interactionism's labeling theory. In that theory, emphasis is placed on societal responses to primary deviance that produce a socially shaped secondary deviance. In this way, chronicity of schizophrenia—its social course as it were—is seen in part as the result of societal responses to symptoms in the creation of disability and barriers to effective treatment.

Yet, this theoretical orientation does not entirely match the illness and disability experiences of patients with depression and most other non-psychotic mental health problems. Here the issue appears to be less about societal response to obvious signs of difference, than it is a question of participants in local worlds feeling especially threatened by the powerful implications of experiences of depression, anxiety, trauma, and suicide, and acting in accord with that intensified sense of threat to widen the perceived difference between themselves and the afflicted. These experiences of serious dysphoria and hopelessness challenge or undermine what is so often locally at stake—from global ideologies of security that support the narcissistic pursuit of happiness through commodities to the efforts to forget or disguise threats of perceived vulnerability and fear of the always real dangers of social life. They also threaten property values and the cultivation of social relations for purely instrumental ends of personal gain and they strike a fear that these experiences of dysphoria and hopelessness not only take time and energy to engage, but may be contagious.

Stigma, seen in this way, is not the social behavioral outcome of some kind of essentialized difference in individuals that produces the brute force of societal censorship and conformity—a view hardly credible in the face of the bewildering heterogeneity of our times. Rather, stigma needs to be understood as a social process in which mental illness becomes dangerous precisely because it threatens the superficial sureties of things as they are and punctures the ideology of distraction and forgetting that covers over the dangers of living, and brings an extra burden to social life that so many seek to avoid in the rush to self-realization. Depression and anxiety clarify the grim aspects of everyday reality and the deep grinding structures of the social world. They force us to the view of the tragedy of historical ontology that even Max Weber could not withstand without himself becoming depressed. By unmasking the practices of forgetting and disguising what is at stake and making demands on lives so tuned to expedience and efficiency, depression and anxiety are unacceptable ways of being in our world, whether the political structure is capitalist or communist or theocratic. Hence the need to see them in euphemized, individualized, medicalized, and biological terms that remove their social sting. Perhaps this is also a comment on the marginality of social science, which so often finds its messages unsettling and unacceptable for perhaps much the same reason. But our analysis needs to include the political realities of local worlds that at particular times make stigma more or less intense, as at moments of political threat, or when the targeting of particular groups easily follows patterns formed by ethnonationalism, religious conflict, and racism.

Because so many campaigns of stigma reduction in the developing and developed world have ended in failure, it is now rather clear that the bald idea that health information alone will change bias (popular, professional, governmental) against mental health problems can no longer be the source of policies and programs. Rather, policies and programs need to focus on the threats to the stakes of social life as a source of fear and hostility that seek out scapegoats among the vulnerable as well as targets among the bearers of images of the real that puncture the myths of ordinary life—or just want to avoid the hassle of engaging people whose suffering is so easily characterized, even in the health professions, as a "burden."

Whether or not I have, in such a compressed space, been able to make the case for another way of viewing stigmas, my point is that a focus on the ethnographic and social historical contexts of local moral processes generates new possibilities for engaging obdurate questions. In an issue of *Daedalus* on *Bioethics and Beyond* (1999) that I had the honor to edit with Renée Fox and Allan Brandt, considerable evidence is provided of the crucial contribution that history, sociology, and anthropology make to the ethics of health and medicine by installing context and providing empirical studies of the social institutions and relationships that frame ethical issues and constrain ethics interventions. The point is not that the moral and political nexus of medicine replaces bioethics deliberation. Far from it. Rather, such deliberation only becomes useful when it is grounded in that nexus, as, for example, in the specifics of the managerial revolution and the political economy of health care as a "market" which is remaking medical practice in HMOs at present. The ethnography of practice in such a setting is a necessary prelude to an ethics of medical practice in managed care. Such an ethnography, which is only just becoming available now, barely evokes the transformation of what is at stake in practice from professional issues of efficacy to managerial issues of efficiency. We have only just begun to do the research needed to more adequately frame the ethics of care in America in our times.[2] And yet, I would contend that the position of the ethnographer betwixt and between local worlds and global discourse is one among many examples of how the moral and the ethical can be accommodated in ways that can enable both to come together into an understanding that is original, relevant, and consequential (Kleinman 1999).

So what are the stakes of social experience and how do they capture the passionate interest of stakeholders? I would argue this is one of the founding questions for ethnographies and social histories and political biographies. Read Ian Kershaw's authoritative biography of *Hitler* (1991), and you come away with a strong sense of the stakes of social experience in Germany in the decades preceding and following the Great War and Hitler's place within them that shaped the Nazi period. Do we possess anything quite like this powerful analytic study in the social sciences that illumines the status of social experience for health and medicine in our times? I am not convinced that we do. Hence, before we deplore the failure of other fields to make use of what we have put on offer, I think we first need to produce the kind of work that will make convincing what is happening to health and medicine in our era due to the global transformation and resistance of local worlds.

The stakes of social experience are mutating. New forms of subjectivity and interpersonal relations emerge from an epochal shift in political economy, cultural representations, and collective experience. There is a sense that voyeurism is a leading edge of consumerism and that compassion is thinning out. Where we do have evidence it shows that in those countries undergoing the greatest societal transformations under the global regime of political economy, substance abuse, violence, family and community breakdown, STDs, HIV/AIDS, suicide, depression, and PTSD (post-traumatic stress disorder) are increasing (Kleinman, Kleinman, and Lee 1999). These problems often run together, especially in the poorest countries and among those in deep poverty who live in rich societies. Contrary to psychiatric assertions, mental illnesses cluster together with social problems. Settings with social breakdown or political violence reveal clusters of substance abuse, depression, PTSD, and the behaviors DSM glosses as anti-social personality disorder (Desjarlais et al. 1995). Emotional processes and norms alter together. Biology is local, with an openness of neurobiology to context and social process pointed out by leading neuroscientists that was not even imagined earlier (Lewontin 1991, Lock 1993). The description of these connections between mind-brain-society may change in a fundamental way how we regard the self and the body. We can already talk of a moral biology that interrelates physiology and molecular processes with meanings and experiences. The fact of these interactions alters our understanding of what is at stake in social experience. This is the kind of line of analysis that is likely to change how ethics is thought about and practiced. But it is also a means of rethinking moral and social theory, an enterprise that has not attracted social scientists of health and medicine to the extent it should. This paper is meant to encourage that development, a development that our honoree also pioneered.

Notes

1. The idea of overwhelming practicality of social life as described by European phenomenologists and American pragmatists is developed in Kleinman and Kleinman (1996). See also Jackson (1997: Introduction), and Nipperdey (1974, 1979).
2. For a telling example of how such ethnographies may reshape our understanding of the ethical issues in medicine, see Tanya Luhrman, *Of Two Minds: American Psychiatry in the New Millenium* (New York: Knopf, 2000), and Alistair Donald, "The Walmarting of American Psychiatry: An Ethnography of Practice in the Late 20th Century," *Culture, Medicine, and Psychiatry* (forthcoming).

References

Bourdieu, Pierre. 1990. *The Logic of Practice.* Stanford: Stanford University Press.

Chen, Lincoln, Arthur Kleinman and Norma Ware, eds. 1994. *Health and Social Change.* Cambridge: Harvard University Press.

Desjarlais, Robert, Leon Eisenburg, Byron Good, and Arthur Kleinman, eds. 1995. *World Mental Health: Perspectives and Problems in Low-Income Countries.* New York and London: Oxford University Press.

Edgerton, Robert B. 1967. *The Cloak of Competence: Stigma in the Lives of the Mentally Retarded.* Berkeley: University of California Press.

Farmer, Paul. 1999. *Infections and Inequalities.* Berkeley and Los Angeles: University of California Press.

Fox, Renée C. 1996. "Afterthoughts: Continuing Reflections on Organ Transplantation," pp. 252-274 in *Organ Transplantation: Meanings and Realities*, edited by Stuart Youngner, Renée Fox, and Laurence O'Connell. Madison: University of Wisconsin Press.

Fox, Renée C. 1974. *Experiment Perilous: Physicians and Patients Facing the Unknown.* Philadelphia: University of Pennsylvania Press.

Fox, Renée C. and Judith Swazey. 1978. *The Courage to Fail: A Social View of Organ Transplants and Dialysis.* Chicago: University of Chicago Press.

Goffman, Erving. 1963. *Stigma: Notes on the Management of Spoiled Identity.* Englewood Cliffs: Prentice-Hall.

Jackson, Michael. 1997. *Things As They Are.* Bloomington: Indiana University Press.

Kershaw, Ian. 1991. *Hitler.* London: Longman.

Kleinman, Arthur. 1988. *The Illness Narratives: Suffering, Healing, and the Human Condition.* New York: Basic Books.

Kleinman, Arthur. 1999. "Moral Experience and Ethical Reflection." *Daedalus* 128(4):69-98.

Kleinman, Arthur and Joan Kleinman. 1996. "The Appeal of Experience; The Dismay of Images: Cultural Appropriations of Suffering in Our Times." *Daedalus* 125(1):1-25.

Kleinman, Arthur, Joan Kleinman and Sing Lee, eds. 1999. *Transformations of Social Experience in Chinese Societies, Culture, Medicine, and Psychiatry* 23 (1).

Kleinman, Arthur, Renée Fox, and Allan Brandt, eds. 1999. "Bioethics and Beyond." *Daedalus* 128(4).

Lewontin, Richard. 1991. *Biology as Ideology*. New York: HarperPerennial.

Lock, Margaret. 1993. *Encounters with Aging: Mythologies of Menopause in Japan and North America*. Berkeley and Los Angeles: University of California Press.

Nipperdey, Thomas. 1974. *Konflikt, Einzige Wahrheitder Gesellschaft*? Osnabruck: Fromm.

Nipperdey, Thomas. 1979. *Theorie und Erzahlung in der Geschichte*, hrsg. Von Jurgen Kockau. Thomas Nipperdey. Munchen: Deutscher Taschenbuch Verlag.

Oakeshott, Michael Joseph. 1933. *Experience and its Modes*. Cambridge: University Press (1978 printing).

IV

Postlude

18

Exploring the Moral and Spiritual Dimensions of Society and Medicine

Renée C. Fox

Your presence at this conference; its multiple sponsorship and generous support; the devoted, hard work that has gone into its organization; the deeply thoughtful way in which its program has been framed; the compact richness of your papers; the vitality of the discussions in which you have engaged; the colleagueship and friendship that underlie this occasion; the sense of mutual respect and affection, of reunion and remembrance, and of thanksgiving and celebration that you have brought to it—and also the festivity and unsolemn fun that it has entailed—imbued this gathering with intellectual excellence, personal pleasure, sentimental significance, and moral meaning. The fact that this conference was a response to my becoming a professor emerita, and that it took place, as the program phrased it, "in [my] honor," makes me the recipient of a gift of such worth that nothing I say or do in response to it—today or in the future—can adequately thank you, in the words of Marcel Mauss (1954), for "the spirit of the thing given." My four-and-a-half decades of research on "the gift of life" import of organ transplantation have heightened my awed appreciation of transcendent gifts like yours, and of their inherently unreciprocal nature.

Although I recognize that I have received more than I can possibly return, I want to try to express my gratitude through some reflections on the topics and themes around which this conference has been structured, and how they are connected to my career as a sociologist and my relationship to you. I hope that I do not sound either sanctimonious or self-congratulatory in saying that my career has been a "vocation" in Max Weber's (1946) sense of the term: an "inward calling" to do social scientific work; questing after knowledge and understanding of what Weber described as the "pulsating reality" of human life and human relations; trying to impart that knowledgeable understanding, and a way of thinking about it, through teaching and writing, with "intellectual integrity" that does not preclude vividness; believing that what is conveyed can contribute to greater clarity and insight about our own lives and the lives of others, and to a "sense of responsibility" and of compassionate caring that extend beyond the parameters of the particularistic enclaves in which we dwell. It is central to "the very *meaning*" of "science as a vocation," Weber wrote, that "we cannot work without hoping that others will advance further than we have." This is not only "our common fate" but "our common goal," he declared. Many of you who have participated in this conference personify for me the fulfillment of that hope and goal. I have much to learn from those whom I once taught.

My professional involvement as a sociologist with health, illness, and medicine began when I was a graduate student in the Harvard Department of Social Relations (1949-1954). Converging biographical, historical, and situational factors moved me in this direction. During my initial graduate school years my mentor, Talcott Parsons, was engaged in drafting what became a founding document of the sociology of medicine—Chapter 10 of his book *The Social System* (1951), entitled, "Social Structure and Dynamic Process: The Case of Modern Medical Practice." He explored the seminal ideas in this chapter with the students, of whom I was one, enrolled in a small seminar that he gave on Social Structure. The interdisciplinary conception of social relations on which the department was founded not only brought students in sociology, anthropology, and personality and social psychology together under the same roof of Emerson Hall; it also meant that we were required to take basic courses in *all* of these fields before we proceeded down the path of intensive training to become a sociologist, anthropologist, or psychologist. My teachers in clinical psychology included a number of distinguished psychiatrists in the Boston area, in an era when psychoanalytic psychiatry was at the height of its development and influence in the United States, and Boston was one of its American meccas. Several of these physicians had been brought into the orbit of the Department of Social Relations by Parsons through his contacts with the

Boston Psychoanalytic Institute, where he had undergone professional training that included a didactic, personal analysis. In turn, they not only provided opportunities for students like myself to learn more about mental health and illness, but also to have first-hand clinical and research experience in psychiatric hospital settings—in my case, at the Boston Psychopathic Hospital, and on the psychiatric unit of the Massachusetts General Hospital. When the psychiatrist-in-chief of the Peter Bent Brigham Hospital asked Parsons if he knew a sociologist who might be interested and qualified to join the interdisciplinary team investigating the biochemical and psychological effects of "stress on man," organized by the metabolic and psychiatric teams of that Harvard Medical School-affiliated hospital, he recommended me. I was hired, and under those auspices, from 1951 to 1954, I conducted my participant observation-based dissertation study of the social world created by the physician-researchers and patient-subjects of the hospital's metabolic research ward, Ward F-Second, in response to the extreme stress that they shared in the face of inexorable illness, human experimentation, uncertainty, physical and psychic suffering, and imminent death. Subsequently, it became my first published book, *Experiment Perilous* (1997a).

Although I could not have predicted it then, my years at the Brigham not only had a determining influence on my enduring interest in patient-oriented clinical research, but also in therapeutic innovation and in organ replacement. For, on Ward F-Second, I witnessed the pioneering development of the artificial kidney machine and of early cardiac surgery; and before I left the Brigham in 1954, the world's first successful human kidney transplant was performed in that hospital.

There were several other aspects of my immersion in the world of F-Second that had a lasting effect on my professional life. Among these were the relationships that I formed with the nurses of F-2—especially with its remarkable head nurse, "Jennie," a young woman of my own age. She and her colleagues had more continuous and closer physical and emotional contact with the patients of F-Second, and the everyday life of the ward, than the physicians. They both cared for and about the patients as individuals, and they recognized and understood the community that the men of F-2 (it was an all-male ward) had fashioned. The nurses grasped and responded to the nature of my research and they became my invaluable teachers, like many other nurses have been over the ensuing years. But there was more to it than that, as the messages the annual Christmas/New Year's cards that I receive from Jennie still express:

> Dear Renée:
>
> Is it 45 or 46 years since we shared the hope and sorrow of those very special patients on F-Second?. . . I've always felt fortunate to be able to share with you my love and frustration of my special "fellas." . . . When you wrote *Experiment Perilous*, you gave me a copy which has been cherished . . . .
>
> When I returned to nursing after years of devoting my time to my family, there were so many philosophical changes, and I never found another Renée to share my frustrations and concerns . . . .

Along with the "hope and sorrow [the] love and frustration," what united Jennie and me was our attunement to what this conference has termed the "moral and spiritual dimensions" of medicine and nursing—especially to the sorts of dilemmas that F-Second embodied, for which there were and are no easy ethical answers or facile practical solutions.

There was another set of experiences at the Brigham that accompanied me over time, in a manner that would shape my sociological future. They grew out of the opportunity that it gave me to meet numerous young European physicians who had come to outstanding American medical centers like Harvard to obtain post-graduate training that they hoped would make them more competent and eligible for academic medical research careers in their own countries. I became interested in the reasons for which so many of them had chosen the United States for their advanced training, particularly in clinical medical research, and why they felt apprehensively unsure about whether they would be able to pursue the careers of their choice when they returned home. These initial observations and questions later plunged me into decades of first-hand research on how social, cultural, and historical factors affected clinical medical research and research careers in a contemporary European society (Fox 1962; 1964; 1978); launched me on no less than forty years of fieldwork in Belgium; and extended my sociological journeying to Zaire (now the Democratic Republic of Congo)—the vast, Central African society that was once a Belgian colony and was still "a frontier and a dreaming space" for Belgians when I first arrived in Kinshasa, its capital, in 1962, two years after it had attained political independence (Fox 1994b).

The fact that at the age of seventeen—only four years before I began my graduate training—I had contracted a severe, life-threatening form of polio that entailed prolonged hospitalization and an extensive process of recovery and rehabilitation, probably heightened my responsiveness to the mixture of serendipitous and not-so-serendipitous forces that involved me as a nascent social scientist in the sociology of medicine before it was a fully recognized and institutionalized field. (It was not until 1960 that the Medical Sociology Section of the American Sociological Association was established, partly as an outgrowth of the Committee on Medical Sociology organized by August Hollingshead in 1955.) But it was neither purely by chance, nor primarily because of my medical history that, as I wrote in an essay on "Talcott Parsons, My Teacher":

> I was profoundly affected by the ideas that Parsons was generating about the importance of health, illness, and medicine to the functioning of a society, their cultural meaning, and their relationship to the human life cycle, suffering and death; about sickness as a social role; about the emotional evocativeness of the physician's role, because of the existential significance of illness, and the physical and psychic intimacies that medical work involves; and by Parsons's special emphasis on the limitations and uncertainty inherent to medicine no matter what its stage of development; the frustrations and strains that these entail for physicians and patients, and the "ritualized optimism"—which he viewed as a form of scientific magic—that physicians and patients develop under these circumstances as a way not only of coping, but of bolstering their confidence. (1997b:408-409)

Parsons's outlook provided a penetratingly deep and broad sociological perspective on health, illness, and medicine that enabled me to identify and appreciate their distinctive attributes, while linking them to other social and cultural phenomena, institutions, and processes. It highlighted the complex and subtle relations between science, medicine, religion, and magic, the interplay of rational and non-rational factors, and the significance of symbols and rituals in a realm of human existence that, irrespective of the advances of modern medicine, remains integrally entwined with what Émile Durkheim termed "la vie sérieuse." It did not minimize the importance of the human body and its biology, or of the roles and organizations that structure and frame illness and medical care. But it gave special weight to the moral components of professions in general, and of medicine in particular. Rather than evading spiritual questions because of their uneasy fit with positivism and secularism, it accorded a central place to the "human condition" aspects of medicine: to its at-once basic and transcendent connections with birth, growth and development, sexuality, aging, and death; to the "problems of meaning" posed by illness and accident, pain and suffering, and by the finiteness of human knowledge and of human life; and to how health professionals as well as patients and their families experience and grapple with these enigmas and limitations.

From the outset, this perspective had resonance for me personally, philosophically, and as a social scientist. But it was not until I began to do firsthand medical sociological research that I realized how powerfully illuminating it could be. Problems of medical uncertainty, of therapeutic limitation, and of meaning, I discovered, were more than theoretical abstractions. They were at the heart of Ward F-Second's "experiment perilous" universe, the reciprocal stresses of its physicians and patients, and the ways of coming to terms with them at which they mutually arrived. The conceptual ideas that I brought into the field not only helped me to perceive and understand this. In some instances, they were concretely observable. I literally saw and heard "scientific magic" in the conference room of F-Second when, accompanied by "serious joking" and highly patterned rituals, the physicians of F-2 recurrently made bets on what the outcome of the highly experimental, danger-fraught drugs and procedures that they were trying on their gravely ill patient-subjects would prove to be (Fox 1997a:82-85, 247).

The theme of medical and moral uncertainty has pervaded much of my reflection, research, and writing: on patient-oriented clinical research in an array of American and European settings; on the education and socialization of medical students; on organ transplantation, dialysis, and the development and implantation of an artificial heart; and most recently, in relationship to the dilemmas-in-action encountered by Doctors Without Borders and Doctors of the World, the two, historically connected medical humanitarian and human rights witnessing organizations that I have begun to study (1995). There are also other leitmotifs that appear and reappear in my work: the concept of "detached concern," for example—the supple balance between objectivity and empathy, equanimity and compassion that health professionals are expected to bring to competent, sagacious, humane patient care; the social dynamics and the symbolic meaning of the gift, especially in the context of organ donation; the courage not only to endure but to try to overcome great medical adversity, risking failure—even death—and the sin of hubris; and the poignant "double effects" of human action—the fact that no matter how noble its intentions or how beneficial its consequences, it is never devoid of undesirable side effects—be they the iatrogenic consequences of medical diagnosis, therapy, and prognosis, the "tyranny" of the unrepayable gift of a donated organ, or the unintentionally harmful repercussions of humanitarian intervention.

Although these themes are imprinted with the influence of my master teacher, with the conceptual approach to sociology in which I was trained, and with my own sense of tragedy and complexity, I do not feel that I have arbitrarily imposed them on the social reality of the empirical situations that I have studied, described, and analyzed. For example, quite early in the course of the participant observation that I did at Cornell University Medical College as a member of the Sociology of Medical Education Project of Columbia University's Bureau of Applied Social Research, I identified and began to trace out what I called the "training for uncertainty" process that "student-physicians" progressively underwent during their medical school years (1957). My theoretical interest in medical uncertainty, and my prior experience in watching the physicians and patients on F-Second struggle with the formidable problems of uncertainty that they faced, probably heightened my awareness of this aspect of the education and socialization of medical students, and my responsiveness to it. But there is cogent evidence that, independently of my attunement to it, training for uncertainty is considered by medical educators and students alike to be a challenging quintessence of becoming a physician, and of practicing medicine. Physician-historian Kenneth Ludmerer (1999) regards what he terms this "elusive ideal" as one of the primary goals of medical education. To this day, in medical as well as social scientific literature, the essay on the training for uncertainty that I published in 1957 is the most frequently cited and quoted of anything that I have written. And despite all of the changes in medical knowledge and the reforms in medical school curricula that have occurred during the past forty years, medical students still give spontaneous testimony to the exceptional importance and the emotional difficulty of learning that "medicine is filled with uncertainty" (Silver 1994).

How can I account for the fact that, again and again, the thematic ideas that hold abiding significance for me have turned out to have high relevance to key empirical phenomena in the social situations that I have investigated? This has been amazingly true of my research on organ transplantation (Fox and Swazey 1974, 1999). When I entered this field of inquiry in 1968 in collaboration with Judith Swazey, I took note of the fact that transplantation had been defined by the medical profession and society at large as a "gift of life" since the first human organ grafts were performed. I had a long-standing interest in the symbolic meaning of the gift and the intricacy of gift-exchange, to which my "growing up Jewish," my immersion in anthropological monographs about societies in Central Africa and Oceania, and my research in Zaire had contributed. In addition, I had not only read Marcel Mauss's essay on *The Gift* (1954) when I was a graduate student, but had re-read it a number of times because I had found it intriguing and enlightening. The iconic status that was accorded to organ donation as a gift in the culture of transplantation activated these associations for me. Nevertheless, I was as surprised as I was fascinated to discover that what Mauss wrote about the triple set of obligations (to give, receive, and repay) that govern all gift exchange; the structural strains that failure to live up to any of these obligations produces for the giver, the receiver, and those connected to them; the bond that develops between donor and recipient; and the sense in which "the spirit" of what is given and received is "alive and personified," literally described what organ donors, recipients, and their families actually experienced.

Something comparable already seems to be happening with regard to the study of Doctors Without Borders and Doctors of the World that I have recently launched. The two organizations, along with other non-governmental and governmental international relief agencies, are undergoing a period of "humanitarian angst" (Weiss 1999). It is a time when they are plunged into deep thought and debate about the moral dilemmas and quandaries they are facing during this post-Cold War era as they try to deliver humanitarian assistance in a way that is consistent with fundamental human rights, in an increasing number of contexts that are euphemistically termed "complex emergencies." These emergencies are the sorts of fratricidal wars of "all against all" *within* states that have occurred in Bosnia, Somalia, Rwanda, Liberia, Afghanistan, Sierra Leone, and Kosovo. The "collective identity crisis" that such humanitarian agencies appear to be undergoing is centered on what one commentator has described as their "loss of innocence about the impacts of aid": painful recognition of "the limits of humanitarianism as a practical philosophy" and of their humanitarian action; conscience-stricken doubts about whether their "engagement makes things better or worse"; the traumatic realization that in the conflict situations to which they are responding, it is very difficult "to do good without doing harm"—that under these conditions, their interventions "can exacerbate the suffering," and "fuel the crises it seeks to alleviate"; and acknowledgement of the inescapability of "moral uncertainty" and "ambiguity" both in providing, and in not providing aid (Anderson 1998). Uncertainty, limitation, moral conundrums and tragic dilemmas, and the harm that accompanies or results from doing or ardently trying to do good—somehow these themes in my past work are manifesting themselves once more in the research that I have just begun.

In part, what I have been describing exemplifies "the bearing of sociological theory on empirical research," to use Robert K. Merton's (1949) phrase: the way that conceptual ideas and the theoretical framework from which they come can provide "a general context for inquiry." In addition, although I do not simply project the themes that preoccupy me onto whatever subject or scene I am investigating, there are elements of "self-fulfilling prophecy" (Merton 1957) and perhaps of obsession that underlie the consistency with which they have surfaced in my research. But I also think these themes recur because they are inherent to a sociology concerned with values, beliefs, and commitment, with the human condition, and with questions of meaning.

My work has been topically as well as thematically focused. For more than forty years I have been involved with matters pertaining to medical research, medical education, and organ replacement; I have spent more than thirty years questing in Belgium (1994b) and following the unfolding of American bioethics (1974; 1976; 1990; 1994a; Fox and Swazey 1984); and from a necessary distance, I have maintained the links with Zaire/Congo that I established in 1962 as best I can. One of my hopes is that, if security conditions permit, I will be able to return to the Democratic Republic of Congo to make a mini-study of medical humanitarian work that Doctors Without Borders is doing there.Its centeredness and constancy notwithstanding, mine has not been a fixed or stationary career. Quite to the contrary, it has involved continuous journeying in a number of ways. The voyaging is closely connected with my perpetual fieldwork. My main methods of research have been ethnographic: prolonged participant observation, detailed in situ interviewing, oral history-taking, and the discovery and content analysis of primary and secondary documents. These forms of research have allowed and obliged me to go wherever my work has carried me—geographically, intellectually, and emotionally—to nearby and faraway places. Colleagues and friends from some of these places—Canada, England, Belgium, France, and Congo/Kinshasa—have graced this conference by traveling great distances to share this occasion with us. My journeying has been vertical as well as horizontal, transporting me into deep layers of the real lives of real people, into real situations, and into the innermost recesses of my own life and psyche. Ethnographic research has been more than a method for me. It has been a way of searching, and as Arthur Kleinman has put it, a "way of being-in-the-world" that has enabled me to move beyond the boundaries of myself and my native land, and become acquainted with societies and cultures other than my own. For a person of my generation, whose graduate training and coming of age in sociology took place in the years immediately following World War II, when many of us who were drawn to social science shared the conviction that cross-cultural knowledge and understanding could contribute to a "one-world" internationalism and a lasting peace, this has had moral as well as intellectual meaning. In addition, fieldwork and the "thickly descriptive" data it yields have given me a medium through which I can personify the individuals who are the flesh-and-blood actors in the situations I study, depict the inner and outer landscapes in which they live their lives, and evoke the atmosphere, mood, and imagery that surround what they are experiencing and feeling. It has invited me to draw on what I think of as the "yearning writer" in me, and put it at the service of a humanistic sociology, that I hope is also humane.

My relationship to the field of bioethics as an observing participant throughout its history has heightened my awareness of some of the premises on which doing social science and my way of being a sociologist rest. The study of the origins, evolution, and significance of American bioethics in which Judith Swazey, Carla Messikomer, and I are presently engaged—especially our examination of the points of tension between the perspectives of bioethics and the ongoing efforts to incorporate more social science thinking and methodology into bioethics—has given me an opportunity to further consider the angle of vision with which I approach my work. Bioethics attaches great philosophical importance to an autonomy-of-self conception of individualism, and to identifying and realizing what is humanly and ethically universal. It does so to a degree and in a manner that have made it difficult to integrate these precepts with notions of community and solidarity, with social and cultural differences, and with what biologist Ernst Mayr (1999) calls the "ubiquity of variation." In addition, a sharp distinction is made between so-called "descriptive" and "normative" ethics in bioethical thought. Drawing this line carries with it the implication that although empirical studies of social reality "as-it-is" may describe how social institutions *actually* work, they do not indicate or affirm how they *ought* to work; and that this kind of immersion in existing reality may insidiously lead to uncritically accepting it as justified and/or unalterable.

In comparison with this outlook, the sociological vantage point that I bring to my work does not dichotomize the individual and the social, or the universal and the particular. Without ignoring what is unique and valuable about every individual, or disregarding the fundamental conditions of being and the rights that are essential to the integrity and fulfillment of self, my conception of the individual has an indwelling social dimension—one that involves relatedness to known and unknown others, and continuous responsibility to them. My sociological view recognizes the omnipresence and importance of social and cultural as well as individual differences among people; considers the diversity that they represent to be an intriguing source of human richness; is respectful of the seriousness and tenacity of these differences; and yet is not oblivious to the ethnocentrism, the prejudice, and even the violence that can accompany certain forms of particularism. Nor does my responsiveness to difference either diminish my awareness of common human qualities and aspirations that transcend borders and boundaries, or my commitment to their realization. In this regard, as in so many others, the discrepancy between the "is" and the "ought" of social reality may be considerable, but I share Alan Wolfe's (1998) sociological and moral conviction that it is not only the "duty of a social scientist to take cognizance of the real world. . .[and] to get it straight," but that in some ways, a "desire for social reform demands" that serious knowledge and understanding of "the existing world . . . come first."

I believe that social science research and teaching, analysis and interpretation can inform social criticism, enlighten social policy, and contribute to social improvement. And I believe that this can be accomplished without becoming ideological or political in the partisan senses of these terms, or violating Max Weber's (1946) dictum that "the prophet and the demagogue do not belong on the academic platform." However, more than occasionally I find myself questioning whether what I have devoted my life to studying is as pertinent to the most crucial social and moral issues associated with health, illness, and medicine as it ought to be—especially the relationship between ill health, poverty, indignity, and social injustice. Long before I ever knew that sociology existed as a discipline and a profession, I wanted to be a social worker; and one of the most meaningful experiences of my youth was the summer I spent as a volunteer at the Henry Street Settlement House on the Lower East Side of Manhattan. The inner voice that reminds me that I have written and spoken far less about the fact that more than 44 million people in this country have no health insurance, including 11.1 million children, and that many more are underinsured, than I have about organ replacement, patient-oriented research, medical education, or bioethics, is associated with this aspect of my story and the family history and social values that underlie it. Without justifying the "rightness" of the paths of inquiry and involvement I have taken, the fact that the specific topics and phenomena on which my sociological work has focused have repeatedly opened onto the themes we have explored together at this conference gives me some reassurance that it has not been unconcerned with important social, moral, and spiritual questions. And the project that I have launched in the seventh decade of my life on Doctors Without Borders and Doctors of the World will bring me as close I ever have been to the kinds of natural and human-made catastrophes, suffering, and needs to which such medical humanitarian and human rights witnessing organizations try to effectively respond.

Of one thing I am absolutely sure: being a teacher has been a bedrock and a wellspring of my life as a sociologist. Forty-one years ago I co-authored an article with Bernard Barber, whimsically entitled "The Case of the Floppy-Eared Rabbits," that contained within it what I have always considered to be a parable about teaching (Barber and Fox 1958). The article examined an instance in which two highly competent medical scientists encountered the same phenomenon in their respective laboratories: the drooping of the ears of the rabbits with whom they were working after the animals received an injection of papain (a proteolytic enzyme extracted from papaya). One of the scientists went on to discover the cause of this floppiness, while the other failed to do so. A number of factors (including "serendipity," in which Barber and I were particularly interested at the time) contributed to the differential outcomes. But the finding that had the most lasting impact on me concerned the revelatory role that teaching had played in this happening. It was not until he examined the "before-and-after-papain" slides of the rabbits' tissues that he had prepared for teaching a class of medical students that the scientist who made the discovery noticed that the enzyme had altered all the cartilaginous structures in the rabbits' bodies, and realized it was the probable cause of the collapse of their ears. This true scientific tale is a living illustration of what I have experienced throughout my career as a teacher: how readying myself to teach a class, presenting what is known—and also what is not—to students, and exchanging ideas with them, could heighten my perception, kindle my insight, and solidify my thinking. All my classes have not soared; not every course has gone well; and it has not been possible to reach and respond to all the students seated in my assigned classrooms, or to profoundly communicate with each student who has crossed the threshold of my office. But taken as a whole, teaching has been a creative, uplifting, and meaning-making experience for me, fulfilling and replenishing, a source of happiness and solace, of identity and of authentication.

A supreme satisfaction of teaching is the privilege of watching the unfolding of persons whom you came to know when they were students and you their teacher—following their professional and personal course, to which you feel linked over time and space by the alchemy of the teaching and learning in which you have mutually engaged. Many of you who have participated in this conference are former students of mine. (I use "mine" in a non-possessive sense.) I have had the opportunity to teach seventeen of the persons who presented papers or chaired sessions—along with the late Herbert

W. Nickens, the physician/social scientist to whom the conference was dedicated—and an even greater number of attendees. Your presence and your contributions, your talents and your accomplishments, have infused this conference with extraordinary quality and surpassing significance; they have leavened my life as a sociologist; and they are helping to make my transition to "professor emerita" a time of renewal rather than of nostalgia.

References

Anderson, Mary B. 1998. "'You Save My Life Today, But For What Tomorrow?'" pp. 137-56 in *Hard Choices: Moral Dilemmas in Humanitarian Intervention*, edited by Jonathan Moore. Lanham, Md: Rowman & Littlefield Publishers.

Barber, Bernard and Renée C. Fox. 1958. "The Case of the Floppy-Eared Rabbits: An Instance of Serendipity Gained and Serendipity Lost." *American Journal of Sociology* LXIV (2):128-136.

Fox, Renée C. 1964. "An American Sociologist in the Land of Belgian Medical Research," pp. 345-391 in *Sociologists at Work*, edited by Phillip E. Hammond. New York: Harper and Row.

Fox, Renée C. 1976. "Advanced Medical Technology—Social and Ethical Implications." *Annual Review of Sociology* 2: 231-268.

Fox, Renée C. 1994a. "The Entry of U.S. Bioethics into the 1990s: A Sociological Analysis," pp. 21-71 in *A Matter of Principles? Ferment in U.S. Bioethics*, edited by Edwin R. DuBose, Ron Hamel, and Laurence J. O'Connell. Valley Forge, Pa: Trinity Press.

Fox, Renée C. 1974. "Ethical and Existential Developments in Contemporaneous American Medicine: Their Implications for Culture and Society." *The Milbank Memorial Quarterly/Health and Society.* 52 (Fall): 445-483.

Fox, Renée C. 1990." The Evolution of American Bioethics: A Sociological Perspective," pp. 210-217 in *Social Science Perspectives on Medical Ethics*, edited by George Weisz. Dordrecht/Boston/London: Kluwer Academic Publishers.

Fox, Renée C. 1997a. *Experiment Perilous: Patients and Physicians Facing the Unknown* (Glencoe, Ill: The Free Press, 1959.) Republished with a new Epilogue by the author, New Brunswick, NJ: Transaction Publishers.

Fox, Renée C. 1995. "Medical humanitarianism and human rights: reflections on Doctors Without Borders and Doctors of the World." *Social Science and Medicine* 41 (12):1607-1616.

Fox, Renée C. 1962. "Medical Scientists in a Château." *Science* 136 (May 11):476-483.

Fox, Renée C. 1994b. *In the Belgian Château: The Spirit and Culture of a European Society in an Age of Change.* Chicago: Ivan R. Dee, Inc.

Fox, Renée C. 1997b. "Talcott Parsons, My Teacher." *The American Scholar* 69(3):395-410.

Fox, Renée C. 1957. "Training for Uncertainty," pp. 207-241 in *The Student-Physician: Introductory Studies in the Sociology of Medical Education*, edited by Robert K. Merton, George Reader, and Patricia L. Kendell. Cambridge, Mass: Harvard University Press.

Fox, Renée C. 1978. "Why Belgium?" *European Journal of Sociology* XIX (2):205-228.

Fox, Renée C. and Judith P. Swazey. 1974. *The Courage to Fail. A Social View of Organ Transplants and Chronic Dialysis.* Second edition, rev., 1978. Chicago, IL: University of Chicago Press. Reissued with a new introduction: Transaction Publishers, 2001.

Fox, Renée C. and Judith P. Swazey. 1984. "Medical Morality Is Not Bioethics: Medical Ethics in China and the United States." *Perspectives in Biology and Medicine* 27(4):336-360.

Fox, Renée C. and Judith P. Swazey. 1992. *Spare Parts: Organ Replacement in American Society.* New York: Oxford University Press.

Ludmerer, Kenneth. 1999. *Time to Heal: American Medical Education from the Turn of the Century to the Era of Managed Care.* New York: Oxford University Press.

Mauss, Marcel. 1954. *The Gift: Forms and Functions of Exchange in Archaic Societies.* Transl. by Ian Cunnison. Glencoe, Ill: Free Press 1954.

Mayr, Ernest. 1999. "Structure for Theories of Biology." *Science* 285 (September 17):1856.

Merton, Robert K. 1949. "The Bearing of Sociological Theory on Empirical Research," pp. 83-96 in Robert K. Merton, *Social Theory and Social Structure: Toward the Codification of Theory and Research.* Glencoe, Ill: Free Press.

Merton, Robert K. 1957. "The Self-Fulfilling Prophecy," pp. 421-436 in Robert K. Merton, *Social Theory and Social Structure* (revised and enlarged edition). Glencoe, Ill: Free Press.

Parsons, Talcott. 1951. *The Social System.* Glencoe, Ill: Free Press, pp. 428-479.

Silver, Marc T. 1994. "The Student Experience," pp. 123-138 in *New Pathways in Medical Education: Learning to Learn at Harvard Medical School*, edited by Daniel C. Tosteson, S. James Adelstein, and Susan T. Carver. Cambridge, Mass: Harvard University Press.

Weber, Max. 1946. "Science as a Vocation," pp. 129-156 in *From Max Weber: Essays in Sociology*, edited by. H. H. Gerth and C. Wright Mills. New York: Oxford University Press.

Weiss, Thomas G. 1999. "Principles, Politics, and Humanitarian Action." *Ethics & International Affairs* 13:1-22.

Wolfe, Alan. 1998. "The Missing Pragmatic Revival in American Social Science," pp. 199-206 in *The Revival of Pragmatism: New Essays on Social Thought, Law, and Culture*, edited by Morris Dickstein. Durham: Duke University Press.

About the Contributors

Elizabeth M. Armstrong, Ph.D., MPA, is assistant professor of sociology and public affairs, Princeton University. Her research interests include the sociology of medicine, social demography, population and health, and the history of medicine and public health. Dr. Armstrong's publications include *Conceiving Risk, Bearing Responsibility: Ideas about Alcohol and Reproduction in the Modern Era* (Johns Hopkins University Press, forthcoming).

Charles L. Bosk, Ph.D., is professor, Department of Sociology and a member of the Center for Bioethics faculty, University of Pennsylvania. His areas of specialization as a medical sociologist include professions and professionalization, deviance and social control, field methods of research, and the sociology of bioethics. Dr. Bosk's publications include *All God's Mistakes: Genetic Counseling in a Pediatric Hospital* (University of Chicago Press, 1992).

Nicholas A. Christakis, MD, MPH, Ph.D., is professor, Department of Health Care Policy, Harvard Medical School. He is an internist and sociologist who has been particularly interested in the role of prognostication in medicine and in the nature of end-of-life care in American society. More recently, he has been examining the health benefits of marriage, and iatrogenesis. Dr. Christakis' publications include *Death Foretold: Prophecy and Prognosis in Medical Care* (University of Chicago Press, 1999).

Renée C. Fox, Ph.D., is Annenberg Professor Emerita of the Social Sciences; fellow, Center for Bioethics, University of Pennsylvania; and a research associate, Queen Elizabeth House, Oxford University. Her areas of teaching, research, and writing have included medical sociology, medical education, patient-oriented clinical research and therapeutic innovation, bioethics, cross-cultural studies in European countries, Zaire, and China, and, most recently, the medical humanitarian and human rights witnessing of Médecins Sans Frontières. Dr. Fox's publications include *In the Belgian Château: The Spirit and Culture of a European Society in an Age of Change* (Ivan L. Dee, 1994), and, with Judith P. Swazey, *Spare Parts: Organ Replacement in American Society* (Oxford University Press, 1992).

Deborah A. Frank, MD, is Pediatrician Director of the Growth and Development Clinic at Boston City Hospital and an associate professor of pediatrics at Boston University School of Medicine. Her clinical work, research, and public service activities have focused on identifying and treating failure to thrive problems in newborns, infants, and young children. Dr. Frank's publications include papers in pediatric and public health journals on subjects such as the effects of prenatal exposure to cocaine and other drugs and of pediatric undernutrition.

Allen Glicksman, Ph.D., is Director of Research and Evaluation, Philadelphia Corporation for Aging. He is also a research associate professor, Buehler Center on Aging, Northwestern University, visiting associate professor at Gratz College, and an adjunct associate professor, School of Nursing, University of Pennsylvania. His work has examined the impact of religion, ethnicity, race, and immigration status on the experience of the Jewish aged, including comparative studies of older Jews born in the United States and in the Soviet Union, and Holocaust survivors. He writings include articles in scholarly, clinical and popular publications on various cross-cultural aspects of elderly immigrants and their caregivers.

Gail G. Glicksman, Ph.D., Rabbi, is Dean of Students and Assistant Professor of Ethics at the Reconstructionist Rabbinical College. She has served as a congregational rabbi, a chaplain, and a consultant on Jewish issues to health and social service agencies. Her research, publications, and professional presentation include studies of ethical issues in the training of health care professionals, prayer and healing, Jewish responses to illness, and Jewish approaches to beginning-of-life issues such as assisted reproductive technology and genetic testing.

Jacqueline Hart, Ph.D., is a postdoctoral fellow in health services research in the Department of Veterans Affairs and University of

Pennsylvania School of Medicine. Her research interests include how the wellness ethic through defining health, risk, and responsibility serves to advantage and disadvantage different groups; sociological and moral aspects of health discourses and policies, including resource allocation; and involving communities in defining their own public health priorities. Dr. Hart's forthcoming publications include papers on the wellness ethic, informed consent, sociological and moral aspects of the listing process for liver transplantation, and the impact of the 9/11 terrorist attacks on identity and definitions of risk and safety.

Jonathan B. Imber, Ph.D., is Class of 1949 Professor in Ethics and professor of sociology, Wellesley College. His research and writings include work on the roles of physicians and medical care, and social and political factors shaping sociology as a discipline. Dr. Imber is editor-in-chief of *Society*, and author of *Trusting Doctors: The Decline of Moral Authority in American Medicine* (forthcoming).

Howard L. Kaye, Ph.D., is professor of sociology, Franklin and Marshall College. His research interests focus on the interrelationships between areas of biology such as genetics and evolution with society and culture, and sociological perspectives on bioethics. Dr. Kaye's publications include *The Social Meaning of Modern Biology* (2d edition, Transaction Publishers, 1999).

Arthur M. Kleinman, MD, is the Maude and Lillian Presley Professor of Medical Anthropology and professor of psychiatry, Harvard Medical School, and professor of anthropology, Harvard University. His work includes research on Chinese society, international mental health, the experience of chronic illness, and social policies concerning the overlap of social and health problems such as suicide, violence, and trauma. Dr. Kleinman's publications include *Writing at the Margin: Discourse Between Anthropology and Medicine* (University of California Press, 1995).

Robert Klitzman, MD, is assistant professor of clinical psychiatry in the College of Physicians and Surgeons and the Mailman School of Public Health, Columbia University. His research and writing has included subjects such as autobiographical studies of professional socialization in medicine and psychiatry, the lives AIDS patients, and a "personal account" of kuru, cannibalism, and mad cow disease. Currently, he is completing a study of physicians who become patients with conditions such as cancer, heart disease, and HIV. Dr. Klitzman's publications include a forthcoming book with Ronald Bayer, *Mortal Secrets: Truth and Lies in the Age of AIDS.*

William R. LaFleur, Ph.D., is the Dale E. Saunders Professor in Japanese Studies and a fellow, Center for Bioethics, University of Pennsylvania. His research has focused on medieval Japan and, more recently, on the nexus between traditional Japanese religious values and contemporary social questions. Dr. LaFleur's publications include *Liquid Life: Abortion and Buddhism in Japan* (Princeton University Press, 1993), and a forthcoming book on bioethical debates in Japan.

Victor Lidz, Ph.D., is assistant professor, Department of Psychiatry, and Acting Director of the Institute for Addictive Disorders, MCP-Hahnemann School of Medicine. He has served on the MCP-Hahnemann Institutional Review Board since 1996 and is currently vice chair. His work in sociological theory has focused on contributions to the theory of action developed by Talcott Parsons. Dr. Lidz's other fields of research and writing include drug abuse and its treatment, and deviance and social control.

David Mechanic, Ph.D., is the René Dubos Professor of Behavioral Sciences and director of the Institute for Health, Health Care Policy and Aging Research, Rutgers University. His research and writing deal with social aspects of health and health care, including areas such as medical sociology, health policy, health services research, and social and behavioral sciences. Dr. Mechanic's publications include *Mental Health and Social Policy: The Emergence of Managed Care* (4th edition, Allyn & Bacon, 1999).

Carla M. Messikomer, Ph.D., is president of The Acadia Institute, a non-profit center for the study of issues in medicine, science, and society. Her research interests include social organizations, formal organizations, the role of religion in health care and medical practice, bioethics, and the career patterns of physicians. Dr. Messikomer is the co-author of two forthcoming books, with Renée C. Fox and Judith P. Swazey on the development and roles of bioethics in American society, and with Judith P. Swazey on the merger of the Medical College of Pennsylvania and Hahnemann University.

Virginia Adams O'Connell, Ph.D., is assistant professor, Department of Anthropology and Sociology, Swarthmore College. Her research interests include medical sociology, professionalizaton, medical education, demography, research methods, gender, and bioethics.

Judith P. Swazey, Ph.D., is founding president and senior scholar, The Acadia Institute, and adjunct professor of social and behavioral sciences, Boston University Schools of Medicine and Public Health. Her areas of research have included social, ethical, and policy aspects of biomedical innovation, bioethics, research integrity, and graduate and professional education. Her publications include (with Renée C. Fox) *The Courage to Fail* (1978; reissued by Transaction Publishers, 2002) and a forthcoming book (with Carla M. Messikomer and Renée C. Fox) on the development and roles of bioethics in American society.

Yves Winkin, Ph.D., is professor of communication at the Ecole Normale Supérieure Lettres et Sciences Humaines, Lyon, France and at the Université de Liège, Belgium. His area of teaching and research is the anthropology of communication. Dr. Winkin's publications, which have been translated into several languages, include *Anthropologie de la Communication: de la Théorie au Terrain* (Le Seuil, 2001).

Index

Abdelhak, Sherif, 74, 82
Abe, Yasuichi, 91-92
Abortion debate, 216, 218-220, 222-223
Abortion: Law, Choice, and Morality (Callahan), 216
Access to medical care, 206-207
Allegheny Health, Education and Research Foundation (AHERF): bankruptcy of, 70, 83; Hahnemann University, acquisition of, 69, 83n1; management, culture of, 74-84; Medical College of Pennsylvania (MCP), acquisition of, 69, 75; secrecy and, 70, 73, 80-81, 83. *See also* Hahnemann University and Medical College of Pennsylvania
Allegheny University of the Health Sciences, 83
American Association of Bioethics, 227
American Medical Association, 211-212, 218-219; Code of Ethics (1847), 218-219; and public relations, 211-212
American Society for Law, Medicine and Ethics, 227
American Sociological Association, Medical Sociology Section, 261
Anspach, Renée, 233
Anti-Semitism, 46, 51-52, 55
Aquinas, Thomas, 218
Armstrong, Elizabeth M., x-xi, 3, 273
Artificial heart. *See* Heart, artificial
Ayala family, 92-93

Barber, Bernard, 268-269
Barnicle, Mike, 162
Barth, Hans, 215
Being Positive: The Lives of Men and Women with HIV (Klitzman), 187-188
Belgium: access to medical care in, 206; Belgian studies, need for, 113-114; "Medical Scientists in a Chateau" (Fox), 110; response to Fox's *In the Belgian Chateau* in, 109-113; sociology in, 112-113; universities in, 113
Belmont Report, 200
Bioethics: Catholicism and, 215-220, 223-224, 229-230; comparative, need for, 92-95; criticism of, 217-218, 227-232; Jewish thought and, 224; the law and, 223; secularization of, 229
Bioethics and Beyond, Daedalus issue, 251
Bioethics in America: Origins and Cultural Politics (Stevens), 221
Biotechnology concerns in Japan, 88
Birth, medicalization of, 12
Birth of Bioethics (Jonsen), 221
Birth-order, in Japan, 92-94
Bone marrow transplantation, 91-92
Bosk, Charles L., x, xiii, xvii, 117, 233, 273
Boston Psychoanalytic Institute, 259
Boston Psychopathic Hospital, 259
Bourdieu, Pierre, 244
Brain death, 88, 199; in Japan, 94-95, 103-105
Brandt, Allan, 251
Bush, Barbara, 104

Callahan, Daniel, 216, 220, 222, 227-232
Caplan, Arthur, 164-165, 227
Capron, Alexander, 228
Catholicism, 47, 211-212, 215-220, 223-224, 229
Le Chateau des Belges. See In the Belgian Chateau
Chernobyl. *See* Chornobyl nuclear disaster
Children, malnourished: cognitive competence in, 166; emergency food for, 162-

167; medical outcomes of, 161, 166; race and, 165-166; statistics on, 165, 165-166
Childress, James, 232
China, 88
Chornobyl nuclear disaster, 46, 53, 57n5
Christakis, Nicholas A., x, xiii-xiv, xvii, 135, 273
Clark, Barney, 99, 199
Clark, Tom C. 214
"The Clinical Moratorium" (Swazey and Fox), 199
Cloak of Competence (Edgerton), 249
Cloning Human Beings (NBAC), 231, 236-239
Coles, Robert, 183
Columbia University's Bureau of Applied Social Science Research, 263
Comte, Auguste, 215, 220
Cooley, Denton, 205
Cornell University Medical College, 263
Council on Bioethics, 224
The Counter-Revolution of Science (Hayek), 215-216
The Courage to Fail (Fox and Swazey), 97, 141, 145-146, 149, 157, 197-199, 244
Crick, Francis, 238

Dawkins, Richard, 238
Death: attitudes toward, in America, 206-207; definition of. *See* "brain death" of organ donors, 152; superstitions about, 65-66
De Decker, Jacques, 111
De Rochemont, Louis, 211
Detached concern, training for, 141-142, 186, 262
DeVries, William, 99
Dewey, John, 244
Doctor-patient relationship: and self-care, 34-35; time spent in, 175; and trust, 170-178, 211
Doctors Without Borders and Doctors of the World, 152, 262, 264-265, 268. *See also* Médicins Sans Frontières
Dodier, Nicolas, 35
Doi, Kenji, 103
Duke University, 201
Durkheim, Émile, 261

Elderly, 43-57, 59-68
Electroconvulsive therapy (ECT), 186
Elsie Venner (Holmes), 213
Emergence of Roman Catholic Medical Ethics in North America (Kelly), 216
Emotional intelligence, 125-126
Erikson, Erik, 43
Ethics, 208-209, 255
Evans, John H., 233
Experience and Its Modes (Oakeshott), 244-245
Experiment Perilous (Fox), 109, 141, 193-198, 204, 208, 243, 259-260

Fletcher, Joseph, 219, 223, 230
Fore group (Papua New Guinea), 188-189
Fox, Renée C., xi, xvi-xvii, 5, 10, 18, 87, 89-90, 92, 95, 97, 99, 101, 109-114, 135, 139-141, 145, 165, 168-169, 189-190, 193-200, 204-210, 225, 227-230, 235-236, 243, 246, 251, 257, 273; and study of Belgium, 109-114, 260, 265; on bioethics 227-228, 235, 266-267; ethnographic field work of, 113, 193, 235-236, 260, 266; on gift exchange, transplantation as, 156-157, 262-264 poliomyelitis of, 153, 209n1, 261; and study of Doctors Without Borders/Doctors of the World, 262, 264-265, 268; on teaching, 153-154, 268-270; on "training for detached concern," 141-142, 186, 262; on uncertainty, medical and moral, 18, 139-140, 196, 262-263, 265; physician training for, 5, 263; on work, 154, 258-270; on Zaire/Congo, 260, 265. *See also The Courage to Fail*, *Experiment Perilous*, *In the Belgian Chateau*, and *Spare Parts: Organ Replacement in American Society*
Frank, Deborah A., x, xiv, 161, 274
Freidson, Eliot, 222

Gardner, Carol Brooks, 9-10
Gaylin, Willard, 224
Geertz, Clifford, 189
Gehlen, Arnold, 244
Genetic determinism, 238-239

"Genetics, Religion, and Ethics" project, 230
The Gift (Mauss), 264
Gift exchange, transplantation as, 262-264; "tyranny of the gift," 156-157, 262-263
Glicksman, Allen, ix-x, xii, xvii, 43, 274
Glicksman, Gail G., x, xii, 59, 274
Goffman, Erving, 5, 17, 249
Guyer, Bernard, 164

Hahnemann University: culture of, 76-77; merger with Medical College of Pennsylvania, 69-85
Hart, Jacqueline, x, xii, 23, 274
Harvard Department of Social Relations, 258
Harvard Medical School, 172
Hastings Center, 224, 229
Hayek, F. A., 215
Health: individual responsibility for, 23-24, 31, 37-38; wellness ideology and, 8-29, 38; World Health Organization's (WHO), definition of, 28-29
Health behaviors, 26-27, 30-33, 38n2, 39n4 and n9; disability claims and, 26-27, 33, 35; values and, 32. *See also* Illness
Health Maintenance Organizations (HMOs), 170-175, 178-180, 207; and efforts to build trust, 178-180; ethnography and, 251; public trust in, 171, 178; wellness program at a, 25-38
Heart, artificial, 101-102, 198-199
"Heroic" medicine and publicity, 198-200
Hippocrates, 3
Hirose, Teruo, 90
Hitler (Kershaw), 252
HIV/AIDS, 187-188, 247, 252
Hollingshead, August, 261
Holmes, Oliver Wendell, 213
Honesty: concept of, 118; surgical residents and, 117-133
Human cloning, 232, 236-239
Human Genome Project, 230
Humanitarianism, 262, 264-265
Hume, David, 218
Hunger, childhood. *See* Children, malnourished
Huxley, T. H., 215

Iatrogenesis, 138-139, 152
Idea of Order (Barth), 215
Illness: class differences and 29-30; de-legitimization of, 33-37; individual responsibility for, 34-36; poverty and, 246-247; in prisons, 247; risk factors for, 23, 27; self-care for, 34-35; sick leave for, in U.S., 36; wellness ideology and, 33-38
Illness Narratives (Kleinman), 246
In a House of Dreams and Glass—Becoming a Psychiatrist (Klitzman), 186-187
In the Belgian Chateau (Fox), x, 109-112
Imber, Jonathan B., x, xv, 211, 275
Immigration: of Soviet Jews to Philadelphia, 45-47; of Ukrainian Protestants to Philadelphia, 47-48
Individual responsibility: for illness, 34-36; of surgical residents for medical mistakes, 122, 130
Institutional review boards (IRBs), 201-205, 232, 234; as seen by their institutions, 202-203; faulted by DHHS, 201-202; work of, 203-205
Internship, 184-185

Jakobovitz, Immanuel, 224
Japan, 87-107
James, William, 244
Jarvik, Robert, 101-102
Johns Hopkins University, 172, 201
Jonsen, Albert R., 221
Judaism, 51-52, 54-55, 59-68

Kant, Immanuel, 218
Kass, Leon, 224, 227-228
Kaye, Howard L., x, xv-xvi, 227, 275
Kelly, David F., 216
Kershaw, Ian, 252
Kleinman, Arthur M., x, xvi, 88, 243, 266, 275
Klitzman, Robert, x, xv, 183, 275
Kluge, Eike-Henner W., 105
Kuru epidemic, 188-189

LaFleur, William R., x-xiii, 87, 276
Lederberg, Joshua, 238

La Libre Belgique, 110
Lidz, Victor, x, xv, 193, 276
Lock, Margaret, 88, 94-95
Ludmerer, Kenneth, 263

Managed care, 169-170, 174, 176, 178-180, 218, 247, 251. *See also* Health Maintenance Organizations
Maquet, Jacques, 113
Massachusetts General Hospital, 259
Mauss, Marcel, 257, 264
May, Rollo, 135-136, 138-139, 142n2
Mayo Clinic, 172
Mayr, Ernst, 267
McFadden, Charles J., 217
Mechanic, David, x, xiv, 169, 276
Medécins Sans Frontières, 152. *See also* Doctors Without Borders/Doctors of the World
Media coverage: of "heroic" medicine, 197-200; of medical institutions, 172; of medical misdeeds, 174; of mergers, 72
Medical College of Pennsylvania: culture of, 76; and merger with Hahnemann University, 69-85
Medical education, 117-133, 184-185; internationalized, 103
Medical Ethics (McFadden), 217
Medical indigence, 205, 207
Medical mistakes, 120, 122, 130, 174
Medical research: Japan, as seen in, 89-90; and religion in America, 99-103
Medicine: Catholicism and, 211-212, 216-220, 223-224, 229; Judaism and, 59-68; professional culture of, 139-140; Protestantism and 211-215, 217; religious influences on, 103, 211-220, 223-224; as a vocation, 211-215
Mental illness, 249-252
Mergers of medical schools, 69-85
Merleau-Ponty, Maurice, 244
Merton, Robert, 140-141, 142n3, 265
Messikomer, Carla M., ix-x, xii, xvii, 69, 276
Metalious, Grace, 213
Mohr, James, 220
Moral theory 245, 249, 251
Morals and Medicine (Fletcher), 219
Moratoria on transplantation, 148, 151, 199-200
Morishita, Naoki, 87-93, 96-99
Mormon Church (Church of the Latter Day Saints), 99-102, 106n7

National Bioethics Advisory Commission (NBAC), 231-232, 236-239
National Commission for the Protection of Human Subjects of Biomedical and Behavioral Research, 200
Neurobiology 252
Nickens, Herbert W., ix, xvii, 270
Nipperdey, Thomas, 244
Noonan, John T., 216

Oakeshott, Michael, 244-245
O'Connell, Virginia Adams, x, xiii, 117, 277
Organ donation: as a gift, 262-263; children conceived for, 90-94; by living donors, 91-94, 151-152
Organs, sale of, 91, 94, 105n4

Papua New Guinea, 188-189
Paré, Ambroise, 3
Paroo, Iqbal, 74
Parsons, Talcott, 34, 193, 209n1, 258-259, 261
Patients: as research subjects, 148-152, 194-208; and trust in physicians, 170-178, 211; and uncertainty, 196
Peter Bent Brigham Hospital (Boston), 109, 259-260
Peyton Place (Metalious), 213-214
Physician assisted suicide, 236
Physician-investigators, 193-210, 259-260
Physician writers, 183, 189
Physicians: advocacy for social change by, 163-168; anger at, 64-65; anxiety of, 135-144, 151; authority of, 211-215, 219, 224-225; Catholic pastoral medicine and, 212, 218; death, attitudes toward, 139-142, 142n5; humanitarianism of, 264-265; medical morality and, 218; motivation of, 152-153; prognosis and, 135-136, 140, 142; Protestant inheritance of, 211-215, 219-221, 223;

socialization of, 225n2; uncertainty and, 138-141, 143n6-7; vocation of, 211-215, 219
Pinker, Steven, 238
Plessner, Helmut, 244
Pope Paul VI, 229
Poverty, 246-247, 252, 268
Pregnancy: advice books, 7, 10-11; chronological quantification of, 13-14, 19n3; commercialization and commodification of, 4, 6, 15-16; group identity and, 14-15; information imperative of, 9-13; Internet and, 8, 10, 13-15, 19, 19n2; as master social status, 5, 11-12, 16-17; maternal-fetal conflict, 17; risks in, 4-5,11-13; tests, prenatal, 5-9, 19n1; uncertainty and, 3-7, 10-12, 18; visualization of, 7-9
Press coverage. *See* media coverage
Principlism, 229, 233-234
Prognosis, 135, 138, 140, 142
Protestantism, 30, 47-50, 102-103, 211-215, 219-220, 223
Public health, 161-168, 200, 207
The Puzzle People (Starzl), 150-151, 155, 158

Ramsey, Paul, 230
Religion and medicine, 59-68, 97-102, 211-226
Religious expression: of Christian missionaries in Japan, 97-102; of Soviet Jewish immigrants in Philadelphia, 51-52, 54; of Ukrainian Protestant immigrants in Philadelphia, 48-50. *See also* Mormon Church
Research, clinical: ethical dilemmas and, 208-209; human subjects of, 101-102, 194-209
Research, clinical, regulation of: *Belmont Report* 200; Data Safety Monitoring Boards and, 200; by Department of Health and Human Services (DHHS), 201; pre-IRB era, 204-205, 210n2. *See also* Institutional review boards
Research subjects, 101-102, 194-208
Residency, psychiatric, 185-187
Residents, surgical: emotional intelligence of, 125-126; risk of attrition by race and gender, 119, 121-124, 127-130, 132; medical mistakes and, 122, 130; response to criticism of, 119-120, 125, 127-128, 130-132
La Revue Nouvelle, 112
Roe v. Wade, 220
Rosner, Fred, 224
Rothman, David T., 221

Saint Augustine, 218
Sakamoto, Masaaki, 99, 101-103
Scheler, Max, 244
Shumway, Norman, 205
Sick role, concept of, 34
Social control: communication as, 80-83; of medical innovators, 205
Social Suffering, issue of *Daedalus,* 248
The Social System (Parsons), 258
Social system identity, 73
Socialization of medical students, 263
Society for Bioethics Consultation, 227
Society for Health and Human Values, 227
Sociological ambivalence, 140
Sociological calendar of academia, 79
Sociology, 112, 215, 221-224, 248-253, 257-271; bioethics and, 221-224, 232-239; consensus and, 215; critique of medical professionalism by, 222-224; moral questions and, 232-235, 248; religion and, 215; values and, 207-208, 223, 248
Le Soir, 110-111
Soviet Union, former, 44-57
Spare Parts: Organ Replacement in American Society (Fox and Swazey), x, 87-102, 149, 197, 204, 244; book jacket design and title of Japanese translation, 95-98; reviews of Japanese translation, 89-91, 94, 99-102
Starzl, Thomas, xi, 103-105, 145-160, 205; on animal research, 147, 150-151; on donor coercion, 151-152; on graft acceptance, 155-158; and kidney transplantation, 146-147, 149, 152, 156; and liver transplantation, 146-150, 156; moratoria on kidney and liver transplants, 148, 151-152; on performing surgery, 151; *The Puzzle People*, 150-151, 155, 158

Stevens, M. L. Tina, 221
Stigma: mental illness as, 249-251; pregnancy as, 17
Strangers at the Bedside (Rothman), 221
Surgery: culture of, 120-121, 131; residency programs in, 117-133
Swazey, Judith P., ix-x, xii-xiii, 87-90, 92, 95-99, 101, 145-146, 150, 153, 156-157, 197, 199, 264, 266
Sweet Charity (Poppendieck), 162

Teaching: Renée Fox on, 153-154, 269-270; in surgical residency programs, 119, 122; Thomas Starzl on, 153
Tillich, Paul, 217, 223
Toulmin, Stephen, 218
Transplantation and transplants, 87-96, 101-105, 145-159, 197-200, 264; cadaveric, in America, 89-90, 102, 104; cadaveric, in Japan, 88-89, 102-105; graft acceptance and, 155-158; immunosuppressive therapy, 146-149; kidney, 146-147, 149, 151-152, 156, 259; liver, 146-150, 156; publicity and, 198-200; recipients of, 156-157
The Trembling Mountain: A Personal Account of Kuru, Cannibals and Mad Cow Disease (Klitzman), 188-189
Trust, public: defined, 169, 171-173; effects on of media coverage, 172, 174; in bioethics, 218; in physicians, by patients, 170-178, 211; in social institutions, 171-174, 178-180
Turner, Bryan, 244

Ukraine. *See* Soviet Union, former
Uncertainty, medical: patients and, 196; physician anxiety and, 139-141; physicians training for, 5, 263; pregnancy and, 3-18; on Ward F-Second, 262
United Network for Organ Sharing (UNOS), 152

Vansina, Jan, 113
Veatch, Robert, 218

Wada, Tsutomu, 94
Wagaman, Samuel M., 212
Ward F-Second. *See Experiment Perilous*
Weber, Max, 223, 233, 236, 250, 258, 268
Wellness ethic, 23-41; attitude and, 29-35; defined, 23-24; health, as defined by, 28-29, 38; illness and, 33-38; sick leave and, 25, 28, 36
What to Expect When You're Expecting (Eisenberg), 4, 7, 10-13
Williams, William Carlos, 183
Wilson, E. O., 238
Winkin, Yves, x, xii-xiii, 109, 277
Wolfe, Alan, 267
Woodruff, Sir Michael, 157
World Health Organization(WHO), 28-29
World War II: and Soviet Jewish immigration, 50-51, 53-54; and Ukrainian immigration to U.S., 47

A Year-long Night: Tales of a Medical Internship (Klitzman), 184-185
Yiddish language, 46-47, 51-52